Handbook of Active Materials for Medical Devices

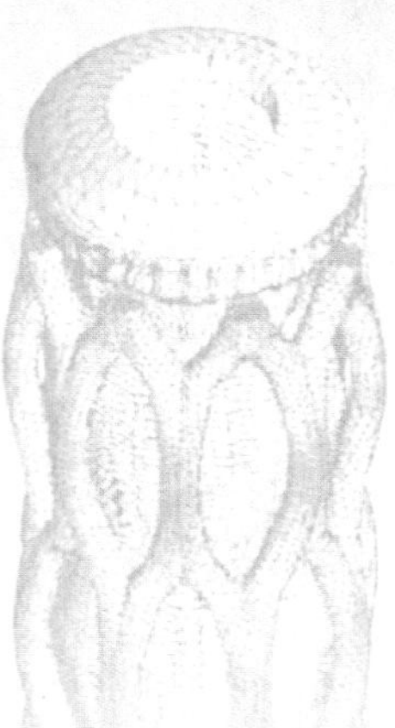

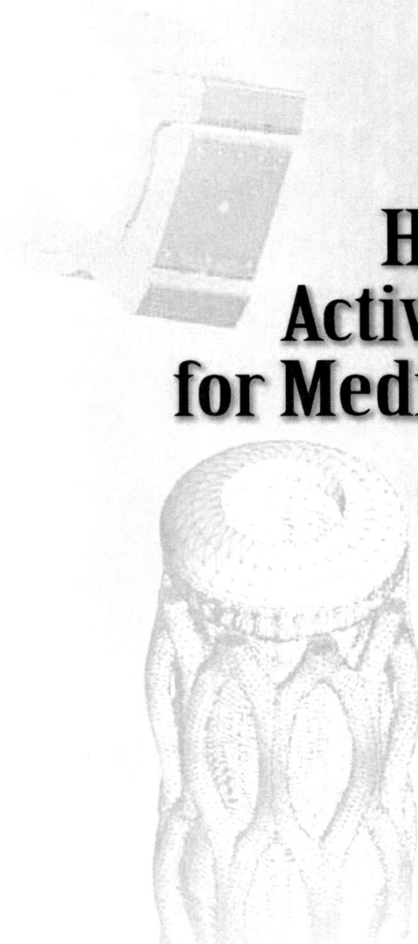

Handbook of Active Materials for Medical Devices

Advances and Applications

Edited by

Andrés Díaz Lantada

PAN STANFORD PUBLISHING

Published by

Pan Stanford Publishing Pte. Ltd.
Penthouse Level, Suntec Tower 3
8 Temasek Boulevard
Singapore 038988

Email: editorial@panstanford.com
Web: www.panstanford.com

British Library Cataloguing-in-Publication Data
A catalogue record for this book is available from the British Library.

Handbook of Active Materials for Medical Devices: Advances and Applications

ISBN 978-981-4303-36-1 (Hardcover)
ISBN 978-981-4303-35-4 (eBook)

Printed in the USA

To my beloved, Melike

When in the chronicle of wasted time
I see descriptions of the fairest wights,
And beauty making beautiful old rhyme
In praise of ladies dead and lovely knights,
Then in the blazon of sweet beauty's best,
Of hand, of foot, of lip, of eye, of brow,
I see the antique pen would have expressed
Even such a beauty as you master now.
So all their praises are but prophecies
Of this our time, all you prefiguring,
And, for they looked but with divining eyes,
They had not skill enough your worth to sing:

For we, which now behold these present days,
Have eyes to wonder, but lack tongues to praise.

William Shakespeare

To our baby, Seda

Caminante, son tus huellas
el camino y nada más;
Caminante, no hay camino,
se hace camino al andar.
Al andar se hace el camino,
y al volver la vista atrás
se ve la senda que nunca
se ha de volver a pisar.

Caminante no hay camino
sino estelas en la mar.

Antonio Machado

Acknowledgements

No book is ever the product of one person's efforts, and certainly this one was no different. This book would never have become a reality without the help and suggestions of many supportive institutions, relatives, friends, and colleagues, only a proportion of whom I have space to acknowledge here.

This book was supported in part by the Spanish Ministry of Science and Innovation, through the Singular Strategic Research Project "IBE — Rapid Manufacturing" (PSE-020000-2009-1), project carried out in collaboration between several industrial partners and universities, including Universidad Politécnica de Madrid (www.upm.es).

I owe a great deal to my colleagues and students at Mechanical Engineering Department (Machines Engineering Division) who encouraged, supported, and enlightened me through their own research, comments, and questions.

Particularly, Chair Prof. Dr Pilar Lafont Morgado, through her guidance during my PhD and with her always bright comments, has deeply influenced my perspective of engineering, research, and teaching. She has helped improve the results of several chapters, with her experience of a career devoted to researching and teaching at university. She has provided the forward-looking approach of a pioneer in several research lines, with multidisciplinary experience in combining CAD-CAE tools and rapid manufacturing for product development, linking the world of microsystems with bioengineering, studying contact phenomena in different media, or applying standards and structured methodologies to machine design.

I am very grateful to Mr Pedro Ortego García, whose expertise has been of great help for the manufacture and trials of many of the prototypes included, as case studies, in the different chapters of book.

I am also very grateful to Prof. John Ollier for his help with the translation of the book, for helping give all the chapters a consistent style, with a great end result.

I would also like to thank the team at PAN Stanford Publishing for their confidence, support, encouraging comments, and help.

Of course, to my parents, Andrés and Piedad, for a whole life of dedication and love, hoping they are proud of their son.

Above all, to my wife, Melike Erol (the essence of joy made person).

A.D. Lantada

Preface

Handbook of Active Materials for Medical Devices: Advances and Applications pays attention to all kinds of biodevices, mainly implantable or quirurgical, for the diagnosis or treatment of different pathologies, which benefit from the use of active materials as sensors or actuators.

Such active or "intelligent" materials are capable of responding in a controlled way to different external physical or chemical stimuli by changing some of their properties. These materials can be used to design and develop sensors, actuators, and multifunctional systems with a large number of applications for developing biodevices and medical appliances.

Current work in these fields entails problems related to synthesis, characterization, modelling, simulation, processing, and prototyping technologies, as well as device testing and validation — all of these have been treated in depth in this book — for the several types of active or intelligent materials covered.

This book is developed for providing support to researchers in physics, materials science, and bioengineering, especially for those working in the field of active or intelligent materials for biological or medical applications. We believe the book can prove to be an interesting and useful reference textbook at the postgraduate or doctoral level, as it covers aspects linked to three (out of four) areas included in the National Science Foundation Report on "Converging Technologies for Improving Human Performance":

- **Biotechnology:** The most important present and forthcoming biological and medical applications of different families of intelligent materials are analysed in depth.
- **Nanotechnology:** The most important properties of active materials are very closely linked to their nanostructure and to the processing conditions for obtaining such structure.
- **Information technology:** The use of computer-based information systems is essential in modelling, simulation, and design tasks related to active materials.

The book discusses in detail the great potential of active or intelligent materials for the development of sensors, actuators, and multifunctional systems linked to applications in the field of biodevices and medical appliances. It also analyses in depth the main biological and medical applications of various families of intelligent materials, including case studies showing complete development processes. The book details the most important aspects linked to the main families of active or intelligent materials, including synthesis, characterization, modelling, simulation, processing, and prototyping technologies, as well as device testing and validation. Ultimately, based on the experiences explained, a proposal of development methodology is presented, so as to help future researches and developments of medical appliances and biodevices on the basis of the capabilities of these novel materials. An extensive bibliography for further reading is provided, together with references to main manufacturers of several families of active materials.

We believe that the researches presented in this book will help future developments of medical devices, based on the additional functionalities that the use of active or intelligent materials, both as sensors and actuators, supplies. We hope that the main results exposed may help in the industrial expansion of this kind of materials as part of more complex systems.

Contents

Chapter 1

Introduction to Product Development and Systematic Methodologies

Andrés Díaz Lantada and Pilar Lafont Morgado
Mechanical Engineering Department, E.T.S.I. Industriales, Universidad Politécnica de Madrid, c/ José Gutiérrez Abascal 2, 28006 Madrid, Spain
adiaz@etsii.upm.es

1.1 An Introduction to Product Development: Basic Concepts

According to the main language academies a "product" (from the Latin *productus*) in its principal meaning is "anything that has been produced", or an expanded definition might be "anything useful manufactured or made that contributes economic value".

If we look more deeply at the meaning of "engineering", we can take the meaning assigned by "Accreditation Board for Engineering and Technology (ABET)", according to which "Engineering is the profession in which a knowledge of the Mathematical and Natural Sciences gained by study, experience and practice is applied with judgement to develop ways to utilise, economically, the materials and forces of nature for the benefit of mankind". In line with this definition and bearing in mind the reality of industry, we can enumerate the main jobs done by engineers in the course of their work:

- Design and calculation of products, processes, facilities and plants in every area of industry

Handbook of Active Materials for Medical Devices: Advances and Applications
Edited by Andrés Díaz Lantada

www.panstanford.com

- Research, development and innovation in products, processes and industrial methods
- Preparing, leading and managing projects in every area of industry
- Managing, planning and supervising multidisciplinary teams
- Strategic planning of quality systems, production systems and environmental management
- Financial management of projects and industrial concerns
- General management or technical work or research and development projects in the plants and factories of industrial concerns

According to the degree of dedication required by the work set out, three types of engineers can be defined for the present-day world:

- **Production engineers**. They produce goods and services. They keep the means of production in working order and manage them efficiently.
- **Design engineers**. They design new products and new processes. They take an active part in research, development and innovation.
- **Management engineers**. They decide and control the techno-economic and political processes on an entrepreneurial level in local, national and global contexts.

In whichever case, many of the problems facing engineers in their jobs are closely linked with the design and development work of new products, a large percentage of which are intended to help solve other more complex problems or evaluate the performance of certain functionalities of a system (as is the case with test equipment and test benches and machines).

In other cases, particularly in research centres and universities, the development process is oriented towards showing the feasibility or usefulness of a new function, geometry, material, technology or process concerning a product.

In these situations, the process usually ends up proving such feasibility or usefulness as a result of a prototype being obtained that is capable of rousing not only the interest of the scientific community but also that of the main companies in the sector concerned that might be willing to start up production and market the concept. Thus, design and development engineers, often called designers, contribute their work finding solutions and developing specific products. They also have important responsibilities as their ideas, knowledge and skills are decisive in deciding the technical, economic and safety aspects of a product.

It is important to emphasise that due to the complexity of modern technology only on very rare occasions can an entire product development process be carried out by an individual organisation. This task usually requires considerable human and technical resources which involve difficulties of organisation and communication.

To increase a new product's chances of success, the development process must be methodically and meticulously planned and systematically executed. Not only must technical and financial feasibility be considered but also concepts like the end safety associated with using the product, and the environmental impact that its use might have in addition to the human factors that can influence the different stages of the design process.

Using wide-ranging information sources and following the recommendations laid down in regulations is also highly recommended for a successful outcome.

A development methodology should, therefore, integrate different issues so that the overall process is logical and comprehensible, as the following section will explain. To achieve this, it is essential for the process to be divided into stages and tasks, each with its own individual method and way of going about the job.

The following section sets out the main stages to be found in most general theories of design engineering and product development (Roozenburg and Eeckels, 1995; Pahl and Beitz, 1996 (ed. Wallace); Muñoz-Guijosa *et al.*, 2005; Ulrich and Eppinger, 2007), also applicable to more complex projects (De Cos, 1999).

Although this work is focused on the design of medical devices, it is important to point out that the main stages of development of these types of products basically coincide with the stages proposed by the systematic methodology about to be explained.

Nevertheless, several additional considerations need to be borne in mind that will be explained later, together with the considerable modifications required that are linked to working with active materials that may help optimise applying this general methodology to the specific case of medical devices with detection or activation capabilities.

1.2 Systematic Methodologies for Product Development

1.2.1 The Need for Systematic Development Methodologies

Depending on the variety of the problems and tasks involved in developing products, design actions have multiple facets. They are dependent not only on basic scientific and technological know-how, but also on the individual experience of different design engineers and their specific knowledge in the area related to the product under development.

It should be remembered that designers have the prime responsibility for a product's technical and economic aspects and also for the efficient development process of its commercial aspects by adapting it to limited schedules and costs. It is therefore important to have designed a process or methodology that will lead to appropriate guaranteed solutions. This methodology must be flexible but at the same time capable of being planned, optimised and verified. However, this approach can only lead to success if all those taking part in the design have the necessary knowledge and work systematically.

It is important to make a distinction between the science of design and design methodology. The science of design uses scientific method to analyse the structure of technical systems and how they relate to the environment, with the purpose of developing rules for these technical systems by taking the system components and examining how they are related.

However, design methodology is a specific way of acting to design technical systems that get their knowledge from the teachings of design science and cognitive psychology as well as from practical experience in different sectors. It includes action plans for connecting the different work and design stages in accordance with content and the organisation envisaged; strategies, rules and principles for reaching general and specific goals; and methods for solving the problems of individual design or partial tasks. In line with this approach, a design methodology should

- Encourage a direct approach to problems
- Foster creativity and understanding

- Facilitate the search for optimal solutions
- Be based on the methodical application of knowledge
- Be compatible with the concepts, methods and discoveries of other disciplines
- Maintain the interest of the participants
- Be easily learned and taught
- Reduce time, costs and errors

The approach set out should lead those involved in design to find possible solutions more quickly and directly than if they were working purely from intuition or experience. These two qualities are obviously important for any design process.

It is important to point out that the use of a systematic methodology is not at loggerheads with intuition or experience, but simply attempts to expand and channel the potential of talented designers while demonstrating that successful solutions do not only depend on intuition or experience but on a whole range of factors.

If the problem and design-linked tasks are structured, we also manage to recognise that existing solutions can be applied to solve concrete problems and speed up the stages of the overall process. It also lets us use powerful computer-aided design tools suited to optimising specific tasks.

These tools will be discussed further on. On the other hand, it is essential to use systematic procedures to properly organise information flows resulting from the design project and to prepare all the paperwork required to start up product production and any after-sales procedures.

Below is an explanation of how the product design process evolves until it reaches the most utilised present-day systematic methodologies, which will then be explained in detail.

1.2.2 A Historic Perspective Up to Present-Day Methodologies

It is difficult to find the origins of what we call "systematic design". To offer but one example, anyone studying the diagrams and sketches of Leonardo da Vinci can hardly fail to observe the depth of his analysis and how he systematically used variations to suggest possible solutions and be able to compare them (Taddei and Zanon, 2006; Bautista *et al.*, 2007).

Up to the Industrial Revolution, product design and development work was essentially linked to art and craft, and only with the gradual mechanization of processes halfway through the 19th century did a need begin to emerge to optimise the use of materials and perform detailed studies on strength, stiffness, wear, friction, assembly and maintenance (Reuleaux, 1875).

However, it was not until the 20th century that a systematic evaluation of these parameters was put forward as a way of gradually reaching an optimal solution (Erkens, 1928). Just before the Second World War a need was beginning to be noticed to rationalise product design processes, but progress in this direction was hampered by the following factors:

- An absence of effective methods for representing abstract ideas
- The widespread belief that design was an art and not a technical activity that could be carried out methodically and not just through creativity

A large-scale use of systematic design methodologies would have to wait for these limitations to be overcome and the introduction of a more widespread use of automation and the appearance of more modern data processing procedures.

Modern ideas on systematic development were given an enormous boost by relevant figures (Kesselring, 1951, 1954; Tschochner, 1954; Matousek, 1957; or Niemann, 1950, 1965, 1975), whose revolutionary ideas continue to suggest ways of solving and dealing with specific tasks related to machine and product design processes (Kaiser and König, 2006).

During the 1940s and the 1950s, Kesserling put forward a method based on successive approaches where each approach optimised different variables in line with technical and economic criteria. He also proposed several principles like "minimal production costs", "minimal weight and volume", "minimal loss" and "optimal functionality and operability".

On the other hand, in the 1950s Tschochner emphasised the importance of four basic design factors: the principles of functionality, material, shape and size, similar to what Matousek would later do, but emphasising the need to consider the principles of functionality, material, manufacture and geometry.

Niemann's approach designed in the 1960s and 1970s consisted in starting out design by defining a general outline for the product with the main sizes to be worked on in greater depth. To this end, the overall design continued to be divided into different parts that could be developed in parallel. The optimal solution was finally reached by a systematic variation of all the possible solutions.

These progressive approaches towards ever more systematic methodologies for product design were mainly performed by university lecturers who had learnt the fundamentals of design and development during their practical class contacts with increasingly complex products. They realised that not only was it possible to apply more mathematical concepts, physical principles, information, theory-based methods and systematic design, but that with the gradual increase in the division of work it was becoming indispensable.

Their designs were evidently strongly influenced by the industries they worked for, but many of their principles suitably modified can be adapted to numerous cases of design in other sectors. The currently accepted principles for effectively carrying out new product development are based on the ideas of the foregoing authors, as well as on the series of design steps that subsequently set apart important researchers (Hansen, 1956; Wächtler, 1967; or Kuhlenkamp, 1971).

In general terms, these researchers talk of "pre-studies", "defining the basic principle", "basic design" and "detailed design" as the main stages. They are also listed in "design guidelines" written by organisations like the "Verein Deutscher Ingenieure (VDI)" or the "International Organization for Standardization (ISO)" in reference to global testing and quality management.

1.2.3 Stages of a Product's Systematic Development Process

The outcomes of previous research, satisfactorily proven through numerous developed products, led to a slightly modified work structure (Roozenburg and Eeckels, 1995; Pahl and Beitz, 1996; Muñoz-Guijosa *et al.*, 2005; Ulrich and Eppinger, 2007) which included planning, conceptual design, basic engineering and detailed engineering, although a clear dividing line cannot always be set between these stages.

Defining objectives and planning

This broadly consists of the strategic decision taken by a company, university or research centre as to which products or ideas must be developed to satisfy the new social needs, taking account of the scientific-technological and socio-economic circumstances of the time. To set about a product idea that will be successful the state of the market has to be fully understood and especially customers and their needs. Thus, market and customer requirements become the major stimuli for developing new products.

However, these stimuli frequently have other origins, the most important of which are politics, the appearance of new technologies, processes, materials, discoveries or research results and environmental issues. Neither should the role played by internal stimuli be underestimated (arising in the company, university or technology centre itself) when it comes to making a decision about a new product. Among these internal stimuli are new ideas or outcomes related to research activity and the implementation of new means of production as well as production being made more rational and diversified.

Depending on the stimuli mentioned, the main tasks to be included in the "defining objectives and planning" stage are:

- **Situation analysis.** By carrying out an in-depth study of the company and its products, together with market analysis and other possible information sources, a thorough analysis can be reached of the starting out point.
- **Drawing up search strategies.** By bearing in mind the companies' aims, strengths and weaknesses, as well as market gaps and needs, certain areas or promising fields can be discovered where ideas can be sought to be applied.
- **Finding product ideas.** From the search in the chosen field for new applications, functions, principles of functionality, geometries, materials, energy management methods and other alternatives, a set of product ideas can be found.
- **Choosing product ideas.** Depending on the company's aims and market needs, the set of ideas found are evaluated in order to choose the most attractive product idea.
- **Defining the product to be developed.** By evaluating the different alternatives against a list of requirements a product proposal or definition is reached together with some initial objectives concerning costs, prices and schedules.

Conceptual design

This is the stage where a decisive global principle is reached or a basis for reaching a satisfactory solution based on identifying crucial problems and choosing the right functional principles that in combination will attain the set objective.

If this stage is to be properly tackled a series of prerequisites must be fulfilled linked to a correct conclusion of the previous stage. The objective must therefore be clearly stated and, in principle, be technically and financially viable. In addition, the designer must be informed of the needs of this conceptual design stage and the existence of possible solutions that allow proceeding directly to the design or basic engineering stage. The scope and depth required for the conceptual design stage must also be pre-established. Related to the above, the main tasks included in this stage are listed below:

- **Abstraction for identifying basic problems.** The decisive designs and principles based on traditional methods cease to provide optimum responses in the face of scientific-technological advances concerning technologies, materials or procedures, which when used in combination usually provide the key to more effective new solutions. On the other hand, every industry, company or research centre has countless experiences, which, although valuable, can lead to prejudice and hinder the creative process. For this reason, particularly at the outset of a new product design, designers must make an effort of abstraction and distance themselves from the influences of conventional ideas and focus on analysing the list of requirements and setting out the fundamental problem or problems in an objective manner.
- **Setting functional frameworks.** Having set out the basic problem to be solved, a global function must be obtained based on energy flows, mass and signals so that a relationship between the inputs to, and outputs from the plant, machine, part or object to be designed can be established. This global function can then be divided into less complex sub-functions and a lower level of abstraction, all of which can be individually dealt with to facilitate the search for solutions. Combining and relating these sub-functions leads to the so-called functional framework. It is advisable to draw up several functional frameworks depending on whether it is wished to optimise costs, functionalities, quality, development time or other factors.

- **Designing functional frameworks.** After establishing the different functional frameworks the principles of functionality for each of the sub-functions need to be sought. When they have been found, they should be properly interconnected to produce all the different possible functional frameworks that fulfil the global function. In line with the different preferences (cost, timeframe, quality and others), a table of choices can be made to choose the most suitable functional frameworks.
- **Obtaining the decisive principle.** By taking the functional frameworks the different decisive principles to be evaluated can be obtained based on the different techno-economic criteria and preliminary calculations that can lead to the choice of the most adequate decisive principle (proposal for a preliminary solution or product concept) that can be worked on.

Basic engineering

When the decisive principle has been arrived at it is time to specify the underlying ideas behind this preliminary proposal for a solution or product concept. During the basic engineering stage (also often called basic design) the design engineers have the task of defining the basic shapes and geometries that characterise the product, and must also choose the preliminary materials and appropriate manufacturing processes. It is at this stage when technical, technological and economic considerations become of vital importance. In other words, the mission of this stage is to provide a definitive general outline of the product to be developed, on which an effective analysis can be performed concerning function, duration, manufacture, assembly, functionality, costs and safety. Unlike the conceptual design stage, the basic engineering stage is subject to numerous checks, which means the work of analysis and synthesis constantly alternate and complement each other. An enormous effort also needs to be made regarding the compilation of information to make it easier to evaluate solutions, identify errors and continuously optimise them.

The complexity of this stage is also greater because many actions have to be performed simultaneously. Sub-tasks need to be repeated when high levels of information are reached and because any change in an area or sub-area has repercussions on all the rest. For these reasons, it is impossible to set a series of steps to be strictly adhered to that will ensure the basic engineering will come to a successful conclusion. However, the following approach may be followed in general terms:

- Choose the requirements that are crucially important in the basic engineering stage.
- Make scale drawings with the existing spatial constraints and evaluate the required free spaces.
- Draw up a basic outline to decide which components will be required to fulfil the main functions.
- Draw up a preliminary design of the parts and components that fulfil these main functions.
- Draw up a basic outline to decide which components will fulfil the remaining secondary functions.
- Draw up the preliminary designs of parts and components that fulfil these secondary functions.
- Evaluate the designs using both technical and economic criteria.
- Decide the overall preliminary design.
- Optimise the chosen design, eradicating any weak points that may have arisen during evaluation.
- Make proposals for improvement and checking if cost and quality objectives are met.
- Prepare a basic preliminary parts and documentation list for production and assembly. This documentation comprises the starting point for the detailed engineering stage.

During the basic engineering stage it is very useful to use checklists to ensure that when designing the different parts intended for the main product functions, all the various aspects have been taken into account. Of these aspects the most important are

- Function
- Principle of functionality
- Design
- Safety
- Regulations
- Ergonomics
- Manufacturing
- Quality control
- Assembly
- Transport
- Operation
- Fault detection

- Recycling
- Maintenance
- Cost
- Timescale

Alongside this stage as part of the work to compare designs and check geometries and functionalities, it is very useful to produce prototypes that will aid decision-making and help reduce the number of design iterations and minimise both the timescales and costs associated with product development.

Currently a distinction is made between virtual prototypes, the result of computer-aided design, simulation, calculation and manufacturing programs ("CAD-CAE-CAM" programs) and physical prototypes that coincide with the traditional concept of "original product sample for testing and checking".

The appearance of support "software" for engineering design work and its gradual incorporation into industry since the end of the 1980s, together with growing operational and calculating capacity, have caused major changes to the way design processes are carried out. Information exchange has become easier, enabling countless effects in combination to be taken into account using multivariable simulations and enabling forecasts to be made concerning the influence of parameters such as the material or the manufacturing process on the end quality of a part or product.

All these "software" tools can be included in a set of computer tools for managing the life-cycle of a product or "PLM – Product Lifecycle Management programs" (Stark, 2004; Saaksvuori and Immonen, 2008). These capabilities enable a company to effectively manage and develop their products and related services throughout their economic life. All companies also need to manage the communications and information with their customers ("CRM – Customer Relationship Management tools or programs"), with their suppliers (programs called "SCM – Supply Chain Management") and company resources (programs referred to as "ERP – Enterprise Resource Planning").

These three groups of software programs together with the PLM programs complete the four cornerstones of the information technology infrastructure that enable the main needs of a company to be addressed.

More directly linked to product development in line with the approach taken here, PLM tools that include the following types of software programs come to the fore for performing tasks like

- **Product and Portfolio Management (PPM).** These programs are aimed at helping determine the optimal combination or sequence for the projects proposed for the company to successfully achieve it's objectives in accordance with its economic and technological strategy and actual market requirements. These tools help analyse resources, costs, investment, production schedules and how one project affects another.
- **Computer-Aided Design (CAD).** These programs support design engineers, architects and other design professionals in their work, which is to make their designs a reality. They usually have 2D and 3D drawing systems for creating files or have all the information on a product's geometry and its different parts, as well as its plans. Changes can be made, symmetries are included, scale designs and numerous operations that can help make changes to the design.
- **Computer-Aided Engineering (CAE).-** These computer programs allow simulating designs that have usually been made with CAD programs, and apply kinematic, dynamic, thermal or fluid mechanic considerations to the geometries designed and, above all, the chosen materials. They allow analysing how changes will affect the product or its parts and help optimise the number of prototypes or tests required.
- **Computer-Aided Manufacturing (CAM).** These programs lend support to prototype manufacturing work and end products by converting the information on part geometry from a CAD program into a code that can be understood by numerical control, manufacturing or rapid prototyping machines. On occasions it has a similar mission to CAE programs, letting part quality be simulated according to the manufacturing process used as well as allowing a study on geometries and materials.
- **Product Data Management (PDM).** These are programs focused on facilitating the records and paperwork of the processes to create, modify and revise any of the parts of a product. The information stored ranges from specifications, CAD file diagrams, plans, manufacturing documents, assembly documents, tenders, test specifications and quality control, as well as financial reports.

In recent years, the boundaries between these types of software are shrinking with the ever more frequent appearance of packs that combine different modules to provide a global response to all the aforementioned needs.

As explained, these technologies can provide assistance at every product design stage as well as production start-up, market placement and after-sales services. The benefits of using them become obvious at the basic engineering stage where their use is even more justified in the detailed engineering stage where the amount of information handled increases rapidly, as will be explained further on.

Regarding prototypes, the industrial importance taken on over the last decade by the so-called "manufacturing and rapid prototyping technologies" should be emphasised.

These technologies enable physical parts to be directly obtained in a short time (hours or a few days) from the designs made with the help of a computer using "CAD-CAE-CAM" programs, as Fig. 1.1 shows.

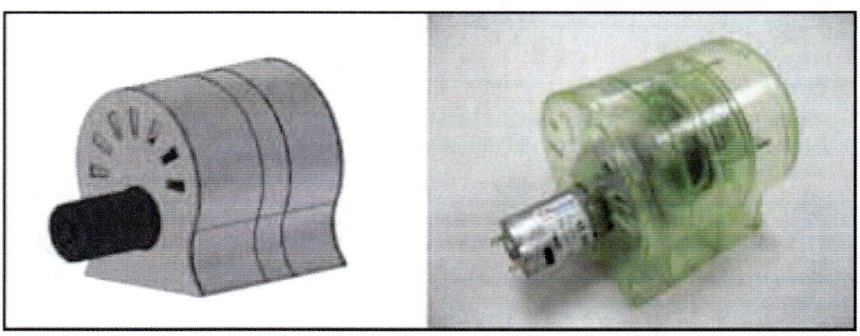

Figure 1.1 Design and prototype of an internal gear assembly pump (Díaz Lantada and Lafont, 2005). Combined use of CAD programs and rapid prototyping technologies.

They are of great help in optimising design iterations, help the early detection of errors and speed up production start-up. They are usually either based on "layer manufacturing technologies" (like laser stereolithography or selective laser sintering) or on material elimination manufacturing processes (high speed numerical control machining). The different technologies available mean that prototypes can be obtained in a wide range of metal, ceramic and polymeric materials with remarkable precision (Freitag and Wohlers, 2003; Kucklick, 2006; Lafont *et al.*, 2007, 2008).

Depending on the objective and the similarity to the end product, the physical prototypes are usually divided into the following three levels:

- **Level "A" prototypes (commonly called "A-samples").** These are demonstration prototypes for analysing shapes, geometries and other more subjective aspects (like aesthetics, visual impact or ergonomics) related to the product under development.
- **Level "B" prototypes (commonly called "B-samples").** These are functional prototypes intended for checking the behaviour of different product parts and their functionalities. Although they are generally made of non-final materials, these tests are usually performed with limits on certain applications.
- **Level "C" prototypes (commonly called "C-samples").** These are prototypes with similar materials and behaviour to the end product although the manufacturing methods used to obtain them do not coincide with the methods used in production. These level "C" prototypes are usually manufactured for final checks, to prepare production start-up and for obtaining official approval as part of the detailed engineering stage which will be dealt with further on.

However, the end of the basic engineering stage and the beginning of the detailed engineering stage cannot be precisely delimited as there is always some overlap that is to the benefit of the overall process.

Detailed engineering

Once the final basic design has been obtained, work must be begun on the requirements of the shape, properties, size and tolerances of the different parts. The final choice of manufacturing and assembly must also be done as well as final cost evaluation. The outcome of this stage is the definitive technical specifications of the product: a list of functionalities, production plans and the specifications including the instructions for assembly, disassembly and operation.

Based on this information or technical documentation, production start-up can be undertaken as well as the placing of the product on the market. According to the above, detailed engineering work can be divided into the following:

- **Finalising the end design.** The different parts are fully defined by means of plans or 3D geometry CAD files, and materials, tolerances, adjustments and other details are specified.

- **Parts integration.** By means of full comprehensive plans or CAD assembly files which define the product as a whole.
- **Finalising paperwork.** For an unambiguous definition of the product and be able to launch production.
- **Final checks.** As to compliance with general regulations and company standards. Precision of size and tolerances, the availability of standard or catalogue parts and other checks.

The basic and detailed engineering stages can often be brought together in one single design stage with a global focus where the level of detail is gradually added. The ever more generalised use of CAD-CAE-CAM technologies and the already mentioned PLM tools has promoted this gradual fusion between stages, which also simplifies any information exchange between the agents involved in product design.

Other authors with a similar outlook to that set out (Roozenburg and Eeckels, 1995) also include production and marketing planning actions in the methodology they put forward, since the overall design of a product requires considerable human resources and materials to be assigned as well as production, distribution and sales strategies and other after-sales services.

Fig. 1.2 shows a full design process diagram with explanations (objectives and planning, conceptual design, and basic and detailed engineering).

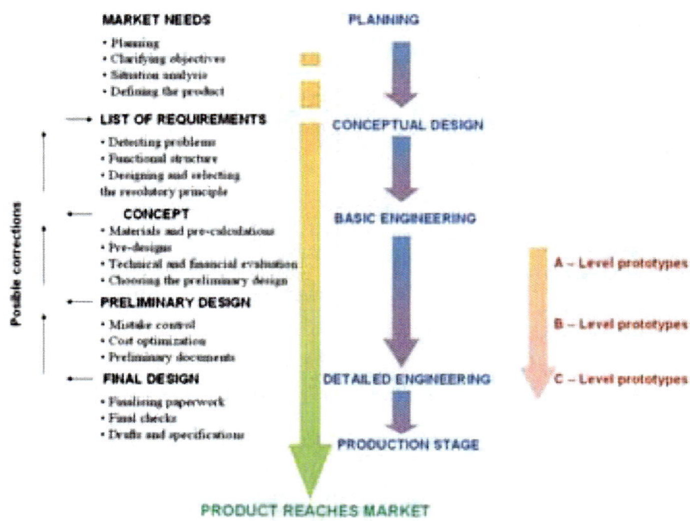

Figure 1.2 Systematic methodology diagram for product design.

1.3 Additional Tools for Ensuring Quality

The history of industrial design usually recognises three quality leaps regarding design approach and the fundamental reasons behind that design; these changes of approach are directly related to the three following concepts:

- **Productivity.** The main objective at the start of the Industrial Revolution since the very existence and survival of emerging industry depended on this concept.
- **Safety.** A concept that has gradually taken on importance throughout the 20th century as society became more aware, with increasing economic growth together with the technological progress that enabled safer systems to be introduced. At first, it was considered to be a factor that hampered production, but later it was shown that productivity and safety contributed synergy, and so, manufacturing safe products safely became paramount.
- **Quality.** A notion that especially over the last three decades has become a basic goal of production processes and developed products. Referring to product design it can be understood to mean "the set of properties of the design process that enables products to be set in production that fulfil the needs envisaged at the outset".

Whatever the circumstances, reaching acceptable levels of quality involves more and more the company as a whole and product design means taking account of quality issues throughout the entire design process already explained.

A good starting point is the ISO 9000 Series set of standards which set out the basis for applying quality procedures in different organisations and the associated tasks, such as product design, production and manufacturing processes and commercial activities. The standards advocate that the best way to attain top quality is to take measures that will avoid failure by systemising processes and quantifying the parameters that have most bearing on quality.

The implications involved in this set of standards and how they relate to the European Union's so-called "New Approach Directives" will be dealt with in the discussion of standards included towards the end of the chapter, with a special emphasis on the design of medical devices.

Another key factor for attaining high levels of quality in product design tasks is to correctly interpret the customers' requirements and be exact in defining the initial specifications.

In principle, the key factors for attaining high levels of quality are

- Systemising the design process by using structured methodologies, as has already been explained
- Identifying potential faults and taking counter-measures
- Identifying any potential disturbances to the input parameters that might affect the output parameters and take counter-measures
- The participation of all departments (design, production, testing, quality, sales, purchases, commercial and any others) in the aforementioned tasks
- Learning based on the defects of previous products

Tools to ensure design quality

To ensure quality throughout the design stage and methodically take account of the key factors, the use of various tools is becoming widespread, of which the most important are

- **"Quality function deployment (QFD)" and related methodologies.** Such tools help to take into account market and user demands when tackling the development of a new product. By using several matrices for quantifying the need of relevant changes linked to the enterprise services and production system, materials and processes used, global quality optimisation is promoted and final results improved. "QFD" is designed to help planners focus on characteristics of a new or existing product or service from the viewpoints of market segments, company strategies or new technology-development needs. It is applied in a wide variety of services, consumer products and emerging technology products.
- **The use of "failure trees".** This is a tool for systemising and enhancing the process and for detecting potential faults and disturbance factors. It is incorporated at the conceptual design stage once the product's functional framework is available with the general function and all the sub-functions involved in the product's proper working, all of which must be checked. The different functions and sub-functions are checked one by one, thinking of how they could fail and searching out any

possible faults and then looking for the possible causes and disturbances that could lead to those faults. When any possible causes of faults have been assessed, counter-measures are designed for each one. If necessary, the concept is redesigned, the design is improved or the procedures for manufacture, assembly, logistics, quality, maintenance and others are modified. As the work required to complete a fault tree for an entire product is considerable, this method is usually limited to decisive issues and critical processes. It is advisable for designers to make this way of working part of their everyday activities and so apply these concepts almost by intuition.

- **"Failure mode and effect analysis (FMEA) method".** This method, originally designed for the "Apollo" program is more powerful than the fault tree since it quantifies the absolute importance of every fault mode by using the so-called "risk number (RN)", which is quantified according to the probability of fault occurrence and the probability of it being detected. Therefore, risks can be classified in order of importance and priorities set for searching and for executing counter-measures. It is widely used nowadays in all industrial sectors. However, the use of this method requires expert staff in all departments. The "FMEA" is usually reviewed several times during product design and possible counter-measures, responsible persons and control dates are set. This method helps ensure the quality but above all the safety of the product right from the design stage, which has previously proven to be of great help in fields such as machine design (Muñoz Sanz *et al.*, 2007).
- **Quality meetings.** Specially designed to avoid difficult-to-solve faults in the advanced stages of development. The starting point is usually a check-list based on questions concerning the experience of previous designs. Members of all departments usually take part in these meetings where counter-measures are suggested and persons are proposed for being responsible for applying the measures in the set timeframe. Once again, it is essential to emphasise the importance of fluid communication between all those involved in the product design process if a successful outcome is to be reached.

***

Having explained the main stages of the most widely used systematic product design methodologies; Chapter 2 will cover some additional issues to be taken into account when the design corresponds to a medical device.

This will be followed by a discussion on the standards to be applied to medical device development, as well as certain issues related to research and questions of ethics that need to be borne in mind and which help in decision-making tasks.

Finally, an analysis is included of how the various additional issues influence each of the design stages of a medical device and how certain changes to these stages can make it easier to integrate the new technologies and materials into the design process for this type of product.

References

Aparicio Izquierdo, F.; González Tirados, R.M.; Sobrevila, M.A. "Formación de ingenieros: Objetivos, métodos y estrategias". Editorial ICE—Universidad Politécnica de Madrid. Madrid, 2005.

Bautista Paz, E.; Bernardos Rodríguez, R.; Ceccarelli, M.; *et al.* "Breve Historia Ilustrada de las Máquinas". Sección de Publicaciones de la E.T.S.I. Industriales. Universidad Politécnica de Madrid. Edición Preliminar, Madrid, 2007.

De Cos Castillo, M. "Teoría general del proyecto. Volumen I: Dirección de proyectos". Editorial Síntesis. Madrid, 1999.

De Cos Castillo, M. "Teoría General del Proyecto. Volumen II: Ingeniería de proyectos". Editorial Síntesis, Madrid, 1999.

Díaz Lantada, A.; Lorenzo Yustos, H.; Lafont, P.; *et al.* "Teaching applications for rapid prototyping technologies". International Journal of Engineering Education, 23(2), 411–418, 2007.

Erkens, A. "Beiträge zur Konstruktionserziehung". VDI-Z Verlag. Integrierte Produktion, 72, 17–21, 1928.

Freitag, D.; Wohlers, T. "Rapid prototyping: State of the Art". Manufacturing technology information analysis centre. Chicago, Illinois, 2003.

Hansen, F. "Konstruktionssystematik". VEB Verlag Technik. Berlin, 1956.

Kaiser, W.; König, W. "Geschichte des Ingenieurs. Ein Beruf in sechs Jahrtausenden". Carl Hanser Verlag. München, 2006.

Kesselring, F. "Bewertung von Konstruktionen". VDI Verlag. Düsseldorf, 1951.

Kesselring, F. "Technische Kompositionslehre". Springer. Berlin, 1954.

Kucklick, T.R. "The medical device R&D handbook". CRC Press, Taylor and Francis Group. Florida, 2006.

Kuhlenkamp, A. "Konstruktionslehre der Feinwerktechnik". Hanser. München, 1971.

Lafont Morgado, P.; Lorenzo Yustos, H. *et al.* "Rapid tooling: Moldes rápidos a partir de estereolitografía". Revista de plásticos modernos, 524, 150-157, 2000.

Matousek, R. "Konstruktionslehren des allgemeinen Maschinenbaus". Springer. Berlin, 1957.

Muñoz-Guijosa, J.M.; Bautista Paz, E.; Lafont Morgado, P.; *et al.* "Proyecto de Máquinas: Apuntes de Clase". Sección de Publicaciones de la E.T.S.I. Industriales - Universidad Politécnica de Madrid. Madrid, 2005.

Muñoz Sanz, J.L.; Leal Wiña, P.; Erades García-Toledano, G.; *et al.* "Metodo cuantitativo para la evaluación de la seguridad en máquinas en la fase de diseño". Actas del 8° Congreso Iberoamericano de Ingeniería Mecánica. Pontificia Universidad Católica del Perú. Cuzco, 2007.

Niemann, G. "Maschinenelemente". Springer. Berlin, 1950, 1965, 1975.

Pahl, G., Beitz, W. "Engineering design: A systematic approach". 2ª Edición Revisada. Springer Verlag. London, 1996.

Reuleaux, F. "Lehrbuch der Kinematik, 1: Theoretische Kinematik". Vieweg und Sohn. Braunschweig, 1875.

Reuleaux, F. "Lehrbuch der Kinematik, 2: Die praktischen Beziehungen Kinematik zu Geometrie und Mechanik". Vieweg und Sohn. Braunschweig, 1875.

Roozenburg, N.; Eeckels J. "Product design: Fundamentals and methods". John Wiley & Sons. New York, 1995.

Saaksvuori, A.; Immonen, A. "Product lifecycle management", 3rd Edition. Springer Verlag. Berlin, Heidelberg, London, New York, 2008.

Stark, J. "Product lifecycle management: 21st Century paradigm for product realisation". Springer Verlag. Berlin, Heidelberg, New York, 2004.

Taddei, M.; Zanon, E. "Atlas ilustrado de las máquinas de Leonardo". Editorial Susaeta. Madrid, 2006.

Tschochner, H. "Konstruieren und Gestalten". Girardet. Essen, 1954.

Ulrich, K., Eppinger, S. "Product design and development", 4th Edition. McGraw-Hill, Irwin, New York, 2007.

Wächtler, R. "Beitrag zur Theorie des Entwickelns (Konstruieren)". Feinwerktechnik, 71, 353-358, 1967.

Chapter 2

General Considerations for Developing Medical Devices

Andrés Díaz Lantada and Pilar Lafont Morgado
Mechanical Engineering Department, E.T.S.I. Industriales, Universidad Politécnica de Madrid, c/ José Gutiérrez Abascal, 28006 Madrid, Spain
adiaz@etsii.upm.es, plafont@etsii.upm.es

2.1 An Introduction to Medical Devices: Basic Concepts

A definition of medical device according to Council Directive 93/42/EEC of 14 June 1993 is "Any instrument, apparatus, appliance, material or other article, whether used alone or in combination, including the software necessary for its proper application intended by the manufacturer to be used for human beings for the purpose of

- diagnosis, prevention, monitoring, treatment or alleviation of disease;
- diagnosis, monitoring, treatment, alleviation or compensation for any injury or handicap;
- investigation, replacement or modification of the anatomy or of a physiological process; and
- control of conception, and which does not achieve its principal intended action by pharmacological, immunological or metabolic means, but which may be assisted in its function by such means".

Handbook of Active Materials for Medical Devices: Advances and Applications
Edited by Andrés Díaz Lantada

www.panstanford.com

According to the U.S. Food and Drug Administration: "A medical device is an instrument, apparatus, device, machine, appliance, implant, *in vitro* agent or other similar or related article, including a component part, or accessory which is

- recognised in the official "National Formulary" or the "United States Pharmacopoeia", or any supplement to them;
- intended for use in the diagnosis of disease or other conditions, or in the cure, mitigation, treatment or prevention of disease, in man or other animals;
- intended to affect the structure or any function of the body of man or other animals and which does not achieve any of its primary purposes through chemical action within or on the body of man or other animals and which is not dependent upon being metabolized for the achievement of any of its primary intended purposes".

The first devices to come to light that fit these definitions date back to Antiquity. Evidence has been found in Ancient Egypt of various surgical instruments for performing trepanations and other surgical operations, as well as instruments intended for use in mummification; splints made of bamboo, cane, wood or the bark of trees. These would most surely have also been used to treat broken bones in living patients. An engraving made around the year 2800 BC at the entrance to the tomb of Hirkouf bears witness to the oldest use of a crutch.

Many of the principles referring to different conditions and their treatment are attributed to the Ancient Greeks (Laín Entralgo, 1973). They may be considered the first to use a scientific methodology and were also the first to describe their history and progress in detail. Homer himself in his epic on the Trojan Wars reveals knowledge of the lesions of that period and the treatments used.

Between 430 and 330 BC, a vitally important Greek text was compiled known as the "Corpus Hipocraticum". It was named after Hippocrates, who was called the father of medicine. Hippocrates was born on the Island of Cos around the year 460 BC and died at a ripe old age in 370 BC. He is known for having endowed medicine with a scientific, systematic methodology and for having defined for the first time the position and role of the doctor in society. Hippocrates possessed a thorough knowledge of fractures. He knew the principles of traction and counter-traction and developed special splints for tibia fractures similar to an external brace. He also designed the Hippocratic bench or "scamnum" to provide a support when realigning fractured bones.

Although many centuries have passed, the Hippocratic Oath continues to occupy a prominent position in medical practice.

Subsequently, Herofilus came to the fore in Alexandria in the 3rd century BC for his study of the human body by dissecting corpses, which up to now had been considered sacred with anatomical studies only being performed on animals. There is a clear proof that during the 3rd to 1st century BC, in Alexandria post mortems were performed for the first time for investigative and diagnostic purposes, and for which very advanced instruments were required.

During the 2nd century BC of the Roman Empire the most important figure of the period was Galen who stood out for his observation of medical phenomena and his attempts to find an answer. He carried out post mortems on dead gladiators in the coliseum at Pergamon. When this empire fell, all scientific progress came to a halt leaving only copyist monks in monastery libraries to act as the transmitters of ancient culture.

Then came the rise and development of Arab culture with its contributions to Medicine and Surgery. Avicenna (980–1037) stood out for his use of cauterization by means of a hot iron, an instrument used to destroy organic tissue by the use of heat and also to stop bleeding. With the onset of the Renaissance, Medicine and Surgery was again given an impulse with the appearance of illustrated treatises on Anatomy like the one by Vesalius (1514–1564). These advances continued throughout the following centuries with the ensuing improvements in surgical techniques as well as methods of anaesthesia.

However, the main advances in medical devices that came about throughout the 19th and 20th centuries were unfortunately as a result of the Great Wars. One example that speaks for itself is that in London alone in the Second World War, it has been calculated that over 260,000 litres of blood were donated.

It is the direct responsibility of those of us who devote our lives to the progress of Science and Technology to make this situation change so that in the future such progress will never again be linked to a country's military might or be driven by the need to find a response to the effects of war, but instead will be devoted to improving the life-quality of human beings as its main objective.

At present, the world market for medical devices is estimated to stand at over 200 billion Euros and shows an annual growth of around 8% (growth only surpassed by the pharmaceutical sector).

The European Union, as a whole, is the second producer with a market share of 30%, with Spain as the fifth producer in the European Union with an EU market share of around 6% (Pammolli *et al.*, 2005).

Different factors and technological advances in recent decades have boosted the enormous growth of this highly economically important industrial sector, whose social impact is equally important. Set out below are the main factors that must drive study in this field and the never-ending search for solutions, as well as the main advances that have led to the rapid industrial expansion of this sector in recent years.

Socioeconomic factors

- The considerable increase in life expectancy in the developed countries has led to a notable increase in the demand for implants, prostheses and orthopaedic devices as the number of patients with degenerative diseases has also increased. According to UN demographers, in around 5 years, there will probably be more people over 60 than children under 15.
- Nowadays, one out of every ten people is 60 or over, but in 2050 it is predicted that these figures will reach one in five, and the number of persons over the age of 80 will multiply 5-fold. Greater longevity must go hand-in-hand with preserving the life quality of this group.
- The rising birth rate in underdeveloped countries together with the difficulty of access to basic needs favours the appearance of epidemics, but whose treatment can be improved by the use of new devices for the controlled delivery of drugs, the use of disposable surgical instruments, birth control devices and other recent or predicted future developments of this industrial sector.

Recent technological advances

- Improvements to purchasing systems, processing, the analysis and telecommunication of physiological signs, which have enabled patients to be more precisely monitored, both in the short term (e.g., during surgical operations and post-ops) and in the long term (studying the evolution of pathologies), by also enabling biological systems to be modelled and contribute physiopathological significance to the parameters found from processing (Deutsch *et al.*, 2007; Cerutti, 2008).

- The development of systems that interact between computers and the nervous systems of living beings based on two-way implants for receiving electric signals from the body and supplying current directly to the nervous system, which will open up new horizons for the treatment of neurological disease (Gasson *et al.*, 2005; Warwick, 2008).
- New micro- and nano-manufacturing techniques, some based on the manufacturing techniques of integrated circuits but applicable to many more materials and shapes, have led to enormous reductions in the end-size of implantable devices with the additional possibility of fitting them with micro-instrumentation to endow them with "intelligence" (Gad-el-Hak, 2003; Schwartz, 2006).
- Optimising the product design process, thanks to a combination of CAD-CAE-CAM and rapid prototyping which speed up the production start-up of devices by reducing intermediate stages and minimizing costs (Kuklick, 2006).
- The development of new bio-absorbable materials that are body-compatible which degrade a certain time after being implanted while only producing non-toxic matter that can be eliminated or metabolised by the body. Outstanding progress has been made in the synthesis of bioabsorbable and biodegradable polymers that can be applied to a large number of devices designed for the controlled delivery of drugs (Lendlein and Langer, 2002), as well as for support tasks for tissue engineering (Freed *et al.*, 1994; Kawanishi *et al.*, 2004).
- The discovery of new active materials that enable functionalities to be inbuilt, open up new horizons for the development of active implantable medical devices, thanks to their potential use as sensors and actuators (Davis, 2003; Wong and Bronzino, 2007; Peterson and Bronzino, 2008). This handbook focuses on these materials and the following sections describe their great importance for the medical device sector.

These advances mutually favour one another and when used in combination can provide multiple novel responses to conditions for which, up to a decade ago, there was no adequate treatment. All this has boosted the development of prototypes for a large number of medical devices, many of which benefit from the use of active materials.

The following section provides an introduction to the systematic process of product development and goes on to examine the further considerations that must be borne in mind should the device under development respond to a medical need. It will then go on to examine the influence of these considerations on the different stages of the proposed systematic process.

2.2 The Development Process of Medical Devices: Additional Issues

2.2.1 Special Difficulties

The design process of medical devices has a series of added difficulties that involve considerable changes and additional issues regarding the systematic methodology for designing the products previously mentioned.

These additional challenges, difficulties or issues can be classified into three different groups set out below:

- **Technical issues.** These are related to the geometries, materials and the principles of functionality that can be utilised in a specific device as they are bounded by the implications involved by their contact with human body tissue. They are also bounded by the influence of the corporeal environment on the in-service performance of the materials used and their progressive deterioration due to this environment.
- **Legal issues.** The direct action on the body of the developed devices and their associated risks increase the responsibility of those involved in the design and gives rise to certain changes to the prescribed methodology. The design process of medical devices is therefore subject to strict rules and care must be taken to adhere to the specific standards if end product safety is to be maximised. The official approval process for these devices also adds to the overall complexity of their development.

- **Human issues.** These are linked to the particular complexity of the design process for these products which require multidisciplinary teams with experts from the different branches of science, particularly, medicine, engineering, biology, chemistry, physics among others, but which can lead to specific communication or coordination problems. On the other hand, it is important to point out that developing a new device should emerge as a result of a real human need, a factor that will be examined more closely further on.

The main additional issues to be taken into account when setting out to develop a new medical device are explained in the following sub-sections. Reference will also be made to the systematic methodology design stages explained previously, together with reflections on how the different issues influence these stages.

2.2.2 The Importance of a Medical Need

New developments and innovations in Medicine and especially in the field of medical device design usually stem from a problem-related need, and then, a technological solution is found to solve the problem and satisfy the need (Kuklick, 2006).

It is true that on some occasions a new technology or material can bring novel diagnostic or therapeutic solutions to concrete problems, but these technologically motivated products (instead of medically) only have an economic or social impact on rare occasions.

Thus, most companies and technology centres given over to the design of medical devices, as well as more effective devices, are based on the application of efficient technologies for resolving very specific clinical or surgical needs. The approach of studying new technologies and examining any possible applications by searching out medical needs is more linked to scientific research projects than with product development, which means that the results are not materialised in the form of commercial products.

However, both approaches have their own advantages and are perfectly valid depending on what the objective is. So, when designing a product, it is usually more effective to start out from a need and look for a technology to solve the problem. However, if it is wished to promote scientific progress the option of developing a new technology and attempting to apply it to solve the needs of many varied sectors probably makes more sense.

Therefore, this handbook looks to both approaches. It shows the development of medical devices based on the use of active materials as sensors or actuators, whose study and subsequent development is motivated by real medical needs requiring a technological solution.

On the other hand, throughout these development processes scientific and technological contributions are made concerning the use of active materials for detection and actuation, novelties that may find a use in future medical applications or even other sectors.

Regarding the development of new medical devices, it is important to emphasise that the need to provide a solution to a medical problem must be kept in mind at the very first "defining objectives and planning" stage. If no such need exists, it is hardly sensible to begin to develop a new product to provide a solution to a problem that does not exist or that is being satisfactorily solved by other means.

One particular skill of entrepreneurs or researchers in the field of medical devices is therefore the ability to search out and understand important clinical or surgical needs. It is a complex issue where it is not enough to carry out questionnaire-based market studies or an analysis of existing products to find gaps in the market. Often, there is no other product for comparison, particularly if the product to be developed is completely new.

All of this, in conjunction with the basic aims to ensure, lengthen and improve patients' quality of life, while at the same time generating economic and social value, complicates decision-making and the search for needs on which to work. Therefore, defining objectives for the development of medical devices is a particularly complex issue.

2.2.3 Biomaterials

As with the concept of medical device, there are various satisfactory definitions for the notion of "biomaterial". The term generally designates any material used in the manufacture of devices that interact with biological systems and that are applied in the different branches of medicine (Wong and Bronzino, 2007; Peterson and Bronzino, 2008). This definition includes materials with very different properties and classifiable into different families, such as metals, ceramics, polymers and composite materials. According to their origin they can also be classified as natural or synthetic. Another possible classification is based on the influence the biomaterial has on the body or the extent of the reaction it produces on surrounding tissues, the following division being generally accepted:

- **Bio-inert materials.** Characterised by their low reactivity in the body, which means they can co-exist with the surrounding tissue without any apparent change to the functions and properties of this tissue. Typical materials of this kind used in implantable devices are tantalum, titanium, aluminium, magnesium and some zirconium oxides.
- **Biodegradable or bioabsorbable materials.** They have the capability to be body-compatible and to degrade a certain time after implant, giving rise to non-toxic products that can be eliminated or metabolised by the body. Some materials of this family are porous hydroxyapatite, the salts of calcium phosphate and some polyurethanes.
- **Bioactive materials.** They have the ability to form direct chemical ties with the surrounding tissue allowing this tissue to grow freely on their surface. Some examples of these materials are high density hydroxyapatite and tricalcic phosphate.

All materials used in medical device development, particularly those that will be in contact with body tissues must meet a set of manufacturing and chemical requirements and properties, and body compatibility requirements, which are mainly mechanical. These are listed in Fig. 2.1 and Table 2.1 shows typical examples of synthetic materials applied to obtain medical devices.

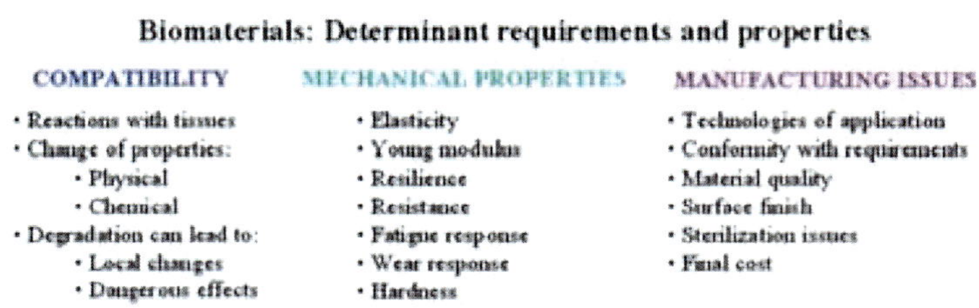

Figure. 2.1 Properties and determining factors for choosing biomaterials.

Table 2.1 Examples of Materials in Medical Applications

Material	Main applications
Metals and alloys:	
Stainless steels	Clamping fractures, stents and surgical instruments
Co-Ti, Ti-Al-V, Ti-Al-Nb, Ti-13Nb-13Zr, Ti-Mo-Zr-Fe	Bone and joint prostheses, clamping fractures, dental implants
Co-Cr-Mo, Cr-Ni-Cr-Mo	Bone prostheses, clamping fractures, dental implants, heart valves.
Ni-Ti	Self-expanding stents, bone plates, clamping fractures, orthodoncy wires
Gold alloys	Dental repairs
Silver products	Antibacterial agents
Platinum and Pt-Ir	Electrodes
Amalgam of Hg-Ag-Sn	Dental repairs
Ceramics:	
Aluminium	Joint prostheses, dental repairs
Zirconium	Joint prostheses
Calcium phosphates	Bone repairs, metal and alloy surface coatings
Glass	Bone prostheses
Porcelain	Dental repairs
Carbon coatings	Heart valves, percutaneous devices, dental implants
Polymers:	
Polyethylene (UHMWPE)	Joint prostheses
Polypropylene	Sutures
PET	Sutures and vascular prostheses
Polyamides	Sutures
PTFE	Vascular prostheses and *in vitro* tissue growth
Polyesters	Vascular prostheses and drug delivery devices

Material	Main applications
Polyurethanes	Devices in contact with blood
PVC	Conducts for pumping operations, drug delivery and others
PMMA	Contact lenses
Silicones	Implants and soft tissue replacement
Hydrogels	Ophthalmology and drug delivery
Composites:	
Bis-GMA with quartz filling	Dental repairs
PMMA with glass filling	Dental repairs and bone cements

2.2.4 Body Conditions

When it comes to choosing suitable materials for a product under development, during the basic engineering stage it is usually essential to consider the environment in which the product is going to act. The particular case of medical devices is no exception and body conditions play a deciding role when choosing materials.

Conditions such as a temperature of around 37°C are not extreme for the materials used in medical devices. However, if active material-based devices are used whose activation is based on a change in temperature, the limits admitted by the body must be taken into account, as will be commented later.

Although temperatures are not usually a big problem, the biomechanical demands and chemical circumstances of the body are usually decisive when choosing the appropriate material for a medical device.

Regarding the mechanical demands, it is essential to bear in mind not only the nominal value of the demand but also the complete load cycle and the number of load cycles to be supported by the device. A typical hip prosthesis may be subjected to 3×10^6 load cycles per year, which in the case of a person of 25, with a 70 year life expectancy, would mean around 108 load cycles in the most unfavourable scenario. Although loads and load cycles depend directly on weight and each specific patient's level of activity, it is patently obvious that the effects of mechanical fatigue in the response of the materials used needs to be taken into account.

On the other hand, any variation in the chemical state of the environment is decisive when choosing a particular material for a device. In this respect, any changes in the pH of the body fluids must be carefully examined.

Blood pH usually remains between 7.38 and 7.41. However, after an operation the pH may increase locally up to 7.8 and then decrease to around 5.5, returning to its normal value after a few weeks.

Infections or haematomas can also give rise to local variations in the pH and situate it between values of 4 and 9.

These variations are important when choosing material (and its processing) for a metal prosthesis where a proper resistance to corrosion must be ensured.

Likewise, the pH of saliva, usually between 5 and 7, is a determining factor when choosing materials for implants or dental repairs.

According to the issues considered up to now, we will summarise the most important requirements to be met by a medical device and the materials of which it is made:

- It must not be toxic or carcinogenic, cause a minimum adverse reaction, and be chemically stable and corrosion-resistant, as will be explained in detail further on in connection with biocompatibility.
- It must be capable of withstanding considerable forces and variables inside the human body, that is to say, in a highly corrosive environment.
- It must be capable of being shaped into complex forms in order to adapt to the geometrical requisites of the body.

From an economic point of view, it is also desirable for biomaterials as well as their manufacturing and transformation processes to be relatively low-cost with a high market availability to avoid dead time during the development process.

Explained below are some of these requirements in relation to the functions that medical devices usually need to perform. Also analysed is the influence of the body on that performance.

2.2.5 Biocompatibility

Like other important scientific concepts that evolve over time, the definition of biocompatibility has gradually changed with the advances made in materials intended for medical devices. Until a few years ago, a biocompatible material was one that did not harm the body. They were basically inert materials "possessing the property of not causing any harm or toxic effects to biological systems".

However, new developments, including those that are active material-based, have made this definition change to, "the capability of a material to properly fulfil its mission in a specific application for a particular patient". The concept thus presents four basic facets:

- Biocompatibility makes no reference to an isolated event or phenomenon. It applies to a set of processes that include diverse mechanisms for an interaction between the material and the surrounding biological tissue.
- Biocompatibility refers to a material's capability to perform a function in the body and not simply to remain inert in the body. Moreover, the material's capability to carry out its function not only depends on the physical-chemical properties inherent to the material but also on its interaction with tissue.
- It is important to take account of the positive response on the part of the particular patient or host of the device. A lack of response is no longer sought but that the response, however slight, should be in accordance with the device's function.
- The most up-to-date definition also makes reference to the specific application. For example, the same material with different geometries or in different organs, in one case can be a final biocompatible application, whereas in the other situation it may fail.

Biocompatibility cannot therefore be considered an intrinsic material property, but must be approached from a more global perspective that involves the whole set; material – application – body.

A good starting point for looking at biocompatibility throughout the different medical device development stages can be found by consulting ISO Standard 10993 on the "biological evaluation of medical devices". It describes a guided process for choosing the tests required to evaluate a device's biocompatibility depending on its degree of contact with body tissue and risks associated with its use. It also includes various procedures for performing specific tests.

In principle, right from the basic engineering stage, it is reasonable to choose materials that have given positive results in other applications, but throughout the detailed engineering stage the material chosen for the new application needs to be checked in every case to ensure that it meets biocompatibility requirements by carrying out the tests (both *in vitro* and *in vivo* tests) described in the Standard.

2.2.6 Mechanical Behaviour

Metal materials are used in implants and prostheses for their remarkable mechanical properties and particularly for their high static and dynamic strength. The main properties to consider when choosing a metal material to withstand mechanical forces are flow tension, tensile strength, elasticity modulus and fatigue resistance. These can be known from the information provided by the suppliers or be obtained through the appropriate tests.

Ceramic materials offer an excellent resistance to compression, for which reason they are used in numerous applications in odonthology. However, their performance in the face of flexion and fatigue are insufficient because the forces appearing cause the cracks to appear and propagate, which leads to a fragile rupture of these materials.

Among the properties to be considered when choosing polymeric materials that are to be subject to forces as part of implants or prostheses is that they should have a remarkable tensile strength, flow tension and fatigue resistance.

Moreover, with polymers the influence of working temperature on these properties must be taken into account when consulting supplier information or carrying out tests to determine such information.

Set out below are certain general issues related to the mechanical aspects that influence the response of different materials in their useful life as component parts of medical devices.

Test-related issues

In ideal conditions, the tests for determining mechanical properties should be performed in an environment identical to the human body where the device is going to work. In practice, due to technical and financial difficulties and timelines, they are normally carried out at ambient temperature and in contact with the air. However, when assessing any possible degradation, tests can be performed in fluids that simulate body properties (isotonic solutions with blood and others).

Fatigue-related issues

Implants and prostheses receive cyclical loads during body movement that promote the appearance of cracks in zones where the tensions are usually concentrated due to irregularities in the microstructure of the material because of surface-finish defects or inappropriate design. Influencing factors on this phenomenon such as shape, material, manufacturing process, surface finish and others make it difficult to measure the fatigue resistance of a specific part in the design stage, which is why test results have to be resorted to. However, testing implants under real load and contour conditions that simulate actual implant performance inside the body is also a very complex and expensive task. Therefore, standardised tests are normally performed with a sample of the candidate materials or the information provided by the suppliers. To assess behaviour in the face of fatigue, the tests described in the documents prepared by the ISO TC164/SC5 committee or those explained in US standards like ASTM F1160, F1440, F1539, F1659, F1717 and F1798 can be used.

Wear-related issues

Resistance to wear is also a decisive criterion when choosing a biomaterial as excess wear cam lead to the premature failure of an implant or prosthesis. It is also important to point out that the residue from the wear must be body-compatible in order to prevent the appearance of infection or long-term rejection. Information on this can be found in ISO Standard 10993 (Parts 13 to 15) which suggests criteria for assessing body-compatibility and wear residue.

Other test methods for assessing the performance of different implant materials and different geometries can be found in the documents prepared by the ISO TC150/SC4 committee or in US standards like ASTM F732, F1714 and F1715.

For example, wear in contact between polymers like UHMWPE and metal alloys or ceramic materials, has been studied for over 40 years. In general, research into material wear for prostheses goes along one of the following three lines:

- The use of test machines to do basic research into wear mechanisms by using samples of different materials.

- Assessing complete prosthetic mechanisms during the *in vitro* test period when they are subjected to static or dynamic loads using simulators.
- Analysing the *in vivo* evolution of prostheses implanted in patients using medical imaging technology.

Elasticity-related issues

As already explained, the need for high static and dynamic strength has led to the extended use of metals and alloys for designing prostheses and implants, particularly cobalt alloys and titanium alloys. However, there are still a number of unsolved problems associated with the use of these alloys, some due to their stiffness being higher than the bones in which they are housed.

Numerous studies show that the bone areas surrounding an implant that receive less load suffer loss of bone mass and therefore mechanical strength (osteoporosis), a phenomenon attributed to the difference in stiffness between implants and the bones in which they are housed, which leads to unequal distribution of forces in the implant-bone contact zone.

Proposals for more flexible solutions to encourage the prosthesis to accompany the bone in its movements and obtain force distributions more like those in a healthy body have led to materials with lower elasticity moduli to be sought and developed.

Composite materials with a polymeric matrix are currently being tested as candidates to replace cobalt or titanium alloys, although problems of degradation and tribological difficulties are hindering its *in vivo* application.

The mechanical issues set out affect different stages of the previously mentioned systematic design methodology. In principle, in the basic engineering design stage the mechanical demands to which the device will be subjected to should be precisely defined.

The family of materials most suited to bearing these loads should also be selected. In the detailed engineering stage the main candidate materials are compared and the final material is chosen.

2.2.7 Corrosion and Deterioration

We have already introduced the problems linked to the body as a corrosive environment and how this has an influence on the final compatibility of devices, as well as being a determining factor for choosing materials during the basic engineering stage.

Some additional issues are examined below that depend on the material family that is to be integrated into the specific device.

Corrosion in metals

The metals used as biomaterials must be noble and resistant to their surroundings (body fluids). Various types of corrosion mechanisms have been observed in the metal materials forming part of implantable devices – general corrosion, local corrosion or "pitting"; corrosion due to a concentration of tensions; corrosion due to fatigue; and intergranular corrosion. In whichever case, for a material to be considered resistant to bodily effects, the annual corrosion rate must be lower than 25×10^{-6} mm/year. A series of standard tests have been developed for assessing behaviour of implant materials in the face of corrosion, such as those set out in ISO Standard 8044 prepared by the ISO TC156 expert committee or those set out in US standards such as ASTM F746, F897, F1801, F1814 and F1875. For assessing the behaviour of coatings in the face of corrosion the tests described in the ISO TC107/SC7 documents can be followed.

Corrosion in ceramics

Corrosion tests for ceramic materials are not habitual as the ceramic oxides normally used in structural implants are very few. However, some ceramics do show certain *in vivo* corrosion which affects their mechanical behaviour. For this reason, in the detailed engineering stage a very exact definition of the manufacturing processes and the transformations required for these materials is very important, as well as specifying the required purity and density (in general, the greater the density the less the porosity and the greater the resistance to corrosion).

Corrosion in polymers

Although the physiological functions and chemical reactions taking place in the body do not occur at high temperatures or with radioactive effects, combining an electrolyte with active biological species, like catalytic enzymes and free radicals, constitutes a particularly reactive environment which leads to a certain degradation of numerous polymers. Of the individual mechanisms linked to polymer degradation in the body (Davis, 2003) there are

- Depolymerization
- Cross-linking
- Oxidation

- Adhesive filtering
- Hydrolysis
- Crack generation and propagation

These mechanisms and their possible effects on the final product must be borne in mind at the basic engineering stage when choosing the most suitable materials for body circumstances as well as for making decisions as to the use of additives that can restrict these problems. The geometries and ways of joining parts can also have an influence on the appearance of these phenomena.

It is therefore important to take notice of the recommendations in the manufacturers' design manuals and technical catalogues for the final material to be chosen in the detailed engineering stage.

Test procedures for evaluating the effects of residue resulting from the corrosion and degradation of polymeric, ceramic and metal materials (and their influence on the biocompatibility of the final materials) can be found in ISO Standard 10993, parts 13, 14 and 15, respectively.

2.2.8 Sterilisation

Sterilisation is also essential for all implanted materials and devices. In medical practice, financial considerations often lead to surgical instruments and costly equipment being used over and over, which means they need to be sterilised after each use with a new patient.

Every sterilisation method must pursue the same objective: to eliminate or destroy living organisms and viruses present in the biomaterial or the medical device to be implanted. This process is usually quantified by the so-called SAL or sterility assurance limit. The details of the sterilisation method are determined from tests until the SAL obtained (the probability that an implant will not be sterile after the process) is less than 10^{-6}. The principal sterilisation methods (Davis, 2003; Simmons, 2004; Kuklick, 2006) are explained below.

Steam sterilisation

Steam or autoclave sterilisation is a simple method based on exposing the device to saturated steam at 120°C for 15 to 30 min (once the entire implant surface has reached 120°C) at a standard pressure of 121 kPa. This is the most widely used method for sterilising metal surgical instruments. The method's main advantages are its effectiveness, rapidity, simplicity and lack of toxic residue. However, the high temperature, humidity and pressure during this type of sterilisation cause the hydrolysis, softening and degradation of many medical grade polymers and problems with any adhesives that may have been used.

When dealing with shape-memory polymers, as will be explained later, the high temperature activates the "memory effect" and the polymer returns to the shape it had before activation, which means this method is unsuitable.

Ethylene oxide sterilisation

This is used as a low-temperature process that is compatible with many materials. The device is placed in a vacuum chamber into which ethylene oxide is injected at a concentration of 600 to 1200 mg/l. The steriliser is usually kept at a temperature of between 30 and 50°C and 40% to 90% relative humidity during the process which lasts from 2 to 48 h.

It is usually used for sterilising a wide range of devices such as surgical sutures, intraocular lenses and devices for repairing ligaments and tendons or heart valves.

The main disadvantage is that ethylene oxide is toxic and possibly carcinogenic, and so, its use in implantable devices is controversial. Eye contact or inhalation of the vapours resulting from the process should always be avoided.

Sterilisation by radiation

Ionising gamma ray radiation from cobalt-60 isotopes is used in dosages ranging from 25 to 40 kGy. The dosage is controlled by a dose meter to ensure the integrity of the device so that it will not be radioactive after the process and can be used immediately.

This is an appropriate process when materials cannot withstand the high autoclave temperatures. It is widely used for sterilising sutures, clips, metal implants, knee and hip prostheses and other implants. It has also been commonly accepted as the most suitable way of sterilising polymeric materials such as polyethylene, polyesters, polystyrenes, polysulphones and polycarbonates. Some exceptions are polytetrafluoroethylene ("PTFE" commonly known as Teflon) because of its extreme sensitivity to radiation.

It is a simple, fast method that can be precisely controlled, but it is not without certain difficulties. In some cases the method can produce a certain oxidation of the polymers sterilised by this method, as has been recorded in some "UHMWPE" implants. This usually leads to an increase in density and crystallinity, as well as a loss of the mechanical properties linked to the greater stiffness acquired.

However, this problem can be considerably reduced by carrying out the process in an inert gas atmosphere (argon, nitrogen) or in a vacuum chamber to reduce the presence of oxidising species and enhance the properties and useful life of "UHMWPE" devices.

New sterilisation techniques

Sterilisation in low-temperature plasma is one method that has given positive results over the last decade, since it is not linked to the use of dangerous products and does not generate toxic waste. Hydrogen peroxide is usually used as the gas to form the plasma and the process is carried out at temperatures below 50°C with cycle times of between 75 min and 3 h.

Ionised gases such as argon, nitrogen, oxygen and carbon dioxide have also been used to destroy surface micro-organisms with low-processing times of between 15 and 30 min. The process has been used to sterilise polymers like polylactic acid ("PLA"), polyglycolic acid ("PGA") and its copolymers ("PLGA").

Carbon dioxide in a supercritical state has also been used to inactivate bacteria in applications including biodegradable polymers such as "PLA" and "PLGA" for drug delivery systems as well as prostheses made of polyester fabric.

So, sterilisation is usually an after-sales activity that is applied to a developed product. However, it also has an influence on the design process since as a prior step to *in vivo* tests in the detailed engineering stage, the device under development must also be subjected to sterilisation with the purpose of minimising any risks associated with these *in vivo* tests.

2.2.9 Regulations

The intrinsically complex process of product development linked to the additional problems already mentioned connected with medical devices, means that consulting the recommendations regarding regulatory standards for the different design stages often marks the difference between a successful design process and an unviable one. The concept of regulatory standards is closely linked to end medical device quality and safety, for which reason it deserves to be dealt with separately in the next sub-chapter.

2.2.10 Multidisciplinary Teams

Product design projects connected with developing a new medical device are probably the ones requiring a team trained by experts from a number of fields, especially if the device incorporates means of detection or can be activated for the diagnosis or active treatment of some condition. A standard design team for these devices is usually made up of doctors, pharmacologists, engineers, computer experts, physicists, chemists and biologists in addition to economics and law graduates to deal with the financial and legal aspects. The design process obviously benefits from such a wealth of approaches and at the same time is a highly attractive working environment.

However, the availability of experts in specific fields can also give rise to problems of communication (misunderstandings, lack of precision, lack of information, false suppositions) that can cause the timescales and costs of specific work to go off course and even lead to personal conflicts that affect the project as a whole.

We need to be aware that working in a global context is ever more usual and that the participation of designers, suppliers and customers from different countries who have a decisive influence on the design process means an increase in communication problems. It is worthwhile making yet another effort to improve understanding as the wide-ranging points of view of multinational teams can be a tremendous help in finding more consistent solutions.

Some strategies for using a common language throughout the design process will be discussed further on (use of documents to define the initial situation, a general use of the International Units System, the participation of experts or communication "facility advisors"), together with certain teaching-related considerations and proposals, a key tool for providing a short-term response to the potential growth of this sector.

2.3 Applicable Standards: Discussion

2.3.1 Standards for Conventional Products Development

As stated earlier on, quality and safety are interlinked and together with productivity constitute the basic issues to be taken into consideration in product design and mark all the difference between successful strategies and ones that are not.

Indeed, the trade promotion sought by the European Union through the Internal Market required additional safety issues for the products commercialised in that market, so that such promotion would not have any negative consequences on the products marketed, particularly industrial products.

This led to a common community policy being adopted based on the "new approach directives", whose application has enabled an homogenised framework of technical references to be established that are valid for all community countries and which hold sway over specific domestic requirements which cannot prevail over the framework. This means an abolition of technical barriers which is coherent with the disappearance of custom barriers.

Therefore, the new approach directives for different product types or sectors set out the basic safety and quality requirements to be met by these products, as well as the checks and tests that must be passed (before duly recognised bodies), before receiving the "CE mark" and being able to be marketed in the European Union.

In order to give "this new approach" solid foundations, the European Union and in particular, the Commission, have used quality techniques applied to the context of product conformity in respect of the applicable European requirements, basing them specifically on the triad of standardisation – certification – accreditation, in order to endow the tests and checks with guidelines and patterns that can be commonly accepted.

Given that standards and quality have come to occupy an important position in the community marketing policy for industrial products, it is not surprising that this official European initiative should end up becoming part of the most widely accepted international standards in the field of quality, to be exact ISO Series 9000 Standards.

It is important to distinguish between directive and standard since the new approach directives are mandatory for placing products on the market in the European Union (obtaining the CE mark), while the standards of organisations like the ISO are proposals or recommendations for working more methodically and effectively.

However, the use of ISO Series 9000 quality standards is recognised by many of the new approach directives as a means of showing conformity with the requirements of these directives and specifically to allow the use of the CE mark.

On the other hand, conformity with the 45000 Series European standards provides organisations with "conformity assessment", the presumption of conformity with the technical criteria set out in the directives.

Thus, the use of 9000 Series or 45000 Series standards is not one of the mandatory requirements of the new approach legislation, but is one possible way of demonstrating conformity.

The directives that apply to the design of medical devices in the European Union are explained further on in greater detail.

2.3.2 Regulations Regarding the Development of Medical Devices

Directives

Regarding the development of medical devices in the European Union there are three directives (with their associated amendments) which must be taken into account in order to be able to market the products under development:

- Directive 93/42/EEC regarding medical devices.
- Directive 90/385/EEC regarding active implantable medical devices.
- Directive 98/79/EC regarding medical devices for *in vitro* diagnosis.

Directive 93/42/EEC regarding medical devices

This directive applies to medical devices and accessories where a "medical device" comes under the definition cited at the beginning of the chapter, which can be summarised as "any instrument, apparatus, tool, material or other article, either used on its own or in combination with others, including the operating system required for it to be properly applied in the way intended by the manufacturer for use in human beings".

A "medical accessory" is an article, which, although is not a device, has been manufactured to be used together with a device in such a way that its use is compatible with the use of the device as intended by the manufacturer.

Medical devices are classified under two headings in line with the classification standards laid down in Annex IX of the directive. The application of these classification standards is governed by the device's intended purpose, the risks associated with its use, the extent of contact with body tissue or the time it will remain in the human body. Therefore, medical devices in order of danger/ increasing responsibility may be: "Class I", "Class II a", "Class II b" or "Class III".

Before manufacturing and placing the device on the market, the manufacturer or its authorised agent in the European Union must subject it to different types of controls depending on how it is classified if the device is to bear the CE mark. These controls are listed below.

For "Class I" Devices:

For sterilised devices and devices with a measuring function the "CE declaration of conformity" must be obtained before placing them on the market and then at the manufacturer or agent's choice

- The "CE verification" by a notified body
- Approval of the "production quality system" by a notified body
- Approval of the "product quality system" by a notified body

Other devices must pass the "internal production control", that is, all the technical documentation necessary for the product's declaration of conformity in line with the requirements of the directives must be prepared and submitted for evaluation.

For "Class II a" Devices:

At the manufacturer or agent's choice these products must obtain

- The "CE declaration of conformity" and depending on the choice
    - The "CE verification" by a notified body
    - Approval of the "production quality system" by a notified body
    - Approval of the "product quality system" by a notified body

These alternative procedures are mandatory for sterilised devices.

As an alternative the manufacturer must receive approval of the "total quality assurance system" by a notified body, with the exception of having to apply the product design examination.

For "Class II b" Devices:

At the manufacturer or agent's choice these products must obtain

- The "CE-type examination" and depending on the choice
  - The "CE verification" by a notified body
  - Approval of the "production quality system" by a notified body
  - Approval of the "product quality system" by a notified body

As an alternative the manufacturer must receive approval of the "total quality assurance system" by a notified body, with the exception of having to apply the product design examination.

For "Class III" Devices:

At the manufacturer or agent's choice these products must obtain

- The "EC-type examination" and depending on the choice
  - The "CE verification" by a notified body
  - Approval of the "production quality system" by a notified body
  - Approval of the "product quality system" by a notified body

As an alternative the manufacturer must receive approval by the "total quality assurance system" by a notified body, including having to apply the product design examination.

For devices intended for clinical research and custom-made devices, the manufacturer must prepare a declaration in accordance with the criteria in Annex VIII of the directive. These research oriented devices should not bear the CE conformity mark.

The directive does not identify any quality system standard but the requirements provided to create the quality system are subject to ISO 9000 Series regarding the total quality system, the production quality system and the end-product quality system. In order to evaluate the technical competence of the notified bodies, the member countries of the EU must implement the criteria laid down in Annex XI of the directive.

Directive 90/385/EEC regarding active implantable medical devices

This directive applies to active implantable medical devices, that is, to say "any medical device (as defined previously) that depends on an electrical power supply to operate it (or any energy source not directly generated by the human body or by the force of gravity) and which must be totally or partially inserted into the human body by surgical or medical means, or into a natural orifice by medical intervention and remain permanently installed after the procedure".

Before placing the product on the market, the manufacturer must subject it to the procedures to evaluate conformity that are laid down in the directive. Except for custom-made medical devices and those intended for clinical research, the manufacturer may opt to

- Follow the procedure laid down in the "CE declaration of conformity" (approval and verification of the total quality system by a notified body) supplemented by the product design examination.
- Subject a model to the "EC type examination" by a notified body in conjunction with one of the following processes:
  - The "EC verification" for devices by a notified body
  - The "EC declaration of conformity"

For devices intended for clinical research and custom-made devices, the manufacturer must prepare a specific declaration. These devices do not have to bear the CE mark. This directive does not identify any quality system standard either, but the requirements provided to create the quality system are subject to ISO 9000 Series standards regarding the total quality system, the production quality system and the end-product quality system.

Directive 98/79/EC regarding medical devices for in vitro diagnosis

This directive covers *in vitro* devices, whose mission is to examine the specimens and samples derived from the human body, reagents, instruments and specimen receptacles linked to these tests. Placing these devices on the market is once again subject to conformity with the directive. In greater detail, for the directive an *in vitro* diagnostic medical device is "any medical device including reagents, calibres, control material, instruments, apparatus, equipment or systems which when used on their own or in combination are intended for *in vitro* use to examine specimens, including blood and tissue, derived from the human body in order to obtain information on pathologies, congenital defects, safety and compatibility with potential receivers or therapeutic measurement monitoring". This definition must be examined in conjunction with what has already been stated for a medical device.

Although these devices do not act directly on the human body, the responsibility connected with their use is still very high as they can be used to supplement the design process of other implantable or active medical devices. In addition, their use in detecting conditions, congenital defects and for monitoring, directly affects the patient, which means the reliability and rapidity of these devices are determining factors. For this reason, *in vitro* diagnostic devices are divided into four classes in order of risk and must be subject to different controls according to the operating instructions in the directive before being placed on the market. The alternatives that can be chosen by manufacturers are similar to what has already been stated regarding the previously mentioned directives and can be examined in more detail by referring to the directive.

Specific regulations

As we have already seen for conventional products, when developing medical devices and sanitary products, in general terms, following the recommendations on quality and procedures laid down in ISO 9000 Series standards, in conjunction with some specific features of ISO 13485 and 13488 standards, although not obligatory, is one way of demonstrating conformity with the requirements of the three specific directives and specifically allow the use of the CE mark.

However, there are certain standards and documents regarding very specific aspects of medical device development which are worth looking at and trying to implement, apart from the ISO 9000 Series, when developing a product from this sector intended for placement on the market, such as

- ISO Standard 10993 on the "Biological evaluation of medical devices".
- ISO Standard 13485 on "Sanitary products. Quality management systems and regulatory requirements" (replaces Standard EN 46001). It lays down the requirements for a quality management system where an organisation needs to demonstrate its ability to design, develop and supply related sanitary products and services that consistently fulfil the customer's needs and the regulations applicable to sanitary products and related services. The main objective of ISO 13485 is to facilitate harmonised regulatory requirements for quality

management systems and sanitary products. Consequently, it includes some specific requirements for sanitary products and excludes some requirements of ISO Standard 9001.

- ISO Standard 13488 on "Sanitary products. Quality management systems and specific requirements for the implementation of ISO Standard 9002" (replaces Standard EN 46002). In conjunction with ISO Standard 9002 it specifies the quality requirements for a company producing, installing and distributing medical devices.
- ISO Standard 14971 on the "Application of risk management to sanitary products". This indicates the process to be followed by designers in order to identify the risks associated with medical devices including those intended for *in vitro* diagnosis, so that these risks can be estimated and evaluated and attempted to be controlled by corrective actions and then verify the impact and effectiveness of such corrective actions. It can be applied to every step of the life cycle of the medical device in question.
- ISO Standard 15223 on the "Symbols to be used with labels, labelling and information to be supplied with medical devices". This identifies the requirements for the design and use of any symbols that may be intended to provide safe, effective information about medical devices.

Together with these general standards referring to the area of medical devices, throughout the design process of these products it can be extremely useful to refer to the specific regulations connected with the methods for characterising and testing the different materials so that objective comparisons can be made of any possible alternatives or be of help in choosing suppliers (depending on the regulations used to verify materials or products).

At the same time regulations are in a constant state of flux as they attempt to adapt to safety and market quality requirements and to cover the latest advances in science and technology that demand changes to product designs. It is therefore important to regularly check updated references (www.iso.org).

The situation in other countries

In general, in order to asses the biocompatibility of a medical device, the strategies complying with what is laid down in Standard 10993 are acceptable both in Europe and Asia (Kuklick, 2006).

However, in the United States the test procedures of the US Pharmacopoeia, used to subsequently request product certification from the Food and Drug Administration (FDA), have certain differences compared to ISO standards. Generally speaking, ISO procedures are stricter, which means that companies intending to market their products both in Europe and the United States must follow ISO requirements.

Nevertheless, in both cases, after applying ISO methods and before placing products on the US market the requirements of the FDA must be carefully checked and if necessary, additional testing be done. It may even be necessary to enlist the help of FDA reviewers to clarify matters.

Research and regulations

As we have seen from our examination of the new approach directives concerning medical devices, for products intended for clinical research and custom-made products, the manufacturer must prepare a declaration in line with the criteria of the appropriate directive.

However, it is not necessary to undergo such strict examinations as for products intended for the market. In fact, medical devices for research or custom-made ones do not have to bear the CE mark.

A certain relaxation as to the application of standards would seem reasonable in the case of research devices as they are often intended to demonstrate the feasibility of a certain functional principal, often as part of the design process of a product to be placed on the market in the long term. This additional freedom is aimed at encouraging a creative spirit rather than rejecting solutions and alternatives because of regulatory difficulties. It encourages technical feasibility (and economic) studies concerning the use of novel materials or technologies.

Finally, it is important to mention the "Helsinki Declaration" enacted by the World Medical Association in 1964 with six subsequent amendments, the latest being in 2008, and currently in force. The declaration is a proposal of ethical principles for medical research in human beings, including the research of human material and identifiable information. It also deals with the ethical issues involved in *in vivo* tests conducted on animals as a prior step to their being conducted on humans.

Although application of the declaration is not mandatory for placing a new device on the market, it establishes a set of ethical principles that can guide and assist researchers to make decisions in medicine-related matters, as well as assisting those of us who are dedicated to "Biomedical Engineering" work. The purpose of these decisions is to ensure the well-being of any person taking part in research, over and above any other considerations, and as a result more effective and safer products are obtained.

The principles of the Helsinki Declaration are also beginning to take on economic (as well as ethical) importance, compliance with which is a *sine qua non* of being awarded biomedical research projects in many countries. This can be seen in calls for the current National I+D+i Plan for the 2008–2011 period and constitutes a strategic point of Spanish policy in matters of research, development and industrial innovation, in a similar way to what happens in other European countries.

2.4 Main Conclusions

Various socio-economic factors are driving the growth of the medical device development industry, all aimed at providing alternative diagnostic and therapeutic, and sometimes more effective solutions than those currently available. This growth will be based on recent scientific and technological progress. However, if this growth is to be given a solid foundation and the proportion of devices finally being placed on the market increased, it is important that systematic product design methodologies are used that have been duly adapted in line with the specific additional considerations required for the medical devices to be properly developed.

After studying the stages usually used in a systematic product design methodology and analysing how the main special considerations mentioned influence this methodology, we can evaluate which steps and considerations require deeper analysis as a result of their greater relative importance.

Table 2.2 quantifies the influence of different special considerations on medical devices in the systematic design process stages. It also includes the device's useful life due to the implications involved in post-production activities.

This table can also be used as a control tool throughout the design process to ensure that the special considerations of greatest influence at each stage have been taken into account before a stage is deemed to have been completed.

Table 2.2 Influence of Different Factors on the Development Process of Medical Devices. Degree of Influence: *Average, **High, ***Very High.

Special considerations	**Medical device development process**					
	Specifications and planning	Conceptual design	Basic engineering	Detailed engineering	Production start-up	Device's useful life
Medical need	***	**	**	*		***
Biomaterials	*	*	***	**	*	***
Body conditions	*	*	**	**		***
Biocompatibility	**	*	**	**	*	***
Corrosion	*	*	**	**	*	***
Mechanical performance	*	*	**	**	*	***
Sterilisation			*	*	*	***
Communication	***	**	**	***	**	*
Regulations	*	*	*	***	***	**
Quality	*	***	***	***	***	***

It should be pointed out that in medical device development projects there are many additional factors that have a decisive impact on the useful life of these devices and which involve special difficulties. However, the use of systematic structured design methodologies, keeping to regulations, and a constant concern for quality and good communication within the design team can help lead to effective, safe end products.

Any projects arising out of clear medical needs (clinical, surgical, diagnostic or therapeutic) where initial requirements are accurately defined will have a far greater chance of success. The basic engineering stage is a particularly critical part of the design due to its being responsible for contributing specific solutions to the devices main functions. On the other hand, adhering to certain ethical standards and principles connected with the direct repercussions to be had on a person's health by using these devices, can also be highly useful throughout the design process, particularly for making decisions or choosing alternatives that cannot simply be based on technical criteria alone.

The last thing to be examined should be any modifications or additions to the stages of the proposed methodology that will make it easier to implement new technologies or materials (especially "active or intelligent materials") to the design of medical devices that will lead to notable clinical, surgical, diagnostic or therapeutic advances. This is essential for promoting the growth of this sector and addressing the ever-increasing needs of society.

References

Cerutti, S. "Multivariate, multiorgan and multiscale integration of information in biomedical signal processing". International Conference on Biomedical Electronics and Devices Biostec 2008 – Biodevices, Keynote Lecture. IEEE Engineering in Medicine and Biology Society. INSTICC Press, 2008.

Davis, J.R. "Handbook of materials for medical devices". ASM International. United States, 2003.

Deutsch, A.; Brusch, L.; Byrne, H. "Mathematical modeling of biological systems. Volume I: Cellular biophysics, regulatory networks, development, biomedicine and data analysis". Series "Modeling and Simulation in Science, Engineering and Technology". Birkhäuser, 2007.

Deutsch, A.; De la Parra, R.; De Boer, R.J. "Mathematical modeling of biological systems. Volume II: Epidemiology, evolution and ecology, immunology, neural systems and the brain, and innovative mathematical methods". Series "Modeling and Simulation in Science, Engineering and Technology", Birkhäuser, 2008.

Freed, L.; Vunjak-Novakovic, G.; Biron, R.J.; *et al.* "Biodegradable polymer scaffolds for tissue engineering". Bio/technology, 12, 689–693, 1994.

Gad-el-Hak. "The MEMS Handbook". CRC Press. New York, 2003.

Gasson, M.; Hutt, B.; Goodhew, I.; *et al.* "Invasive neural prosthesis for neural signal detection and nerve stimulation". Proceedings of the International Journal of adaptive Control and Signal Processing, 19(5), 365–375, 2005.

Kawanishi, M.; Ushida, T.; Kaneko, T.; *et al.* "New type of biodegradable porous scaffolds for tissue-engineered articular cartilage". Materials Science and Engineering: C, 24(3), 431–435, 2004.

Kuklick, T.R. "The medical device R&D handbook". CRC Press, Taylor and Francis Group. Florida, 2006.

Laín Entralgo, P. "Historia Universal de la Medicina". Salvat Editores S.A.. Madrid, 1973.

Lendlein, A; Langer, R. "Biodegradable, elastic shape-memory polymers for potential biomedical applications". Science, 296(5573), 1673–1676, 2002.

Lendlein, A.; Kelch, S. "Shape-memory polymers as stimuli-sensitive implant materials". Clinical Hemorheology and Microcirculation, 32, 105–116, 2005.

Pammolli, F.; Riccabonni, M.; Oglialoro, C.; *et al.* "Medical devices competitiveness and impact on public health expenditure". Study prepared for the Directorate Enterprise of the European Commission. University of Florence, 2005.

Peterson, D.; Bronzino, J. "Biomechanics. Principles and applications". CRC Press, Taylor and Francis Group. Florida, 2008.

Schwartz, M. "New materials, processes and methods technology". CRC Press, Taylor and Francis Group. Florida, 2006.

Simmons, A. "Sterilization of medical devices". Business Briefing: Medical Device Manufacturing & Technology, August, 2004.

Warwick, K. "Outthinking and enhancing biological brains". International Conference on Biomedical Electronics and Devices Biostec 2008 – Biodevices, Keynote Lecture. IEEE Engineering in Medicine and Biology Society. INSTICC Press, 2008.

Wong, J.; Bronzino, J. "Biomaterials". CRC Press, Taylor and Francis Group. Florida, 2007.

Standards Summary

Main organisations:

- International Organization for Standardization "ISO" (www.iso.org)
- The World Medical Association (www.wma.net)

"New approach" directives related to the Medical Industry:

- Directive 93/42/EEC related to "medical devices"
- Directive 90/385/EEC related to "active implantable medical devices"
- Directive 98/79/EC related to "medical devices for *in vitro* diagnosis"

Standards related to the development of medical devices:

- ISO 10993 standard on "biological evaluation of medical devices"
- ISO 13485 standard on "sanitary products, quality management and regulatory affairs"
- ISO 13488 standard on "quality systems, medical devices, sanitary products and special requirements for applying ISO 9002 standard"
- ISO 14971 standard on "application of risk management to medical devices and sanitary products"
- ISO 15223 standard on "symbols used for labelling and information provided together with medical devices"

Standards and associations related to medical imaging:

- DICOM standard: Digital Imaging and Communications in Medicine: Strategic Document (http://medical.nema.org)
- Medical Imaging and Technology Alliance (www.medicalimaging.org)
- NEMA: The Association of Electrical and Medical Imaging Equipment Manufacturers (www.nema.org)

Additional documents of interest:

- Council of Europe "Convention for the protection of Human Rights and dignity of the human being with regard to the application of biology and medicine: Convention on Human Rights and Biomedicine" (1994).
- UNESCO "Universal Declaration on the Human Genome and Human Rights" (1997) and "Guidelines for Implementation" (1999).
- World Medical Association "Declaration of Helsinki. Ethical principles for medical research involving human subjects" (current revised edition 2008).

Chapter 3

Active Materials in Medical Devices

Andrés Díaz Lantada and Pilar Lafont Morgado
Mechanical Engineering Department, E.T.S.I. Industriales, Universidad Politécnica de Madrid, c/ José Gutiérrez Abascal 2, 28006 Madrid, Spain
adiaz@etsii.upm.es, plafont@etsii.upm.es

3.1 An Introduction to Active Materials

Numerous active, multipurpose or "intelligent" materials have appeared in recent decades, all capable of responding in a reversible and controllable way to different external physical and chemical stimuli to change some of their properties. Due to their sensitivity or action, these materials can be used to design sensors, actuators and multipurpose systems with a wide range of applications for medical device design (for both surgery and implants).

One of the most remarkable advantages of integrating multiple functions into a system is the ensuing reduction in size, the increase in production runs and the reduction in costs in materials and processes. Active materials will play a decisive role in numerous future applications as they all embrace electrical, thermal, chemical, optical, magnetic and mechanical properties.

These materials present different features: inorganic, metallic and organic, both natural and synthetic, and are sensitive to a wide range of physical and chemical phenomena. Figure 3.1 outlines the main families of active materials used in the different fields and the coupling between their physical–chemical properties.

Handbook of Active Materials for Medical Devices: Advances and Applications
Edited by Andrés Díaz Lantada

www.panstanford.com

Although there are other active material families with electrochromical, thermochromical, or electrochemical couplings, those shown in the figure are ones that have led to the largest number of applications in different fields of science and engineering.

The industrial importance of these materials for the development of medical devices, as well as the most prominent prototypes based on such materials, is set out in the following sections.

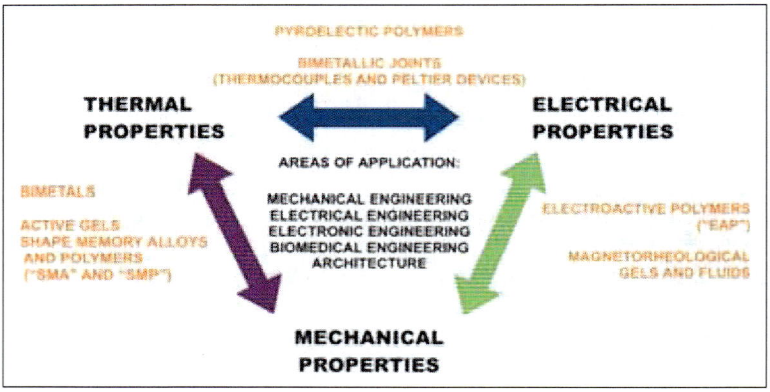

Figure 3.1 Families of active materials and coupling between their properties.

In addition, the following chapters will cover in depth the most relevant of these active material families, as well as the current capabilities, main challenges and future trends, linked at every moment with the new diagnostic and therapeutic possibilities which multifunctional materials provide.

Some final chapters will provide additional information on other families not included in this chapter, due to their novelty and shortage of present industrial applications, but with great potential, especially when combined with actual methods of micro- and nano-manufacturing.

3.2 The Importance of Active Materials in Medical Device Development

As a means of evaluating the scientific and industrial impact of the different families of active materials and their advantages as a support for designing medical devices capable of activation or detection for diagnostic or therapeutic ends, various searches were carried out at the beginning of August 2008 with the aid of the ISI Web of Knowledge electronic tool (Copyright© 2008 Thomson Reuters).

This portal provides access to, and enables searches to be conducted in data bases containing the world's most important scientific documents, in the form of books, journals, annals, conferences and patents.

The initial search was aimed at finding patents concerning the use of active materials for medical applications and devices. To achieve this, the combination of "Active Material AND Medical Device" or "Active Material AND Medical Application" were entered in the search: 725 patents referring to active materials for medical applications and devices were found (615 of which were for proposals for medical devices, the remaining documents being related to the use of drugs and other therapeutic procedures). These patents were also grouped by year of publication to obtain a historical perspective, which is shown in Fig. 3.2.

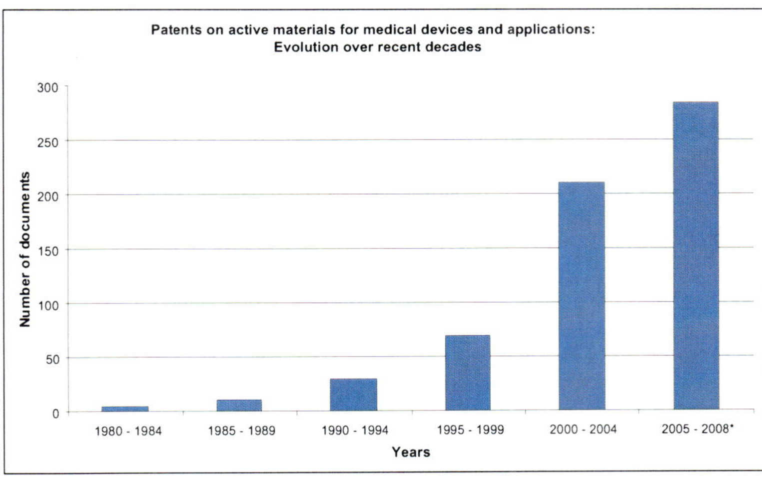

Figure 3.2 Evolution of patents for active materials for medical applications and devices.

*It must be borne in mind that the last period is only 4 years long.

It is important to emphasise that the pronounced growth shown by this field over the last decade is partly due to the scientific progress made in other areas that have boosted the use of these materials as medical device components, as was explained in the preceding section.

This growth is especially outstanding in the last decade concerning the proposals for utilising the different families of active polymers, mainly electroactive polymers and shape memory polymers, as will be explained further on.

For each of the main families of materials a search for scientific documents related to synthesis, processing, characterisation, modelling, simulation and applications was also conducted by entering the name of the family as the document topic in the search criteria field; between 1300 and 15000 documents were found for the different types of materials.

The historical evolution of the number of impact scientific documents published for the different types of materials considered is shown in Fig. 3.3. The growth over the last decade has been particularly outstanding concerning the two kinds of active polymers (electroactive polymers and shape-memory polymers).

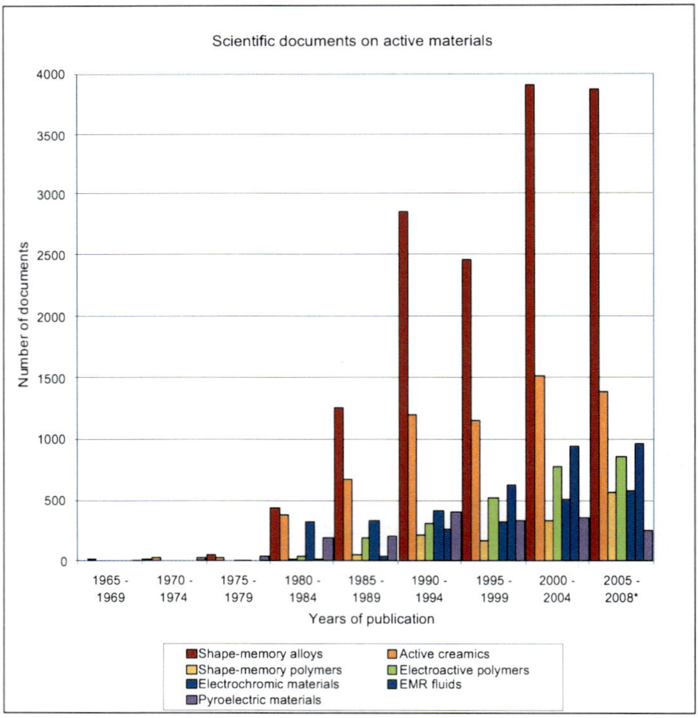

Figure 3.3 Evolution of scientific documents of the different families of active materials.

*It must be borne in mind that the last period is only 4 years long.

3.3 Main Developments of Medical Devices Based on Active Materials

Explained below are major proposals for active material-based medical device design, most of which have been tested *in vivo* in laboratories. Marketing these devices after conducting the *in vivo* tests and obtaining the requisite official approvals, is in some cases subject to achieving the objectives set out at the end of the chapter. The proposals have been grouped together in material families.

3.3.1 Shape Memory Alloys

Alloys with "shape memory" are metal alloys, which after an apparently plastic deformation of around 8% between both geometries return to their original shape, and this can be reversible and repeatable (although with considerably lower recovery rates of around 1% that result in more fragile devices). Within a certain range of temperatures these same materials can be deformed by up to 10% and recover their original shape when discharged, a property known as "superelasticity". Both effects are due to a change of phase called "thermoelastic martensitic transformation". The memory effect can be used to develop actuators while the superelasticity property is suitable for storing energy.

Of all shaped memory alloys, the Nitinol family (acronym of Nickel Titanium Naval Ordnance Laboratory, discovered by Buehler and his team in 1962) is the one for which the greatest number of applications has been found. It contains nickel and titanium in almost identical proportions as well as other elements added to vary the properties. The active properties of Ni–Ti alloys are far ahead of other alloys like Au–Cd and Cu–Zn, discovered up to present. This gave an enormous boost to its use as did its properties of biocompatibility, resistance to corrosion, cycle stability and its ability to recover from major deformations. The main applications developed are listed below.

Self-expanding "stents"

There are different commercial stent designs for treating arteriosclerosis made from shape memory alloys which are folded before being inserted into the human body and then are caused to expand by body temperature until, they become fixed in the artery destroying the atheromatous plaque that caused the initial obstruction (Duerig *et al.*, 1997; Rapp, 2004).

"Amplatzer" devices

By using self-expanding meshes made of shape memory alloy Amplatzer devices have been developed, like those tested in the Heart Centre of Columbus Children's Hospital or those developed by AGA Medical Corp., to treat septal defects that join the right heart cavities with those of the left, either at an auricular or ventricular level, as well as for blocking other blood pass points (Ha and Calagnano, 2005).

Thrombectomy devices

Devices for treating brain ischemia based on catheter ends made of shape memory alloy (like the prototype MERCI X6) which, with slight geometric changes, manage to trap and remove thrombi (Smith *et al.*, 2008).

Active catheters

By using shape-memory wires twisted in a spiral around polymeric catheters, the ends of these catheters can be controlled to make them reach parts that are difficult to access. All that is needed to achieve this is to send an electric current through the shape memory alloy filament to heat it and bend the catheter in a specific direction (Mineta *et al.*, 2002).

3.3.2 Active Ceramics

Besides the benefits linked to the ceramic coatings of numerous prostheses, either to increase the resistance to wear or to enhance body compatibility, also worthy of mention is the use of active ceramics with piezoelectric properties, mainly as component parts of medical devices capable of detection or activation (Cheremisinoff, 1990; Haertling, 1999; Davis, 2003; Schwartz, 2006). Some of the most implemented active devices are calcium titanates, barium or lead, lead zirconate-titanate ("PZT") or tungsten and bronze compounds.

On the other hand, being able to deposit them in the form of thin layers in combination with polymer or metal substrates also endows these materials with numerous capabilities (Sakamoto *et al.*, 1998; Albella *et al.*, 2003, Janas and Safari, 2005). Some major applications are listed below, firstly looking at their applications as sensors and then as actuators.

Pressure sensors

In order to evaluate the pressure or contact forces between different parts of the body, suitably prepared piezoelectric ceramics can be used to measure footstep pressure for use in rehabilitation or high-performance physiotherapy (Pons *et al.*, 2007).

Active orthopaedic devices

Their use as transducers in inertial sensors has been tested for various orthopaedic devices, such as motorised leg orthosis that require real-time electronic control by means of information from inertial sensors (Moreno *et al.*, 2006).

Compact rehabilitation systems

Piezoelectric ceramics possess the capability to be used in small-size rehabilitation systems that send the patient mechanical requests by means of various piezoelectric actuators. Their use has also been put forward for exoskeletons intended to control degenerative illnesses like Parkinson disease (Pons *et al.*, 2007).

Medical imaging systems

Piezoelectric ceramics have been used for some time as precision actuators to move medical imaging systems and in electronic and atom force microscopes (Mc Keighen, 1989). In order to expand the movement achieved/applied voltage ratio, multilayer ceramic stacks can be used to pass from around 1 to 5 nm/V to values of 1 μm/V.

Drug delivery systems

There are different types of micropump designs, with and without valves, for the controlled delivery of drugs based on the use of a piezoelectric ceramic actuator (usually PZT) which operates a membrane whose job is to absorb and then drive the fluid in question (Feng and Kim, 2004; Qiu *et al.*, 2006). The flow volume can vary depending on the operating frequency and the flows can reach levels as small as 1 to 10 μL/min.

3.3.3 Shape-Memory Polymers

Shape-memory polymers (SMPs) are active materials that present a mechanical response to external stimuli, usually changes in temperature. When these materials are heated above their "activation" temperature, a radical change takes place from rigid polymer to an elastic state, which in some cases allows deformations of up to 400%. After being manipulated, if the material is cooled with the imposed deformation, this structure is "frozen" and returns to a rigid but "unbalanced" state. When the material is once again heated above its glass transition or "activation temperature" it returns to its initial non-deformed state.

The cycle can be repeated numerous times without any degradation to the polymer and most suppliers can formulate different materials with activation temperatures of between −30 and 260°C, according to the use required.

Among the polymers developed that possess shape memory, the most important are epoxy resins, polyurethane resins, cross-linked polyethylene, styrene-butadiene copolymers and other formulations (Lendlein and Kelch, 2002, 2005; Liu *et al.*, 2007).Some of the major applications put forward are

Self-expanding stents

Like the stent designed by Boston Scientific Corporation using the polymer from CRG Industries, known as "Veriflex" under its trade-name, to treat the problems arising when the arteries become narrow or obstructed and also for removing obstructions from other "tube-shaped" body parts, like the urethra and the bronchial tubes. The stent is inserted in its temporary form (reduced) and the body's own heat causes it to dilate and become attached to the artery. They may well be used to replace stents based on shape memory alloys such as Nitinol when the appropriate biocompatibility studies have been carried out. Designs of self-expanding stents have also been presented in injected polyurethane (Wache *et al.*, 2003).

Intelligent sutures

Like those developed at the Forschungszentrum in Karlsruhe by Lendlein's team and at the M.I.T. by Langer's team, which have a temporary linear shape and a permanent shape in the form of a knot, with the change in geometry being activated by the body's own temperature.

They have numerous applications in minimally invasive surgery and as they are biodegradable they have advantages over the use of textile sutures and metal clips (Lendlein *et al.*, 2002, 2005).

Thrombectomy devices

With the recent discovery that the thermal effect of shape memory can be activated by a laser, part of whose energy is absorbed by the polymer, devices have been proposed for removing clots (Wilson *et al.*, 2005.

The polymer is shaped in a spiral mould and then heated and stretched to give it its temporary shape. When the laser is passed over the polymer, the shape memory effect is activated and the device recovers its spiral shape trapping the clot which can then be removed.

Active catheters

By using shape memory polymers for the distal point of catheters together with a subsequent activation of the effect by laser light or body heat, different drugs and antitumoural agents can be released. The presence of an active catheter point can also help reach zones that are difficult to access in minimally invasive surgery work (Yakacki, 2008.

Drug release devices

If biodegradable shape memory polymers are used for implantable medical devices, drug supply reservoirs can be incorporated into the device itself. After implant, the polymer begins to be absorbed by the body and the drug is released. Patents have been taken out in this respect for self-expanding coronary stents or intra-urethral stents (Boston Scientific Co. and Surmodics Inc.). The possibility of obtaining temporary geometries with micro-reservoirs for drug storage has also been studied. The drugs would then be released on activation of the shape memory effect by body heat (Gall *et al.*, 2004).

Active annuloplasty rings

Aimed at obtaining a progressive postoperative treatment of mitral insufficiency, they are based on the use of a polymeric ring with resistances distributed around the inside to activate the shape memory effect by heating. This activation must allow the cross-section of the mitral ring to be gradually increased to reduce the degree of insufficiency. Prototypes of these rings have been developed and tested *in vitro* in pigs' hearts (Díaz Lantada *et al.*, 2008).

The different devices explained will provide considerable therapeutic benefits compared to conventional passive devices due to their capability to act inside the body given by the use of shape-memory polymers.

3.3.4 Electroactive Polymers

Since the beginning of the 1990s, new polymers have been obtained that respond to electrical stimuli with considerable changes in shape or size, which has been a big step forward in the use of polymeric materials. They are called electroactive polymers (EAPs), although they also go by the name of "Artificial Muscles" due to the similarity of their behaviour with animal muscles (electric impulse-based mechanical activation).

The large differences in properties between the different kinds of electroactive polymers enable them to be used as sensors and actuators contributing versatility to device development. The main designs proposed for medical device development will be now explained.

Pressure sensors

A precision sensor has been designed by Madrid Polytechnic University that has uses in odonthology for diagnosing and treating bruxism (Lafont *et al.*, 2008), based on the use of PVDF piezoelectric laminate. These laminates are sold with the electrodes already in place, usually Au or Pt ones, by companies like Piezotech S.A. or KTech Co. Piezoelectric polymers are also used inside special footwear that enable the user's footsteps to be analysed to detect any problems and check how improvements could be made with orthopaedic apparatus or prostheses.

Micropumps for drug delivery

Based on existing designs of piezoelectric micropumps or diffusers or diaphragm micropumps, by replacing the traditional ceramic activator component (usually PZT, zirconate-titanate or lead zirconate) by dielectric electroactive polymers, micropumps can be had that can be used to deliver drugs. They have also been proposed for use in the treatment of glaucoma and hydrocephaly. Such micropumps have been developed by Medipump LLC Inc. and Ophthalmotronics Co. and utilise a dielectric electroactive polymer laminate as activation element.

Microanastomosis devices

Anastomosis is an operation for reconnecting communication between vessels, ducts and nerves. The smaller the diameter of the vessel, the more difficult the operation. Micromuscle AB enterprise has designed a cylindrical device made of electroactive polymer on the outside and biocompatible material on the inside. This means an operation can be done simply as the cylinder can be made to dilate or contract by applying a voltage.

Devices for minimally invasive surgery

Electroactive polymers can be used as guides for active catheters; by applying opposite voltages the catheter bends in one direction or the other thereby allowing access to more inaccessible areas. Once the catheter is in position, drugs can be supplied through it or optic fibre inserted to perform an inspection. They can also be used in other minimally invasive surgery work such as removing intravenous (IV) clots or to help in positioning stents.

Fluid system micro devices

The development of electroactive polymer-based active microvalves and microchannels are being used to design controlled drug delivery devices. They can also be used in lab-on-a-chip devices, and Microsystems that integrate various laboratory functions in a few square centimetres. They can be used for blood analysis, DNA sample extraction, perform antigen-antibody reactions and others; all of this in the fastest, most controlled, cheapest way. In these designs the polymer generally acts as an agitator to speed up the chemical analysis process (Cardoso, 2008).

Haptic devices

Teleoperators are operators that control tools remotely and in these cases the contact resistance forces need to return to the teleoperator. This is called "haptic teleoperation". When these devices are user-operated by means of computer-guided simulation, it is important to provide the return force that could be felt in real operations. As the objects being handled do not exist in reality, the haptic forces generated (by the computer) as return force must be such that they give a feeling as to the surroundings. Haptic simulators are currently widely used for training in surgical operations. They are useful when attempting to minimise damage caused by the use of invasive procedures (invasive laparoscopy/radiology) and let operations be performed remotely.

Electroactive polymers have been used as the active part that generates the return force in these devices in various research centres such as the Jet Propulsion Laboratory NASA (Bar-Cohen, 2004 or the Research Centre of EAP Devices in Switzerland.

3.3.5 Electrochromic Materials

These materials possess the property to change the absorption spectrum, and usually their colour, when they change their state of oxidation or change their particle orientation in dispersion at the core of the material, by applying an external potential difference (Granqvist *et al.*, 2004; Avendaño *et al.*, 2006.

They have major industrial uses such as optical memory information panels, the windows that attenuate the intensity of the light and solar energy entering vehicles and offices, and anti-dazzle rear-view mirrors that make for safer driving. They also have uses for medical device design which are currently being developed, among which the most important are

Active protective eyewear

The ability to change colour possessed by these materials can be used to design protective glasses whose lens change their colour or degree of transparency according to the intensity of the light (Ma *et al.*, 2006). They are of great use to patients with eye trouble, and even implants could be contemplated with lens made of electrochromic material or active contact lens.

Visors for radionuclide scanners

Recently (Hempel, 2006), Siemens AG company has patented the use of a controlled opacity visor aimed at reducing the problems of claustrophobia suffered by many patients when they need a radionuclide scan, particularly when the upper part of the patient is inside the body of the machine. The visor could be activated to let the patient see the room from inside the machine and so reduce their anxiety or fear during these examinations.

3.3.6 Electro/magnetorheological (EMR) Fluids

These are 0.1 to 100-μm particle suspensions in an isolating base fluid that undergo major changes in viscosity when subjected to an electric or magnetic field. When subjected to the field, the particles go into alignment due to the dipolar moment produced and form chains along the field lines. This causes drastic changes to properties such as viscosity and the yield stress of the ERF or MRF, changing from fluid behaviour to behaving like viscoelastic gel. The application of a magnetic field of around 100 mT in air is sufficient to align the fluid particles and make them form temporary column-like structures that increase the viscosity of the fluid while also producing anisotropic behaviour. The phenomenon is considered to be practically reversible and almost instantaneous with response times of around 10 ms.

Its uses in engineering are many, mainly in simplifying hydraulic control mechanisms. It has been successfully used in active suspensions, clutches and variable flow pumps.

However, the particles in suspension are particularly abrasive, which combined with the need to ensure a hermetic seal encumbers a prolonged use of devices based on these fluids. Various medical applications of these fluids have been tested and these are detailed below.

Haptic devices

As explained previously, haptic devices support telesurgery and computer-aided surgery. Active dampers have been developed based on the use of these fluids, whose incorporation into haptic systems lets a very precise control be had over the sensations reaching the operator (Bar-Cohen *et al.*, 2001; Neelakantan *et al.*, 2002; Rizzo *et al.*, 2007).

Rehabilitation devices

Making the best of the benefits provided by stiff dampers and controllable dampers using these fluids, training systems can also be built (static bicycle-type machines) with variable resistance to movement depending on the patients' degree of recovery (Dong *et al.*, 2005).

Possible cancer therapy

The use of these materials has also been proposed as a way of blocking the blood that reaches tumours so as to cut off their food supply and destroy the harmful cells (Flores *et al.*, 1999).

Such blocking systems have been tested *in vitro* with favourable results. However, its *in vivo* use will need to take account of safety aspects for the surrounding tissues as well as compatibility with the rest of the patient's body.

Braille readers/translators

A possibility to design a panel with a surface whose rigidity could be modified locally could be used to develop Braille reading and writing systems to help the blind without any need to store information in physical external supports (like punched or embossed cards). The use of electro/magnetorheological fluids for this purpose have been demonstrated in the laboratory (Bansevicius and Virbalis, 2007), although, to date, there are no commercial devices.

X-ray collimator

Lens prototypes have recently been developed that contain magnetorheological fluids and have been used to collimate X-rays in dental radiography equipment with some preliminary positive results (Dyszkiewicz *et al.*, 2009).

3.3.7 Pyroelectric Materials

Pyroelectricity is the change in polarisation of a material subjected to changes of temperature. This type of phenomenon can be observed in dielectric materials that contain spontaneous polarisations produced by oriented dipoles.

These effects have been known to man for many years in ceramic and metal oxide materials and it was Brewster who gave them their name in 1824. But research into pyroelectricity in polymers is relatively new and dates only from the middle of the 20th century, with a few initial results that had little commercial attraction.

Giant leaps forward came about with the discovery of pyroelectric effects in polyvynilidene fluoride or "PVDF" (Bergman, 1971), and only after the discovery of piezoelectricity in the same material (Kawai, 1969).

The most common types of this material are triglycine sulphate, lithium tantalite, strontium niobate and barium or polyvynilidene fluoride.

The main industrial uses are linked to the development of temperature sensors, presence detectors, humidity, leaks or other phenomena that go hand-in-hand with temperature changes. Their use in medical devices is also notable as the following examples will show.

Thermographic cameras

The sensor matrix of a thermographic camera is usually based on using pyroelectric materials as infrared sensors. The medical applications of these apparatuses are many, the most important being to detect tumours or subcutaneous defects and evaluate the progress of muscle or bone injuries (Schindel, 2007). They can be also used as a support tool for other medical devices based on active materials with thermomechanical coupling (Paumier *et al.*, 2008).

Biometric systems

These materials can be used as the component parts of real-time footstep pattern biometric systems used to examine persons recognised by security systems or in more medical spheres, to study the evolution of injuries affecting the patient's mobility (Fang *et al.*, 2007).

Assisted surgery

These materials have been used to measure blood temperature during operations to implant coronary stents, in order to correlate temperature profile with blood flow and as a tool for controlling the surgical process (Mochi *et al.*, 2004).

Flow volume sensors

Dymedix Co. has developed nasal flow detectors using PVDF, which, besides their pyroelectric properties enable temperature changes to be detected. This means problems like sleep apnoea or cot death in the newborn can be actively controlled. These devices are placed in the nasal orifices and the patient's respiration induces charges in the polymer according to a particular pattern. If the patient stops breathing the sensor detects the pattern change and through a microcontroller activates an alarm that wakes the patient or alerts their family.

X-ray intensity detectors

The fact that human body tissue heats up through the absorption of X-rays (during X-ray examinations), pyroelectric sensors can be used to estimate the dose of radiation absorbed and assess risk situations. The phenomenon has been tested *in vivo* during mammogram tests with results showing high precision and high sensitivity (De Paula *et al.*, 2005).

Following on from these devices and other proposals contained in the annexes in data base form, the following section sets out an analysis of the current state of technology concerning the use of active materials in the development of medical devices. At the end of the work there is a set of proposals for future action to increase the scientific, industrial and social impact of these multifunctional materials.

3.4 An Analysis of the Current State of Technology

All the devices mentioned in the preceding section together with many additional proposals for the use of active materials to develop medical devices have been brought together in a data base that is attached as an annex. This annex has been used to prepare an analysis of the current state of technology, which is set out below.

The data base contains about 100 medical devices based on different active materials belonging to the families already dealt with. These devices have been compiled and classified for study in line with the following parameters:

- Purpose of the device
- Active material used
- Function of the organ affected by using the device
- Organ affected by using the device
- Associated pathology
- Associated medical speciality
- Extent to which the idea is developed (patent, *in vitro* tests, *in vivo* tests, placed on the market)

Information on the most important patents and publications linked to each proposal for use is also included, as well as the main companies, technology centres and universities where these proposals are being developed. The main outcomes of the analysis conducted from the information compiled is summarised in Figs. 3.4 to 3.9, which will now be examined.

As may be gathered from the results in Fig. 3.4, the active material types with the largest number of proposals for use in the Medical Industry are electroactive polymers, shape memory alloys and shape memory polymers. These three families of materials cover almost 70% of the total medical applications put forward for active materials.

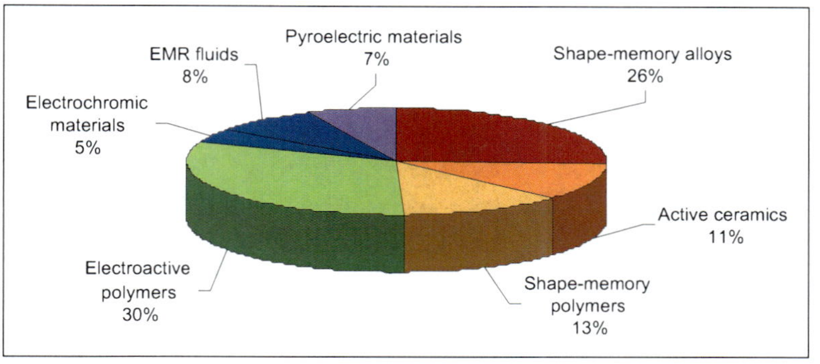

Figure 3.4 Types of active materials in medical devices. Percentage classification according to current usage.

The percentage of applications for active ceramics is not inconsiderable, even though their use as piezoelectric sensors is being prejudiced by the better properties possessed by some other piezoelectric polymers, generally less fragile and with a higher generated signal/applied force ratio. However, active ceramics still have many advantages in their use as actuators due to their inverse piezoelectric effect, particularly in micropositioning tasks and as mechanical impulse generators (Piezo Film Sensors, *Measurement Specialties*).

Nevertheless, of the three active material families with the largest number of proposed uses, it should be pointed out that only in the case of shape memory alloys does the percentage of designs passing through the *in vivo* testing or marketing stage supersede 50%. When it comes to shape memory polymers and electroactive polymers over 70% of the designs have only reached the patent or *in vitro* testing stage.

This situation is undoubtedly due to the shape-memory alloys having been discovered in the 20th century with the first medical devices based on these alloys beginning to be placed on the market in the 1980s. For this reason, the development of these alloy-based devices is much more advanced. At the same time the processes of prototype synthesis, characterisation, modelling, simulation, transformation and manufacturing have been studied in greater detail.

With active polymers (especially shape memory polymers and electroactive polymers) the most promising discoveries regarding their properties were made in the 1980s and 1990s, which means the scientific-technological knowledge of these materials has not yet reached the same degree of maturity as available for other materials.

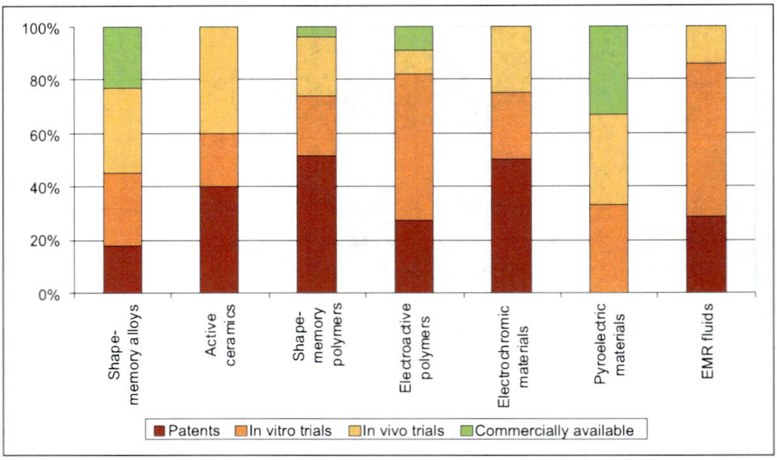

Figure 3.5 Types of active materials in medical devices. Percentage classification according to the proposed usage.

The families of electrochromic materials, electro/magnetorheological materials and pyroelectrical materials (except some isolated cases, such as their use in infrared thermography) have not yet resulted in commercial medical devices. The preliminary results of the numerous devices tested *in vitro* and *in vivo*, however, hold promise for the coming decade.

It should also be emphasised that, according to Fig. 3.6, 73% of the uses proposed for active materials basically seek the actuation capability of these materials, while only 17% focus on the possibilities of these materials as sensors.

The use of activation and detection capabilities, in some cases combined with different types of active materials accounts for 7% of the uses proposed for medicine.

On the other hand, from Fig. 3.7 it can be seen that some active material families are mainly used when the material is intended for activation tasks (alloys and shape-memory polymers), while in other cases (pyroelectric materials) the material is mainly used for its detection properties. In this regard, the most versatile family of materials are electroactive polymers, among which, the very large difference in properties broaden their range of applications meaning they can be used individually or in combination of activation and detection.

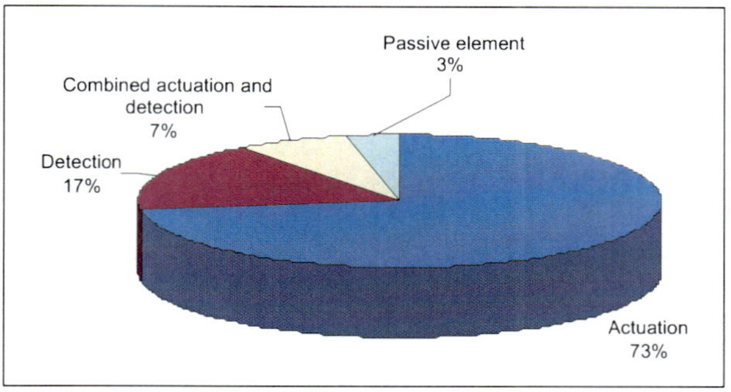

Figure 3.6 Types of active materials in medical devices. Classification according to the active material's role in the device.

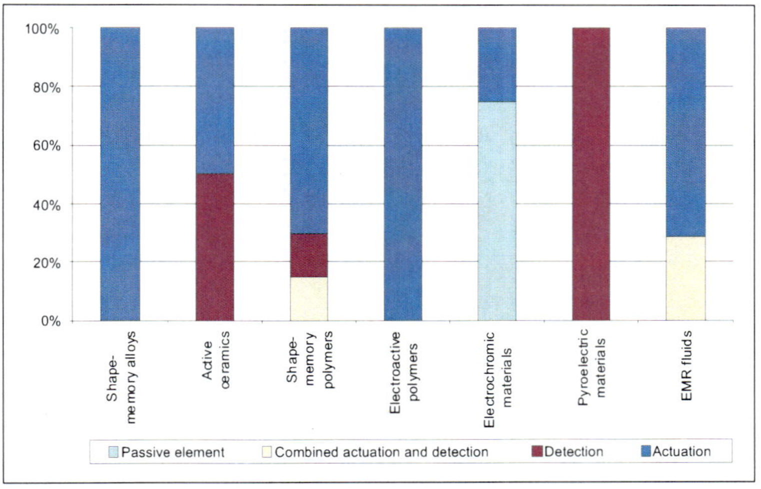

Figure 3.7 Types of active materials in medical devices. Classification of material families, according to the active material's role.

Regarding the medical uses put forward, Fig. 3.8 shows a percentage classification according to the functions of the organism wished to be modified by the use of active material-based medical devices. Most proposals are related to cardiovascular functions (25%) and musculoskeletal functions (20%). There are also numerous devices that can be used to support various functions (17%), as is the case with all devices intended to enhance surgical instrument capabilities or chemical analysis systems.

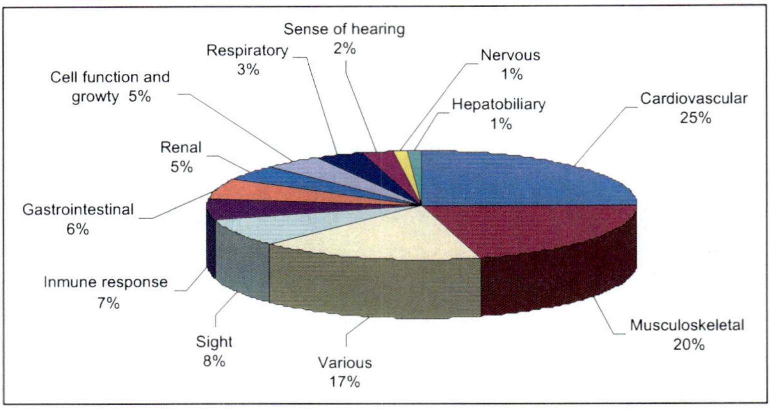

Figure 3.8 Active material uses in medical devices. Classification according to the function of the organism associated with the device.

Moreover, the classification according to related organ, reflected in Fig. 3.9 reveals that the heart, eyes, bones and the joints at the end of the arms and legs practically cover 30% of the proposed uses. In all, we have discovered proposals for using multipurpose materials for treating at least 17 organs. As with classification according to their use, there are also many ideas for devices (41%) that can be used (with slight modifications) to treat different organs beyond those specifically enumerated.

The classification of uses, according to the medical specialities, as shown in Fig. 3.10, makes it clear that cardiology and orthopaedic surgery are the areas of medicine for which there has been the largest number of proposals for active material-based devices (attaining 34% between both). At the same time 10% of the devices fall into different areas and 9% support general surgery, obviously with various purposes.

It needs to be underlined that currently at least 17 medical specialisations could directly benefit from a more generalised use of active materials in medical device development. Other multidisciplinary specialisations, like General Surgery, could benefit indirectly from such new approaches and developments based on active materials for diagnostic and therapeutic purposes.

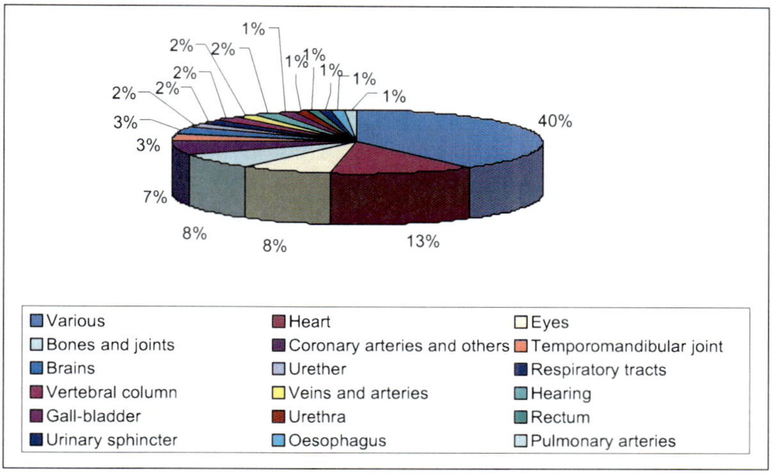

Figure 3.9 Active material uses in medical devices. Classification according to the function of the organism associated with the device.

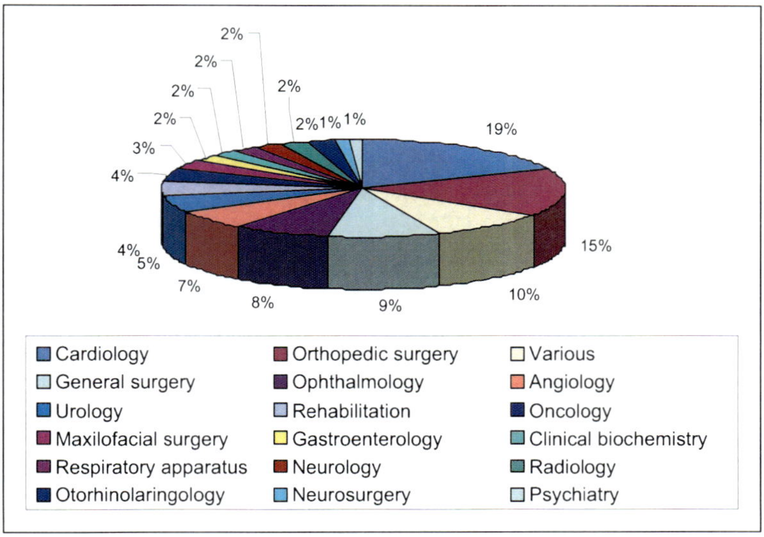

Figure 3.10 Active material uses in medical devices. Classification according to the medical speciality associated with the use of the device.

However, to achieve this generalised use of multifunctional materials in the Medical Industry, various fields of study need to be examined more deeply and some of the difficulties set out in the next section need to be overcome.

3.5 Main Study Trends and Challenges to Overcome

This section examines the main fields that need to be looked at more closely in order to promote the industrial expansion of active materials as component parts of medical devices.

3.5.1 Synthesis and Transformation Processes

Generally speaking, the families need improvements to some of their properties if more effective end devices are to be had. It is being attempted to achieve these improvements by testing the synthesis between new formulations and different subsequent transformation processes. Listed below are the main drawbacks to the main active material families taken into consideration:

- **Shape of memory alloys.** By varying the proportion of Ni and Ti, together with other materials, changes can be obtained within the activation temperature range and in the ability to recover from deformations. This ability to recover from deformations is particularly low in these types of active materials, usually up to a maximum of 8%. This turns out to be a limiting factor compared to the deformations to be got by using shape memory polymers or electroactive polymers (De la Flor *et al.*, 2006; Bar-Cohen, 2004.
- **Active ceramics.** The main problem for developing small-size long-lasting sensors is the fragility of the active ceramic layers, especially for uses intended for measuring pressure. For this reason, complex manufacturing techniques are being used to integrate them into structures that provide greater strength (Sachau *et al.*, 1999).
- **Electroactive polymers.** Most electroactive polymers developed require the use of strong electric fields for activation that are unacceptable to the body (electronic electroactive polymers) or in cases where admissible fields

can be used (ionic electronic polymers), they are only capable of overcoming very small forces during activation. This means their use in implantable devices is limited, although recent advances have been promising (Bar-Cohen, 2004.

- **Shape-memory polymers.** Their uses are limited by the tiny forces they are capable of overcoming during activation (around 4 MPa) and the need to achieve activation temperatures that are not harmful to body tissue. Enormous progress is being made regarding the synthesis of these materials, testing different proportions of monomers and formulations to improve these aspects (Lendlein *et al.*, 2002, 2005, 2006).
- **Electrochromic materials.** Since these are multilayer micrometric thick glass structures, they are usually rigid and fragile. These properties limit their use as component parts of complex systems in combination with other more flexible materials. Studying the processes of synthesis, transformation and deposition linked to obtaining the multilayer structure is important if these limitations are to be solved (Granqvist *et al.*, 2004; Avendaño *et al.*, 2006.
- **Electro/magnetorheological materials.** Their remarkable properties as actuators are limited by their corrosive action, which deteriorates their casings and makes it difficult to use them in living organisms (Mavroidis *et al.*, 2001; Hafez, 2006).
- **Pyroelectric materials.** These are beset by the problems of aging which lead to greater fragility (especially pyroelectric polymers) and the depolarisation of the dipoles. On the other hand, sudden changes of temperature can produce high voltages that affect the polarisation of the material. These effects are generally borne in mind by designing appropriate electronic conditioning to avoid overload, while the effects of aging can be modelled and corrected (Lines and Glass, 2001).

If detection and activation properties are to be improved, a greater understanding of the fundamental physical-chemical principles behind these phenomena is required and how the end results are affected by changes to the synthesis and transformation processes.

To this end, computational models can be used that help combine the uses of knowledge concerning material science, thermodynamics, heat transmission, mechanics (classic and quantum) and electromagnetism (Deutsch *et al.*, 2007, 2008; Conti, 2007).

3.5.2 Modelling and Simulation

From the data obtained from characterisation testing (both materials and specific uses), performance models can be had that facilitate the development of new applications with the same material or similar applications with other active materials from the same family.

Being able to use the ad hoc models developed in a combined way together with multivariable simulations that let finite element calculation be used, can be of tremendous help in simplifying the design of auxiliary systems and making it easier to integrate these active materials into complex devices (Liang *et al.*, 1996;; Bar-Cohen, 2004; Hafez, 2006).

Taking the simulation and programming tools commonly taught as part of the technical university educational programs such as Matlab, Maple, Simulink, ANSYS and others, it would be a very positive step (to encourage the industrial expansion of these materials) if experts in the characterisation, modelling and simulation of different active material properties could get together to create programming libraries.

In this way, a whole lot of phenomena to be found in different active materials could be placed at the disposal of the scientific community. Such phenomena might be represented in graphic form as block diagrams that would enable the responses of these materials under different circumstances to be predicted and then integrated into multivariable systems to provide support for development tasks.

Combining all this with the recent progress in modelling and simulating biological systems and their response to external stimuli (Kohl *et al.*, 2000; Deutsch *et al.*, 2007, 2008; Cerutti, 2008), would result in a considerable optimisation of the processes for creating new active medical devices, speed up production start-up and minimise the costs associated with *in vitro* and *in vivo* tests.

3.5.3 Stability of Properties

The body is an aggressive environment for implantable devices as these implants are in permanent contact with aqueous salt solutions, which can lead to degradation and corrosion, particularly in metals and alloys (Rondelli, 1996; Davis, 2003).

On the other hand, the properties of polymeric materials change with the passage of time, usually resulting in greater rigidity and fragility accompanied by an increase in their glass transition temperatures (Plazek and Andrekanic, 1995; Cernosek *et al.*, 2002. This change in properties has strong financial implications since it affects in-service performance. Particularly in the case of shape memory implants, any change in the glass transition temperature (activation) can lead to problems in activating the required geometric changes. In the case of electroactive polymers certain increases in rigidity can come about that limit their speed and activation capability or their behaviour as sensors.

Therefore, the changes in the mechanical properties (surface and internal) of these materials (such as elasticity modulus, hardness and strength) due to their being implanted in the human body need to be studied so as to be able to predict any possible changes in response right from the design stage. The effects of using protective coatings or appropriate transformation processes can also be very positive for obtaining longer-lasting stability.

3.5.4 Safety Issues

Biocompatibility

Although various active material-based medical devices have already been marketed, biocompatibility continues to be paramount for new designs based on these ideas, since such biocompatibility does not depend only on the material used, but also on factors such as implant geometry and surface, the zone where it is implanted and other factors (Davis, 2003).

For instance, many shape-memory polymer formulations are toxic. However, some of them have been shown to be compatible (Cabanlit *et al.*, 2007; Sokolowsky *et al.*, 2007), which brings a ray of hope for future designs based on this family of active materials. Electroactive polymers are in a similar situation; although many are toxic some formulations have been found to be compatible and could be used in contact with tissue without any problem (Kamalesh *et al.*, 2000; George *et al.*, 2004).

In whatever the case, the use of protective surface coatings (using physical or chemical "PVD" or "CVD" vapour deposition techniques) can be extremely helpful for improving this situation and obtaining safer end devices (Albella, 2006).

Sterilisation

Before an *in vivo* implantation of active implantable devices, they must be sterilised by using some of the methods generally used with ceramics, metals or polymers [steam, ethylene oxide, gamma radiation, low temperature plasma (LTP) or the Noxilizer process]. The process must be carefully chosen so as not to affect the integrity of the devices or their detection or activation capabilities (Simmons, 2004).

For example, when dealing with shape memory polymers and alloys, of all the methods that can be used, it is preferable to choose low temperature sterilisation (LTP, ethylene oxide or the Noxilizer method) in order to avoid activating the memory effect. Other polymers may also require low-temperature processes while active metals and alloys may require gamma radiation-type processes to avoid their deteriorating in the presence of oxidising agents.

It is important to examine the influence of these methods on the toxicity and thermo-electrical-mechanical response of different active materials. A study of this has been begun with promising results for some types of alloys and active polymers (Thierry *et al.*, 2000; Yakacki *et al.*, 2008).

Regulations

In order to optimise devices based on these materials it is mandatory to comply with the guidelines of the "European Directive on Medical Devices – 93/42/EEC" and the "European Directive on Active Implantable Medical Devices – 90/385/EEC".

It is also advisable to follow the recommendations contained in ISO Standard 13485 on medical device quality, as well as specific rules applying to material characterisation tests (ISO and ASTM Standards).

However, the increasing use of active materials in medical devices may lead to new more specific standards being drawn up aimed at making it simpler to get safer end designs.

3.5.5 Structured Development Process

In order to promote the development of marketable medical applications based on these devices, it would be advisable to ensure a better degree of cooperation among all those involved in the various development stages. In this way, they could all get together to establish a structured development process combining tasks such as material synthesis, characterisation and processing, mechanical design, electronic design, prototype manufacture, *in vitro* and *in vivo* testing, official approval and the subsequent production start-up.

Similar proposals are being successfully applied to promote electroactive polymer-based device development (EAPs) (Bar-Cohen, 2001, 2004. Dealing with different active materials in an all-embracing manner that takes account of their mutual strengthening properties and their combined use as a source of solutions for diagnostic and therapeutic problems, would be of tremendous help for expanding the industrial use of these materials.

3.6 Conclusions

Different families of materials showing great potential have emerged, especially over the last decade that have led to medical device prototypes being developed with special features and activation capabilities that were up to now unattainable. Acknowledgement must also be made of the help contributed by the progress made in other fields of science and technology.

The principal active material families have been introduced as well as their most prominent uses in the Medical Industry, almost all of which have emerged in recent years. All have been developed on a test prototype level although there are around 700 to 800 active material-based medical device patents which herald a considerable social and economic impact on the sector.

The development of biosensors and bioactuators using these materials currently requires progress in various aspects of science and technology if their possibilities are to be optimised. Thus, it will be possible to obtain marketable medical devices that meet all mechanical, diagnostic and therapeutic requirements such as stability and safety.

There has recently been progress in international cooperation regarding active materials with specific forums having been set up such as Scientific.net, Biomat.net and others, which help the dissemination of results and the exchange of opinions.

However, it would be of great interest to set up a specific forum on "Active Materials for Medical Devices", where researchers, universities and enterprises could come into contact to be able to match technology supply to market demand, which would be particularly important for the Medical Industry.

While the new capabilities of these materials give rise to expectations that many medical devices will be more effective for diagnostics and therapy, considerable effort still needs to be put into research and development to produce more accurate sensors and more robust, rapid and effective actuators.

References

Albella, J.M. "Preparación y caracterización de recubrimientos y láminas delgadas". PhD Program "Ciencias Físicas de la Universidad Autónoma de Madrid - Instituto de Ciencia de los Materiales de Madrid (CSIC)", Teaching Resources. Madrid, 2006.

Albella, J.M.; Gómez-Aleixandre, C.; Ojeda, F.; Martí, F.J. "Síntesis de materiales cerámicos mediante técnicas químicas en fase de vapor (CVD)". Boletín de la Sociedad Española de Cerámica y Vídrio, 42(1), 27–31, 2003.

Avendaño, E.; Berggren, L.; Niklasson, G.A.; *et al.* "Electrochromic materials and devices: Brief survey and new data on optical absorption in tungsten oxide and nickel oxide films". Thin Solid Films, 496(1), 30–36, 2006.

Bansevicius, R.M.; Virbalis, J.A. "Two-dimensional Braille readers based on electro-rheological fluid valves controlled by electric field". Mechatronics, 17(10), 570–577, 2007.

Bar-Cohen, Y. "Electroactive polymer actuators as artificial muscles: Reality, potential and challenges". SPIE Press. Washington, 2001.

Bar-Cohen, Y. "Electroactive polymer (EAP) actuators as artificial muscles: Reality, potential and challenges". SPIE Press, 2nd Ed. Washington, 2004.

Bar-Cohen, Y.; Mavroidis, C.; Bouzit, M.; *et al.* "Virtual reality robotic telesurgery simulations using MEMICA haptic system". Proceedings of EAPAD, SPIE's 8th Annual International Symposium on Smart Structures and Materials, Newport, CA, 4329–4347, 2001.

Bar-Cohen, Y.; Sherrit, S.; Shyh-Shiuh, L. "Characterization of the electromechanical properties of EAP materials". Proceedings of EAPAD, SPIE's 8th Annual International Symposium on Smart Structures and Materials, Newport, CA, 4329–4343, 2001.

Bergman, G.J.; Mc Fee, J.H.; Crane, C.R. "Pyroelectricity and optical second harmonic generation in polyvinilidene fluoride films". Applied Physic Letters, 18, 203-205, 1971.

Cabanlit, M.; Maitland, D.; Wilson, T.; Simon, S.; *et al.* "Polyurethane shape-memory polymers demonstrate functional biocompatibility *in vitro*". Macromolecular Bioscience, 7(1), 48–55, 2007.

Cardoso, V.F.; Rocha, J.G.; Soares, F.O.; *et al.* "Lab-on-a-chip fluid acoustic microagitation: Piezoelectric polymer beta-PVDF used as ultrasonic transducer". International Conference on Biomedical Electronics and Devices Biostec 2008 – Biodevices, 2, 262–267.

Cernosek, Z.; Holubova, J.; Cernoskova, E.; Liska, M. "Enthalpic relaxation and the glass transition". Journal of Optoelectronics and Advanced Materials, 4(3), 489–503, 2002.

Cerutti, S. "Multivariate, multiorgan and multiscale integration of information in biomedical signal processing". International Conference on Biomedical Electronics and Devices Biostec 2008 – Biodevices, Keynote Lecture. IEEE Engineering in Medicine and Biology Society. INSTICC Press, 2008.

Cheremisinoff, N. "Handbook of Ceramics and Composites". Marcel Dekker. New York, 1990.

Conti, S.; Lenz, M.; Rumpf, M. "Modelling and simulation of magnetic shape-memory polymer composites". Journal of Mechanics and Physics of Solids, 55(7), 1462-1486, 2007.

Davis, J.R. "Handbook of materials for medical devices". ASM International. United States, 2003.

De la Flor, S.; Urbina, C.; Ferrando, F. "Constitutive model of shape memory alloys: Theoretical formulation and experimental validation". Materials Science and Engineering: A, 427, 112–122, 2006.

De Paula, M.; Carvalho, A.; Brassalotti, A.L.; *et al.* "Microcontrolled pyro-electric instrument for measuring X-ray intensity in mammography". Medical & biological engineering & computing, 43(6), 751–755, 2005.

Deutsch, A.; Brusch, L.; Byrne, H. "Mathematical modeling of biological systems. Volume I: Cellular biophysics, regulatory networks, development, biomedicine and data analysis". Series "Modeling and Simulation in Science, Engineering and Technology". Birkhäuser, 2007.

Deutsch, A.; De la Parra, R.; De Boer, R.J. "Mathematical modeling of biological systems. Volume II: Epidemiology, evolution and ecology, immunology, neural systems and the brain, and innovative mathematical methods".

Series "Modeling and Simulation in Science, Engineering and Technology", Birkhäuser, 2008.

Díaz Lantada, A.; Lafont Morgado, P.; Lorenzo Yustos, H.; *et al.* "Treatment of mitral valve insufficiency by shape memory polymer based active annuloplasty". International Conference on Biomedical Electronics and Devices Biostec 2008 – Biodevices, 1, 17–22.

Díaz Lantada, A.; Lafont Morgado, P.; Lorenzo Yustos, H.; *et al.* "Active annuloplasty system for mitral valve insufficiency". Chapter from: "Biomedical Engineering Systems and Technologies 2008" editado por Springer Berlin Heidelberg Verlag. I.S.B.N.: 978-3-540-92218-6 (press) 978-3-540-92219-3 (online). Among series: "Communications in Computer and Information Science" I.S.S.N.: 1865-0929 (press) 1865-0937 (online), Vol. XXV.

Dong, S.; Lu, K.; Sun, J.; Rudolph, K. "Rehabilitation device with variable resistance and intelligent control". Medical Engineering and Physics, 27(3), 249–255, 2005.

Duerig, T.; Pelton, A.; Stöckel, D. "Superelastic nitinol for medical devices". Medical Plastics and Biomaterials Magazine, 30–43, March, 1997.

Dyszkiewicz, A.; Polec, P.; Zajdel, J.; *et al.* "Collimation of X-Ray Diagnostic Bundle by Means of Steering Ferrofluid". International Conference on Biomedical Electronics and Devices Biostec 2009 – Biodevices, 1, 441–447. Special Session on Active Materials for Medical Devices.

Fang, J.S.; Hao, Q.; Brady, D.; Guenther, B.; Hsu, H. "A pyroelectric infrared biometric system for real-time walker recognition by use of a maximum likelihood principal components estimation (MLPCE) method". Optics Express, 15(6), 3271–3284, 2007.

Feng, G.H.; Kim, E.S. "Micropump based on PZT unimorph and one-way parylene valves". Journal of Micromechanics and Microengineering, 14, 429–435, 2004.

Flores, G.; Sheng, R.; Liu, J."Medical applications of magnetorheological fluids: A possible new cancer therapy". Journal of Intelligent Material Systems and Structures, 10(9), 708–713, 1999.

Gall, K.; Kreiner, P.; Turner, D.; Hulse, M. "Shape memory polymers for MEMS systems". Journal of Microelechtromechanical Systems, 13(3), 472–483, 2004.

George, P.; Lyckman, A.W.; La Van, D.A.; *et al.* "Fabrication and biocompatibility of polypyrrole implants suitable for neural prosthetics". Biomaterials, 26, 3511–3519, 2004.

Granqvist, C.G.; Avendaño, E.; Azens, A. "Advances in electrochromic materials and devices". Materials Science Forum, 455, 1–6, 2004.

Ha, C.D.; Calagnano, D. "Amplatzer Vascular Plug to occlude the internal iliac arteries in patients undergoing aortoiliac aneurysm repair". Journal of Vascular Surgery, 42(6), 1058–1062, 2005.

Haertling, G.H. "Ferroelectric ceramics: History and technology". Journal of the American Ceramic Society, 82(4), 797–818, 1999.

Hafez, M. "Polymer based actuators as artificial muscles". FSRM Training in Microsystems Course. Teaching Resources. Zurich 2006.

Hempel, E. "Medical diagnosis or therapy apparatus with an electrochromic display for the patient". Siemens AG. Deutsches Patent und Marken Amt - DE102006021355, 2006.

Janas, V.; Safari, A. "Overview of Fine-Scale Piezoelectric Ceramic/Polymer Composite Processing". Journal of the American Ceramic Society, 78(11), 639–640, 2005.

Kamalesh, S.; Tan, P.; Wang, J.; *et al.* "Biocompatibility of electroactive polymers in tissues". Journal of Biomedical Materials Research Part A, 52(3), 467–478, 2000.

Kawai, H. "The piezoelectricity of polyvinylidene fluoride, Japanese Journal of Applied Physics 8, 975-976, 1969.

Kohl, P.; Noble D., Winslow R.L.; *et al.*.- "Computational modelling of biological systems: tools and visions". Philosophical Transactions A of the Royal Society London, 2000.

Lafont Morgado P.; Díaz Lantada, A.; Lorenzo Yustos, H.; *et al.*- "Sistema activo de anuloplastia para tratamiento de la insuficiencia mitral y otras patologías cardiovasculares". Oficina Española de Patentes y Marcas (OEPM) – Documento de Patente P200603149, 2006.

Lafont Morgado P.; Díaz Lantada, A.; Lorenzo Yustos, H.; *et al.* "Active annuloplasty system for the progressive treatment of valvular insufficiencies and other cardiovascular pathologies". World Intellectual Property Organization (WIPO) – International Bureau – Patent Document WO/2008/071817 – PCT/ES2007/000719, 2007.

Lafont Morgado, P.; Díaz Lantada, A.; Martínez Álvarez, A.; *et al.* "System for the detection and treatment of bruxism and other occlusal conditions". World Intellectual Property Organization (WIPO) – International Bureau – Patent Document WO/2009/013371 – PCT/ES2008/000498, 2008.

Lafont Morgado, P.; Díaz Lantada, A.; Martínez Álvarez, A.; *et al.* "Instrumented splint for the diagnosis of bruxism". International Conference on Biomedical Electronics and Devices Biostec 2008 – Biodevices, 2, 216-222.

Lendlein, A.; Hiang, H.; Jünger, O.; Langer, R. "Light-induced shape-memory polymers". Nature, 434, 879–882, 2005.

Lendlein, A; Kelch, S. "Shape-memory polymers". Angewandte Chemie International, 41(12), 2034–2057, 2002.

Lendlein, A.; Kelch, S. "Shape-memory polymers as stimuli-sensitive implant materials". Clinical Hemorheology and Microcirculation, 32, 105–116, 2005.

Lendlein, A; Kelch, S; Kratz, K.; Schulte, J. "Shape-memory polymers". Encyclopedia of Materials: Science and Technology, 1–9, 2005.

Lendlein, A; Langer, R. "Biodegradable, elastic shape-memory polymers for potential biomedical applications". Science, 296(5573), 1673–1676, 2002.

Liang, C.; Sun, F.; Rogers, C.A. "Electro-mechanical impedance modeling of active material systems". Smart Materials and Structures, 5, 171–186, 1996.

Lines, M.E.; Glass, A.M. "Principles and applications of ferroelectrics and related materials". Oxford Classic Text in the Physical Sciences Series. Oxford University Press, 2001.

Liu, C.; Mather, P.T. "Thermomechanical characterization of a tailored series of shape memory polymers". Journal of Applied Medical Polymers, 6(2), 47–52, 2002.

Liu, C., Qin, H.; Mather, P.T. "Review of progress in shape-memory polymers". Journal of Materials Chemistry, 17, 1553–1558, 2007.

Ma, C.; Taya, M.; Xu, M. "Smart sunglasses and goggles based on electrochromic polymers". Center of Intelligent Materials and Systems, University of Washington. American Chemical Society Meeting, 2006.

Ma, C.; Taya, M.; Xu, M. "Smart sunglasses based on electrochromic polymers". Polymer Engineering and Science, 48(11), 2224–2228, 2008.

Mc Keighen, R. "Optimizing transducer design for medical imaging". Proceedings of the IEEE Engineering in Medicine and Biology Society 11th Annual International Conference, 2, 404–404, 1989.

Mineta, T.; Mitsui, T.; Watanabe, Y.; *et al.* "An active guide wire with shape memory alloy bending actuator fabricated by room temperature process". Sensors and Actuators A: Physical, 97, 632–637, 2002.

Mochi, M.; Giovanetti, G.; Francesconi, R.; Hartwig, V. "A study for a portable IR sensor to detect the blood temperature during coronary bypass implantation". CNR – University Pisa. Technical Report, 2004.

Moreno, J.C.; De Lima, E.R.; Ruíz, A.F.; Brunetti, F.J.; Pons, J.L. "Design and implementation of an inertial measurement unit for control of artificial limbs: Application on leg orthoses". Sensors and Actuators B: Chemical, 118(1), 333–337, 2006.

Neelakantan, V.; Washington, G.N.; Wolf, R.K. "Force feedback system using magneto-rheological fluids for telerobotic surgery". Smart Structures and Materials 2002: Industrial and Commercial Applications of Smart Structures Technologies. Proceedings of the SPIE, 4698, 509–518, 2002.

Paumier, G.; Siv, S.; Bancaud, A.; Sudor, J.; Gué, A.M. "Thermoresponsive polymer-based microdevice for nano-liquid chromatography". International Conference on Biomedical Electronics and Devices Biostec 2008 - Biodevices, 1, 178–181.

Plazek, D.; Andrekanic, R. "Keynote Lectures in Selected Topics of Polymer Science", 117-138. CSIC (Riande, E. ed.). Madrid, 1995.

Pons, J.L.; Rocon, E.; Forner-Cordero, A.; Moreno J. "Biomedical instrumentation based on piezoelectric ceramics". Journal of European Ceramic Society, 27, 4191–4194, 2007.

Qiu, C.; Zhao, Q.; Zhanj, H.; et al. "A valve-less PZT micropump with isosceles triangle cross-section diffuser elements". First International Conference on Nano/Micro Engineered and Molecular Systems, 200–203, 2006.

Rapp, B. "Nitinol for stents". Materials Today, 13–13, May, 2004.

Rizzo, R.; Sgambelluri, S.; Scilingo, E.P.; Raugi, M. "Electromagnetic modelling and design of haptic interface prototypes based on magnetorheological fluids". IEEE Transactions on Magnetics, 43(9), 3586–3600, 2007.

Rondelli, G. "Corrosion resistance tests on NiTi shape memory alloy". Biomaterials, 17(20), 2003–2008, 1996.

Sachau, D.; Wierach, P.; Monner, H.P.; Schönecker, A. "Smart structures based on thin piezoceramic plates". Functional Materials, Euromat 99 Series, 520–524, 1999.

Sakamoto, W.; Shibatta-Katesawa, S.; Kanda, D.; *et al.* "Piezoelectric effect in composite polyurethane-ferroelectric ceramics". Physica Status Solidi, 172(1), 265–271, 1998.

Schindel, B. "Thermographie in der Theorie und Praxis". Online book 2007.

Schwartz, M. "New materials, processes and methods technology". CRC Press, Taylor and Francis Group. Florida, 2006.

Simmons, A. "Sterilization of medical devices". Business Briefing: Medical Device Manufacturing & Technology, August, 2004.

Smith, W.; Sung, G.; Saver, J.; *et al.* "Mechanical thrombectomy for acute ischemic stroke: Final results of the Multi MERCI Trial". Stroke, 39(4), 1205–1212, 2008.

Sokolowsky, W.; Metcalfe, A.; Hayashi, S.; Yahia, L.; Raymond, J. "Medical applications of shape memory polymers". Biomedical Materials, 2, 23–27, 2007.

Taya, M. "Hierarchical modelling of active materials". Nippon Genshiryoku Kenkyujo JAERI, 19-25, 2003.

Thierry, B. Tabrizian, M.; Trepanier, C.; Savadogo, O.; Yahia, L. "Effect of surface treatment and sterilization processes on the corrosion behavior of NiTi shape-memory alloy". Journal of Biomedical Materials Research, 51(4), 685–693, 2000.

Wache, H.; Tartakowska, D.J.; Hentrich, A.; Wagner, M.H. "Development of a polymer stent with shape memory effect as a drug delivery system". Journal of Materials Science – Materials in Medicine, 14(2), 109–112, 2003.

Wilson, T.; Small IV, W.; William, B. J.; Bearinger, J.P.; Maitland D.J. "Shape memory polymer therapeutic devices for stroke". Smart Medical and Biomedical Sensor Technology III. Proceedings of the SPIE, 6007, 157–164, 2005.

Wörgerbauer, H. "Die Technik des Konstruierens". Oldenbourg. München, 1943.

Yakacki, C.M.; Lyons, M.B.; Rech, B.; Gall, K.; Shandas, R. "Cytotoxicity and thermomechanical behaviour of biomedical shape-memory polymer networks post-sterilization". Biomedical Materials, 3, 015010, 2008.

Yakacki, C.M.; Willis, S.; Luders, C.; Gall, K. "Deformation limits in shape-memory polymers". Advance Engineering Materials, 10(1), 112–119, 2008.

Chapter 4

Shape-Memory Alloys for Biodevices

Andrés Díaz Lantada
Mechanical Engineering Department, E.T.S.I. Industriales,
Universidad Politécnica de Madrid, c/ José Gutiérrez Abascal 2,
28006 Madrid, Spain
adiaz@etsii.upm.es

4.1 Brief Introduction to Shape-Memory Alloys

Shape-memory alloys or SMAs are metal alloys that can be subjected to an apparently plastic deformation (up to deformation figures of around 8%) and recover their original shape through subsequent heating. This is commonly known as the "shape-memory effect". Under certain conditions, some of these alloys can also be subjected to deformations of up to 9% to 11% under load and then recover their original geometry when the load is removed. This is commonly known as "superelasticity".

Both effects and other similar ones are a consequence of the so-called "austenite-martensite" transformations (rapid displacement transformations regardless of diffusion) and the special facility of these materials to transform themselves into and from a martensite form. These transformations and their effects will be dealt with in more detail throughout the chapter, as we consider the main kinds of shape-memory alloys and their different properties and ways of working and methods of activation.

Since these alloys respond in a controllable way to temperature changes and mechanical forces, they can be classified as part of

Handbook of Active Materials for Medical Devices: Advances and Applications
Edited by Andrés Díaz Lantada

www.panstanford.com

the "intelligent" materials group and have numerous applications for actuator development (with shape-memory properties) or for energy storage devices (in the case of superelastic alloys). Many of these alloys are suitably resistant to body fluids as they are bioinert, which means they are relatively easy to use to produce biocompatible devices. This makes them particularly ideal intelligent materials for medical applications.

The first major research into these kinds of shape-memory alloys was linked to the study of superelastic effects in Au-Cd alloys (Ölander, 1932) and the observation of martensite transformations in Cu-Zn alloys that were reversible by thermal effects (Greninger, 1938). However, the most important discovery and the most remarkable properties were achieved through the development of a Ni-Ti alloy, approximately 55% and 45%, respectively, at the Naval Ordnance Laboratory and was given the name of Nitinol (Buehler, 1962). The use of certain additives has gradually led to a whole family of Nitinol-based alloys, although the original continues to be the most commercially widespread due to its good thermomechanical properties as well as an excellent resistance to corrosion, especially in the presence of body fluids.

Some excellent works on this kind of alloy, with particular reference to aspects of modelling and thermomechanical characterisation are included in the references in the chapter (De la Flor, 2005; Boohan, 2006). However, we believe that the approach taken here contributes something new as it focuses on some specific aspects of the analysis and synthesis of medical devices based on these shape-memory materials.

4.2 Main Medical Device Applications

Biomedical applications of these kinds of "intelligent" materials are related to their being used as actuators for surgical tasks or for tissue geometry modification, as explained further on. Some of the most remarkable examples of application are included in this sub-chapter.

Self-expanding "stents"

There are different commercial stent designs for treating arteriosclerosis made from shape-memory alloys which are folded before being inserted into the human body and are then caused to expand by body temperature until they become fixed in the artery destroying the atheromatous plaque that caused the initial obstruction (Duerig *et al.*, 1997; Rapp, 2004).

"Amplatzer" devices

By using self-expanding meshes made of shape-memory alloy some Amplatzer devices have been developed, like those tested in the Heart Centre of Columbus Children's Hospital or those developed by AGA Medical Corp., to treat septal defects that join the right heart cavities with those of the left, either at an auricular or ventricular level, as well as for blocking other blood pass points (Ha and Calagnano, 2005). Some vena cava filters with similar working principles have been *in vivo* tested with positive results.

Thrombectomy devices

Devices for treating brain ischemia based on catheter ends made of shape-memory alloy (like the prototype MERCI X6) which, with slight geometric changes, manage to trap and remove thrombi in a minimally invasive way, as has already been proven *in vivo* (Smith *et al.*, 2008), present a promising expansion throughout the industry.

Active catheters

By using shape-memory wires twisted in a spiral around polymer catheters, the ends of these catheters can be controlled to make them reach parts that are difficult to access.

All that is needed to achieve this is to send an electric current through the shape-memory alloy filament to heat it and bend the catheter in a specific direction (Mineta, 2002).

Microvalves for fluid devices

These are various fluid and microfluid devices used in the medical industry, particularly volumetric pumps for drug delivery, in which a rotational or flexible component (gears, blades, membranes etc.) pumps fluid from suction to propulsion. They work with less loss if input and output valves are used whose opening and closure are synchronised with the pumping cycle. In these small devices, using intelligent materials as actuators helps reduce the end size. Different microvalve designs have been developed using SMA wires as active components to help control opening and closure (Krulevitch *et al.*, 1996; Suzumori *et al.*, 2005; Asao *et al.*, 2005 among others).

Devices for treating infantile scoliosis

The conventional treatment of infantile scoliosis is to place growth braces on the spinal column or ribs to attempt to correct these anatomical problems (with better results than the more traditional spinal braces, which sometimes cause respiratory problems).

However, shape-memory alloy braces have appeared recently. These can be easily bent when cold to facilitate implanting and when gradually heated they recover their original shape and force the spine into a more correct position.

These solutions were successfully tested on four 15 to 40 year old patients for the first time in December 2008 at the Hospital de la Paz, Madrid, as part of the pre-commercialisation *in vivo* validation tests (Sánchez Pérez-Grueso, 2010).

Bone splints

To aid the recovery of patients after complex operations and provide stable solutions bone splints are frequently used in conjunction with conventional geometry parts like clips, plates, bridges, screws and other implants. The use of these kinds of components made of shape-memory alloy that can easily be bent without heating makes implanting easier. When they are exposed to body heat, they force the surrounding bones into the right position. This is a particularly outstanding alternative to conventional passive splints, as was described when dealing with new solutions for infantile scoliosis.

These shape-memory solutions are used in maxillofacial surgery and neurosurgery to aid craneoplasty and jaw reconstructions, which are usually the result of traffic accidents. Superelastic Nitinol wire is often used in dentistry, particularly in orthodoncy to join different braces and progressively align the patient's teeth, since these superelastic wires are fitted when stretched and tend to shorten with the passage of time.

***

These materials were discovered before other families of active materials, and have produced promising results since the 1940s and particularly remarkable results since the 1960s with the appearance of Nitinol. Therefore, these "intelligent" alloys have been subjected to decades of research concerning their synthesis, processing, characterisation, modelling and simulation. This has led to the progressive appearance of commercial devices that range from surgical instruments to numerous implants.

Thanks to this, since the 1980s they have come into general use in different areas like heart surgery or dentistry and are probably now the most widely-used family of materials in health sciences.

However, it must be mentioned that other more recently discovered families of active materials, which will be dealt with in the following chapters of the handbook, also have a marked potential, especially for medical device development. However, research efforts need to be made like those that were dedicated to the field of shape-memory alloys in the last 40 years of the 20th century (and which are still being made).

The following sections provide a more detailed explanation of certain aspects, like the synthesis, processing, modelling, simulation and integration of these materials into more complex devices. We will then proceed to analyse the major current research trends and present needs regarding the use of these materials in the Medical Industry.

4.3 Current Capabilities and Recent Advances

Set out below are some of the main advances achieved in the last decades concerning shape-memory alloys and the technologies associated with their use. We will begin by describing the main types and the standard methods of activation, as these depend on the composition and the conditions under which they are synthesised and processed, and then go on to an in-depth examination of their characterisation, simulation and integration into devices for use as actuators.

4.3.1 Main Types of Shape-Memory Alloys

Depending on their properties, operating conditions or the kind of stimulus applied, shape-memory alloys can behave differently, which we will now explain.

In principle, an "intelligent" 1:1 proportion nickel-titanium alloy behaves as shown in Fig. 4.1. When subjected to mechanical forces, it reaches a so-called "deformed martensite" (DM) phase. When it is heated during this phase, the atoms become rearranged and the material passes on to the so-called "austenite" (A) phase in which the material contracts.

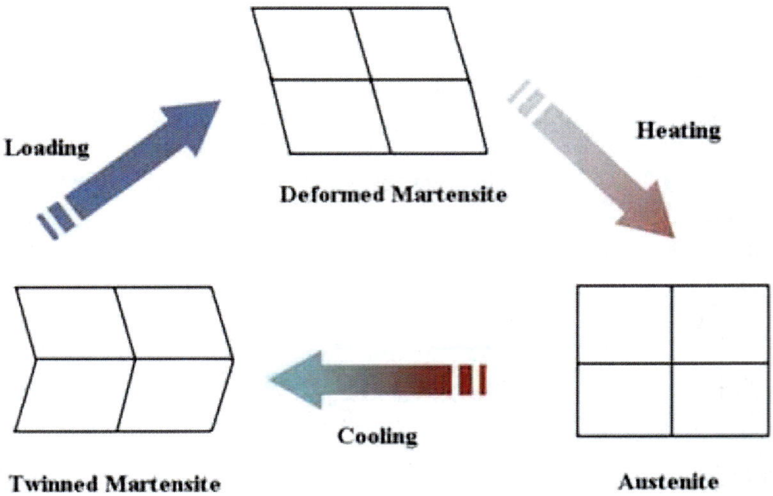

Figure 4.1 Scheme of thermoelastic martensite transformation.

The austenite phase is the phase that the material usually "remembers", as it is a more symmetrical phase than the martensite one. This means that at high temperatures the material tends towards a single minimum energy state. As it cools, the austenite passes to a "twinned martensite" state (TM), which on a macroscopic scale presents the same shape and size as the austenite phase, so there is no visible change in the material when it cools.

We have stated that the most stable shape depends on load and temperature conditions as well as on the composition of the material. The schematised diagram in Fig. 4.2 outlines the shapes adopted by the material under different load and temperature conditions. The diagonal lines represent the temperatures at which each phase begins and ends. So, A_s and A_f mark the beginning and the end of the transformation from a martensite to an austenite phase. On the other hand, M_s and M_f are the temperatures at which the transformation from austenite to martensite begins and ends.

The different cycles (A, B, C and D) marked on the diagram will help detail the different behaviours of shape-memory alloys. Cycle A shows an "intelligent" wire that is heated and passes from deformed martensite to austenite, shortening its length (as Fig. 4.3 illustrates). It is then cooled until it becomes twinned martensite, without any apparent change. The martensite is more elastic, and when subjected to stress it can deform (stretch) until it becomes deformed martensite.

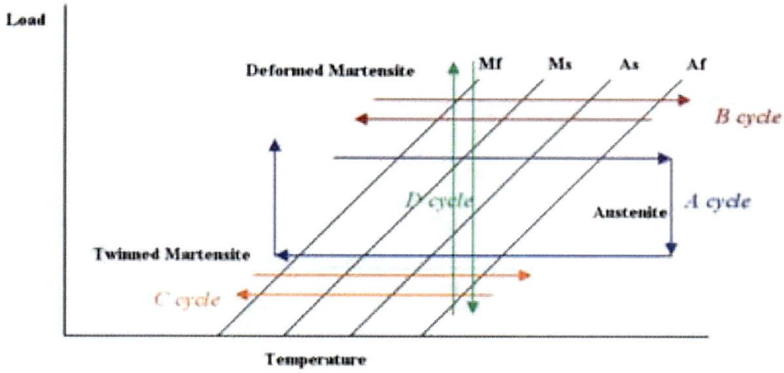

Figure 4.2 Different transformations depending on the relative situation between the temperatures M_f, M_s, A_s, A_f and room temperature and the loads applied.

On the other hand, the B cycle shows the effect of keeping a load applied to an "intelligent" SMA. If the wire is heated, it shortens as it passes from deformed martensite to austenite and when heating stops the wire becomes longer as it is transformed into deformed martensite. In this way, bistable actuators are obtained through thermal effect, which have applications in the development of the medical devices that have been described.

The slope of the lines helps appreciate the effects of thermal hysteresis produced in the course of the cycle. It can be seen how at the end of the DM → A transformation it does not coincide with the beginning of the A → DM transformation. Likewise, the temperature on completion of the A → DM transformation does not coincide with the temperature at the beginning of the DM → A transformation.

The C cycle shows the behaviour of the so-called two-way alloys, in which the stable phase at room temperature is the deformed martensite phase, even without a load. On heating, it becomes austenite and on cooling goes back to deformed martensite. The difference between temperatures at which the phase changes on heating and cooling takes place can also be seen. This explains the hysteresis phenomena observed when these materials act.

The D cycle shows the typical behaviour of a superelastic alloy in which the austenite is the stable phase at room temperature.

Applying a load produces deformed martensite and removing it causes the material to go back to austenite (the remembered shape, as Fig. 4.7 shows). In this way, bistable actuators are obtained through mechanical effect. This has applications in the development of many medical devices, mainly regarding the production of small-size temporary geometries that are ideal for minimally invasive implants, as we have stated previously.

The behaviour of different shape-memory alloys and the temperatures at the beginning and end of the austenite-martensite transformations under different load conditions obviously depends on the alloys used as well as the synthesis and processing conditions.

Described below are the different types of alloys with these properties and the influence of the various alloys on the end properties.

Although the Ni-Ti system, in different proportions is the most widely studied one and the one that has led to the largest number of medical applications, it can sometimes be recommended to incorporate some alloying components to change some specific characteristics, such as the attainable deformations, the start and end temperatures of the transformations and the thermal hysteresis. In order to shorten the hysteresis range, Cu is usually added, whereas to lengthen it, Nb is frequently used. To reduce the transformation temperatures, alloying components such as Fe, Co, Cr or Al are usually added, and to increase them, Hf, Zr, Pt, Au or Pd are used (Schwartz, 2006)

Other Cu (Cu–Al–Ni, Cu–Al–Mn, Cu–Al–Zn)-based alloys also present shape-memory properties (Calvo, *et al.*, 1990) with transitions at different temperatures depending on the composition. This is beneficial for many industrial applications. In the case of Ni–Ti alloys the activation temperatures that are close to body temperature are an additional positive point for their use in medical devices.

It is important to point out that transformation temperatures are particularly sensitive to changes of composition. Variations in a component of less than 1% can cause changes of temperature of over 100 to 150°C. Some of the most popular shape-memory alloys in industry, including data on standard attainable deformations and activation temperatures, are shown in the following Table 4.1.

When selecting a specific alloy for a specific application it is recommended to look closely at the suppliers' characteristics sheets or discuss the problem directly with them in order to obtain more accurate and clear information for design work and prototype production (the data in the various property Tables for each system, either from the references or those included here, are for guidance only).

It is also important to perform one's own tests to validate the behaviour required before proceeding to any *in vivo* test, either with samples, on receipt of the material or *in vitro*, once the SMA actuator has been incorporated into the end device.

Table 4.1 Comparison of Different Industrial Shape-Memory Alloys

Alloy	Composition (% weight)	Ms (°C)	Hysteresis (°C)
Ni-Ti	50–55 Ni; 50–45 Ti	−180 → 110	20–40
Ni-Al	50 Ni; 50 Al	+50 → +550	40–60
Au-Cd	45–50 Au; 55–50 Cd	+25 → +110	15–20
Cu-Zn-Al	5–30 Zn: 5–10 Al	−200 → +100	approx. 10
Cu-Al-Ni	11–15 Al; 3–5 Ni	−150 → +200	30–50
Cu-Al-Be	9–12 Al; 0.3–1 Be	−100 → +100	6–8
Fe-Mn-Si	approx. 62 Fe; 32 Mn; 6 Si	−200 → +200	approx. 100
Fe-Pt	approx. 75 Fe; 25 Pt	−150 → −100	approx. 5–10

4.3.2 Synthesis and Processing

These materials are usually obtained by vacuum alloying, generally by induction or electric arc, and then subjecting the alloy to a heating process, usually extrusion, laminating or forging in order to strengthen the shape, memory properties or superelasticity required. Carrying out the processes in a vacuum helps prevent impurities getting into the core of the material as this could negatively affect the end properties (since the activation temperatures and the hysteresis ranges are very sensitive to any variations in composition), and also helps prevent unwanted or even dangerous oxidations.

After the hot processing it is important to carry out some subsequent cold operations (usually cold laminating and cold extrusion) that help attain the mechanical properties required. This cold operation results in the final geometry and is a determining factor for the surface finish and microstructure obtained. On occasions, the material is subjected to various alternative hot and cold processes in order to favour some specific aspects.

The different thermomechanical processes described in the references enable an optimal training or teaching of the simple shape-memory effect, the dual shape-memory effect or the superelasticity of the material, which usually involves performing different load and unload cycles a considerable number of times.

Manufacturers normally supply these alloys in the form of small diameter wires, tubes or sheets, which makes the geometries of the respective actuators especially simple. The material usually comes already "trained" with a specific, usually very simple, linear, tubular or flat remembered geometry. If a new "remembered" geometry is required the materials can be cold-worked again and given subsequent thermal processing. This should be done as indicated by the suppliers' references and data sheets depending on the alloy used and the effect required.

To obtain more complex actuators, soldered joints, shaped joints or adhesive joints are often used (usually with epoxy-based adhesives), depending on the specific alloy and the properties required for the joint, as well as machining to attain the required final geometry. Laser processes are also used, but taking care to minimise the heat affected zone (HAZ), either by adjusting the designs or the operating conditions or performing subsequent thermal processing to help reduce the differences between the original alloy and the joint area.

Closely related to active polymers, in future chapters we will see how casting in "rapid" moulds produced by rapid tooling technologies is a very convenient and effective process for obtaining complex geometries for more specific actuators. However, casting shape-memory alloys is usually discarded as a processing method, particularly for alloys containing titanium, as the slightest presence of oxygen can dramatically oxidise the titanium.

So, for producing complex geometry shape-memory actuators machining processes are usually used (mainly laser) with the aid of CAM tools (computer aided manufacturing) that help guide the cutting tool in line with the required geometry that is stored in the control computer as a 3D CAD file.

4.3.3 Characterisation and Modelling

When characterising thermoactive shape-memory materials (both alloys and polymers) it should be borne in mind that magnitudes like stress, deformation and temperature are very closely linked, for which reason it is highly positive to use more complex test methods than the usual tensile tests.

It is customary to use heated tensile machines for constant tests under constant stress and variable temperature as well as other combinations that can be PC-controlled, like the MTS series machines from Alliance, to name just one of the many excellent manufacturers.

DSC (digital scanning calorimetry) tests are also useful (as is the case when studying polymer materials) for the precise measurement of the temperatures at which the phase changes take place and the DMTA (dynamic thermomechanical analysis) tests for evaluating additional thermal and mechanical effects. This information is suitable for designing exact behaviour models based on thermodynamic calculation models where the energy released (or absorbed) in the different transformations and transitions plays a predominant role (Besseghini and Villa, 2005).

When evaluating the composition and the phases occurring in a specific alloy, the use of X-ray diffractometry is also very appropriate as previous research has shown.

To begin working with these kinds of materials and to learn about testing, property characterisation and modelling, there are some excellent teaching kits available like those supplied by MUTR, a spin-off of Middlesex University, (www.mutr.co.uk) that is working on teaching and publicity activities linked to a wide range of innovative materials and new technologies.

The following images show the characterisation test results of different actuators manufactured from shape-memory alloys, according to some of the activation cycles described in Sec. 4.3.1. Thus, Fig. 4.3 shows a clear example of phase change due to heating from deformed martensite to austenite, whose transformation is shown schematically in Fig. 4.4.

Figure 4.5 depicts an example of a two-way alloy-based spring actuator whose shape at high temperature (austenite) is open, and whose low temperature shape (deformed martensite) is closed.

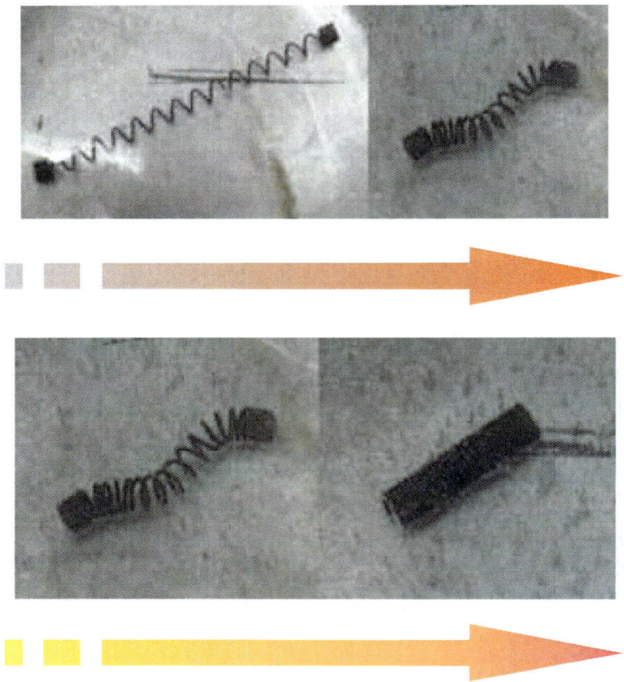

Figure 4.3 Example of shape change in thermal activation of NiTi. Initial stretching to temporary geometry and contraction to original shape. Top photographs: Heating in water from 25°C up to 70°C. Bottom photographs: Heating in water from 70°C up to 85°C.

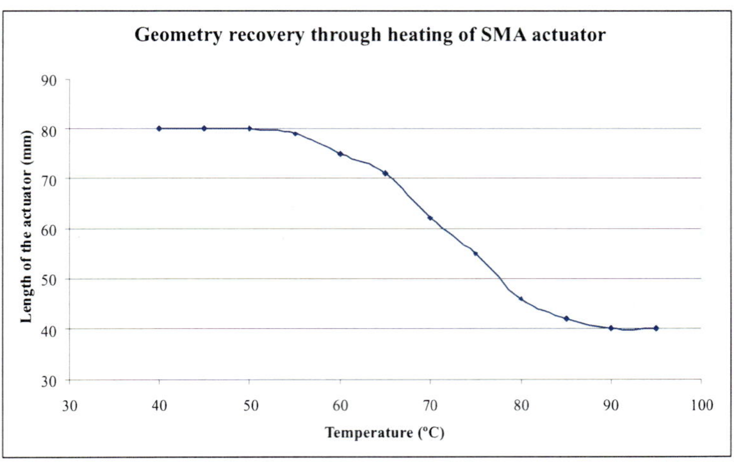

Figure 4.4 Example of geometry recovery in SMA actuator. Transformation from deformed martensite to austenite.

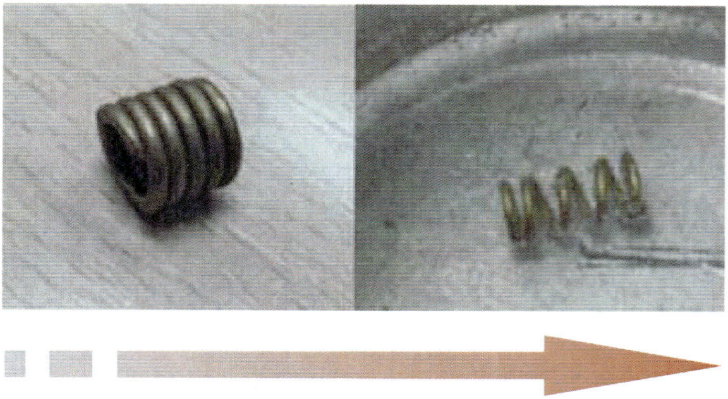

Figure 4.5 Example of shape change through thermal activation of SMA spring. Initial compression to temporary geometry and expansion to original shape. Heating in water from 25°C up to 90°C.

The hysteresis of this kind of actuator is shown in the graph in Fig. 4.6, an effect that needs to be taken into account when designing devices as it can limit some applications, particularly in medical device development where the variations in environmental temperature and the device itself must be very small in order not to damage surrounding tissues.

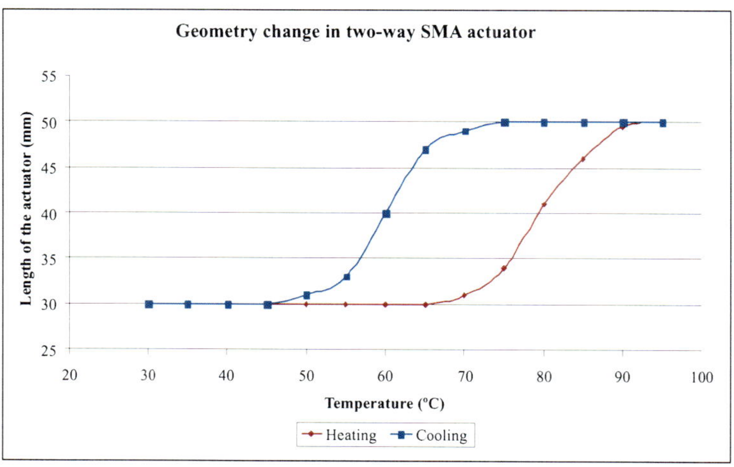

Figure 4.6 Example of behaviour of a "two-way" actuator. Transformation from deformed martensite to austenite through heating and from antenite to martensite through cooling.

Figure 4.7 also shows the behaviour of a superelastic wire that can be bent with amazing ease (up to deformed martensite), and recover its original shape (austenite) when the force is released.

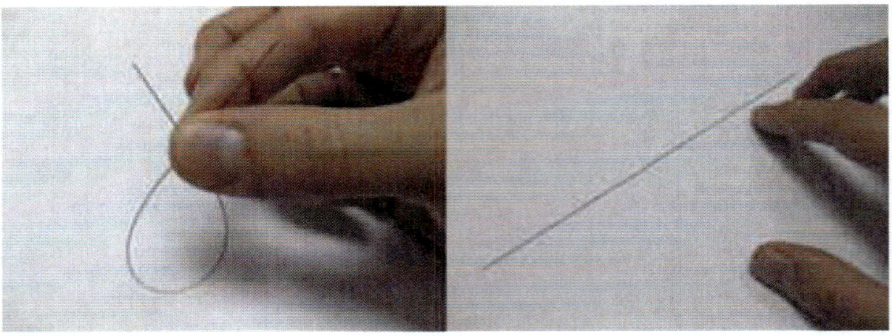

Figure 4.7 Example of superelasticity at room temperature in SMA wire.

It needs emphasising that different activation principles can be applied to make optimal use of the different effects mentioned; particularly shape memory, dual shape memory (two-way) and superelasticity.

Depending on whether we need an easily implantable device (passive after the implant) or a device that can act on surrounding tissues once implanted, we can use some alloys or others depending on the effects required but always bearing in mind the limitations inherent to medical devices due to the considerable heat restrictions and the need to find solutions that will finally be biocompatible.

It is also important to emphasise the need to look carefully at how to normalise and standardise the testing and characterisation of these materials so that the information furnished by suppliers can be better understood and compared. This will aid selecting shape-memory alloys for specific devices without having to be an expert in the matter. Such standardisation would also encourage researchers to publish their findings under more universally acknowledged guidelines and formats, which would also make data taken from scientific publications more meaningful.

Therefore, by taking the outcomes of thorough characterisation and following standardised procedures, more basic models can be achieved that can be used to simulate how different types of shape-memory alloys respond and so assist device design work. Much detailed work has been done in this respect, but it falls outside the scope of this short introduction. However, it should be consulted by researchers who wish to delve more deeply into this field (De la Flor, 2005).

4.3.4 Simulation Tools to Assist Device Development

As previously stated, the use of CAD-CAE-CAM tools for design, calculation and computer-aided manufacturing is on the rise and is contributing to the steady increase in productivity and end quality in every kind of engineering project. These tools are also of major use in the development of active medical devices, as can be seen from the following examples.

The designs and simulations described below were done with the aid of the "Design" and "Advanced Simulation" models of the "NX-6" program from Siemens PLM Software Solutions, whose NX-7 version has just appeared on the market. One of the main advantages of this package is that it can perform finite element simulations directly from the geometries designed by the program itself, eliminating the need to convert formats, which often leads to a lack of accuracy and a loss of information.

On the other hand, the FEM module is linked to a Nastran solver that enhances the end quality of the results. As will be seen throughout the different examples included in the handbook, such quality of results is linked to there being a similarity between the values resulting from the simulations and those attained in the subsequent stages of prototype manufacture and working trials. This does not only depend on implementing the right model for the problem to be dealt with or the right choice of load and boundary conditions, but also on the solver used being able to properly handle the equations given by the model.

The first example shown refers to the design of a balloon-mounted stent for treating coronary conditions. These devices consist of a metallic mesh that is compressed on an expandable balloon or ball. The initial geometry (shown in Fig. 4.8) makes implanting easier as it has a very thin thickness that can be guided with the aid of a catheter to the place where the artery has an accumulation of fat (or some other defect).

When it has got to the right spot the balloon or ball is inflated, which plastically deforms the metallic mesh until it becomes firmly attached to the artery wall, providing the wall with rigidity and returning it to its original cross section. The balloon is then deflated and the catheter withdrawn, while the mesh remains implanted.

The design was made following the standard measurements of these devices, although for the balloon a somewhat simplified shape was adopted. The properties of the materials chosen in the finite-elements model (also included in Fig. 4.8) are those of standard balloon elastomer and those for a similar alloy to that used in actual stents (usually Ni-Ti system- based).

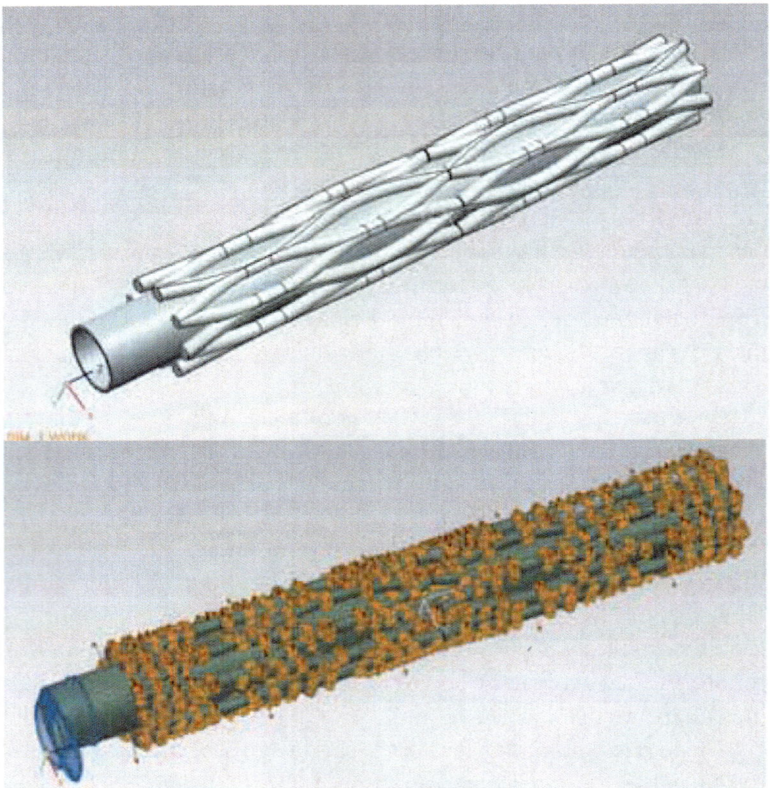

Figure 4.8 CAD design and FEM model of an expandable balloon-mounted stent.

The finite-elements model includes a "contact surface" boundary condition between the balloon and the metallic mesh so that during the deformation of the balloon (in response to the pressure of the air forced inside) the mesh expands along with this balloon to the size finally required. So, in accordance with material properties and device geometry, these simulations help estimate the power pressure needed to achieve the required expansion.

The images in Fig. 4.9 show the results of the displacements and stresses reached in the stent and in the expandable balloon during the activation that implants the stent in the artery. It can be checked that the stress limits of the materials are not being exceeded, in order to prevent any of the device components from breaking.

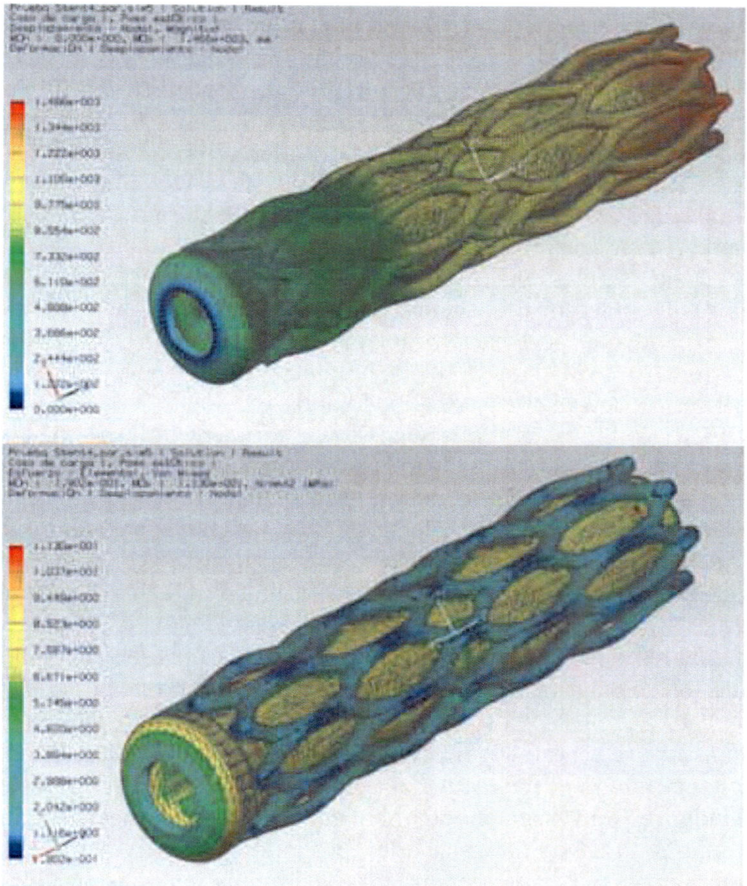

Figure 4.9 Simulation of displacements and stresses attained in the stent and the expandable balloon during the activation that implants the stent in the artery.

In this kind of simulation where the materials (in this case, the metallic mesh) are forced to their point of plastic deformation, it is important to include the material's stress-deformation curve (standard for tensile tests) in order to be able to take account of these effects. It is also advisable to make calculations under the hypothesis of "major deformations", especially when the deformations reached exceed figures that are 5% to 10% of the standard size of the system studied, as in this way, the calculation program updates the system stiffness matrix in each calculation iteration.

The model and the simulations shown can also be completed by including a new tubular part that is representative of the artery on which the metallic mesh is to be implanted, so that any possible mechanical effects of applying overpressure to the balloon, which must be validated with *in vitro* tests (using biological, synthetic or real tissues), can be analysed before carrying out the *in vivo* tests. One example of the effects of prosthetic devices on biological tissues is included in Chapter 5, to complement the design of a shape-memory ring actuator for heart valves.

These simulations of balloon-mounted stent activation can be easily adapted to evaluate the working of Mc Kibben muscles or expandable electroactive polymers. These comprise a hollow elastomeric structure that can be inflated by electrovalve-controlled pneumatic power, as described in Chapter 6 ".

Therefore, these tools, whose use for conventional medical device development has been proven (like the balloon-mounted stents that have been in common use since the 1980s), can also be of great help in analysing the use of active or "intelligent" materials as component parts of more innovative medical devices. These are closely examined in various examples included in the handbook for different families of multifunctional materials.

Analysed below is the behaviour of a stent that is self-expanding due to it being made of shape-memory alloy. The device can be activated when it comes into contact with the body and reaches body temperature. These kinds of devices are replacing the traditional balloon-mounted stents due to their greater simplicity and the avoidance of any problems of the balloon bursting. The ideal situation would be to have FEM calculation programs that included specific components for shape-memory material simulation. However, these kinds of special finite elements are not available in most commercial software but are usually the "individual fruit" of research centres that are devoted to characterising and modelling these materials.

One possible alternative, though, to measure the behaviour of these shape-memory alloys as actuators in a specific device, is to use finite elements with another kind of coupling with which the behaviour of the SMA can be imitated by taking the results of more simple characterisation tests.

Below is an example of a design for a self-expanding stent made of shape-memory alloy. It was modelled and simulated with NX-6, which is not equipped with specific finite elements for simulating these very singular alloys. However, the program does allow the use of elements with thermo-mechanical coupling (where thermal loads induce deformations). The data from SMA manufacturers' characterisation sheets describe deformations of up to 8% during thermoelastic martensite transformation, in heating ranges that vary from around 10 to 20°C.

A metallic material with mechanical properties similar to Nitinol was applied to the FEM model to emulate this effect and with a modified thermal expansion coefficient to achieve this 8% increase in length in the principle directions, since the temperature increases the interval just enough for the martensite transformation to take place. A temperature rise of 20°C was applied to the whole device as a heat load, and as a boundary condition one end of the device was secured to simulate the catheter on which it was mounted during implantation. The results can be seen in the Fig. 4.10.

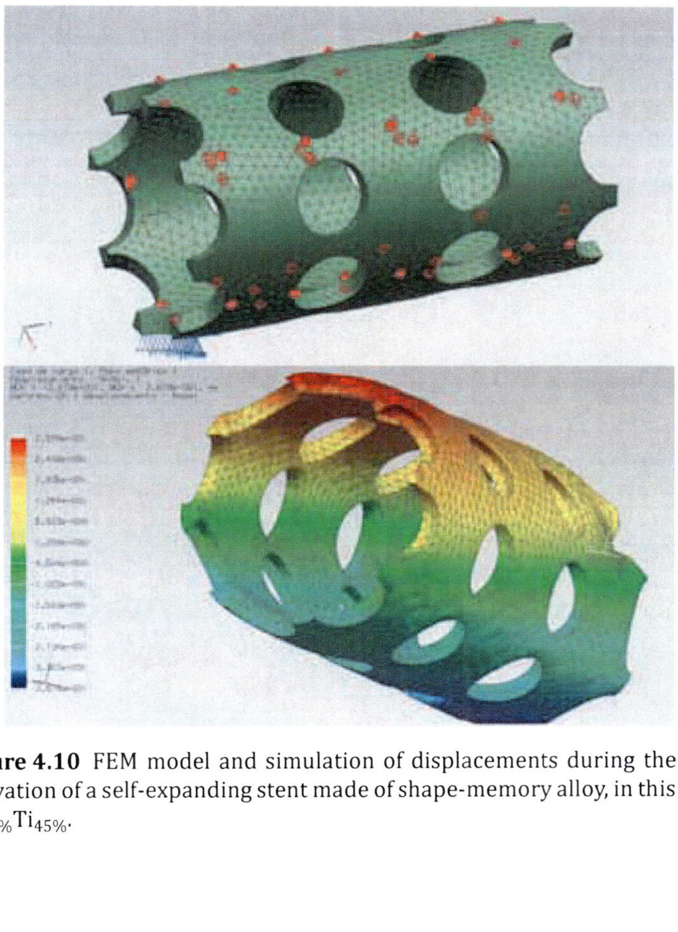

Figure 4.10 FEM model and simulation of displacements during thermal activation of a self-expanding stent made of shape-memory alloy, in this case $Ni_{55\%}Ti_{45\%}$.

One's own simulation codes can of course be used (Lagoudas, 2008), especially if work is being done in advanced materials simulation groups, but approximate approaches, like that shown here can be highly useful while commercial FEM programs are gradually including elements and models that enable these materials to be more accurately simulated.

4.3.5 Integration into Devices: *In vitro* and *in vivo* Tests

The integration of SMA actuators into the core of active devices to boost their activation capabilities, especially during minimally invasive surgical operations, can benefit from the use of structured design methodologies similar to those that can be applied to other active materials.

So, it is usually a good practice to work on a potentially valid preliminary design, like the one in Fig. 4.11 which shows elastic tweezers that can act as an active catheter end. With the aid of FEM calculations and simulations, we can choose the optimal zone for placing an actuator to cause the tweezers to open and evaluate the force that must be exerted by the actuator and the deformations it is required to induce depending on the opening (in this case, either to deposit some kind of solid drug or other object or as an aid to other surgical work).

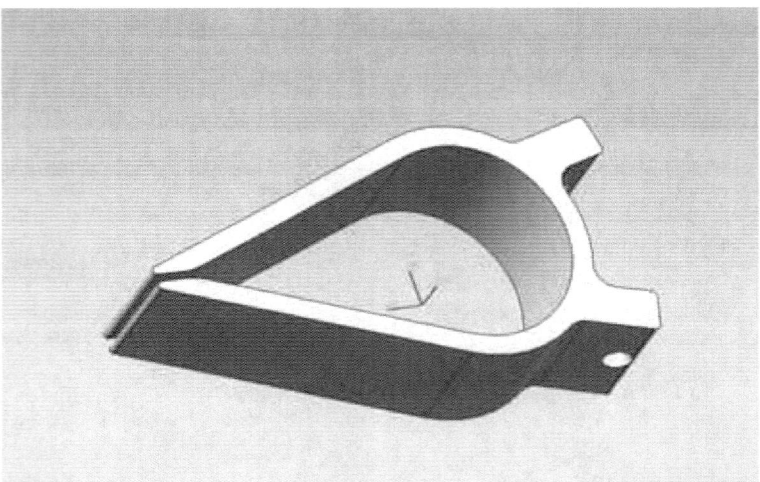

Figure 4.11 CAD design of elastic polymer tweezers as a catheter end.

Figure 4.12 shows a finite-elements model for simulating the displacements achieved in the polymer tweezers after their activation by using a shape-memory alloy "muscle wire" in its lower part. As boundary conditions, one of the tweezers' sides was fixed while on the other side the force applied was gradually increased (as if it were a shape-memory actuator), until the tweezers had opened as required.

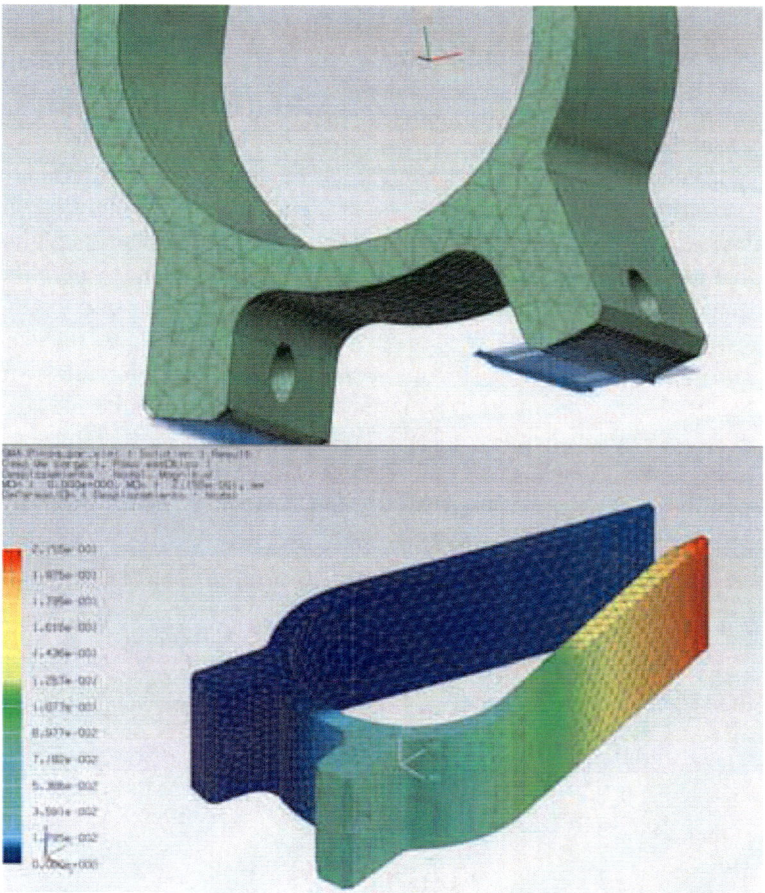

Figure 4.12 FEM model and simulation of displacements obtained in the tweezers after activation using a "muscle wire" with a shape-memory alloy in their lower part.

This lets us analyse if the structure of the tweezers is sufficiently flexible for the target task. Moreover, the values found concerning the force and deformation to be achieved by the actuator are a valuable aid to choosing the type of actuator and it basic dimensions from the shape-memory alloy manufacturer's characterisation sheets or from the data obtained from one's own characterisation tests.

The information obtained can also used to produce redesigns of the "potentially valid" initial design by varying its geometry and dimensions to obtain tweezers with a stronger or softer or more or less flexible grip, as well as for selecting or validating the most suitable material for the tweezers themselves. Other design details, like housings to clamp the actuator can also be verified using these tools, usually by carrying out design iterations which are made much simpler thanks to the CAD-CAE tools and the possibilities for parametric design that these entail.

If calculation and simulation tools are to be complemented, it is essential to use prototypes whose designs can be validated (*in vitro* or *in vivo*). This is causing the so-called "rapid prototyping & manufacturing" technologies to come to the fore in industry, particularly for product development-related research work.

As an example of their use, Fig. 4.13 illustrates several tweezer prototypes manufactured by laser stereolithography technology in which a laser beam photopolymerises an epoxy resin and builds the parts layer by layer, following the CAD design guidelines fed into the computer to guide the movement of the laser. In this case study the manufactured prototypes correspond to the design in Fig. 4.11.

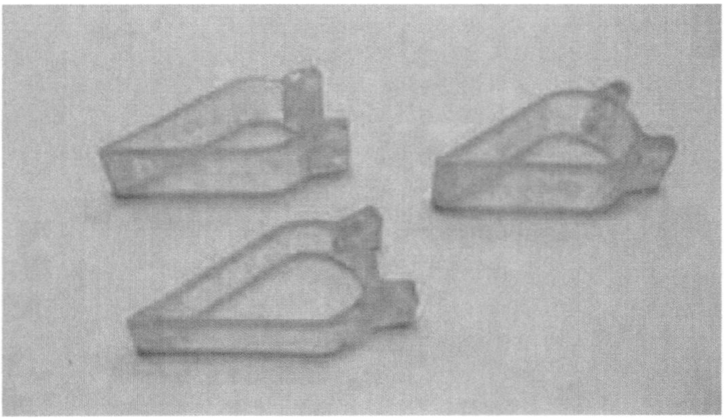

Figure 4.13 Rapid prototypes for active catheter ends.

They are extremely versatile manufacturing technologies for a fast, cheap production (on a prototype scale) of a whole range of complex geometry parts for obtaining not only devices but also casings and accessories for testing the device or for constructing test benches.

When the prototypes have been produced, the shape-memory actuator is integrated into the zone designed for such. In this case, the actuator is fitted in its stretched shape (deformed martensite phase), as the upper image in Fig. 4.14 shows. Heating the actuator, either by sending an electric current through it or using some contact resistance causes the actuator to shorten, enabling its suitability for opening the tweezers to be validated.

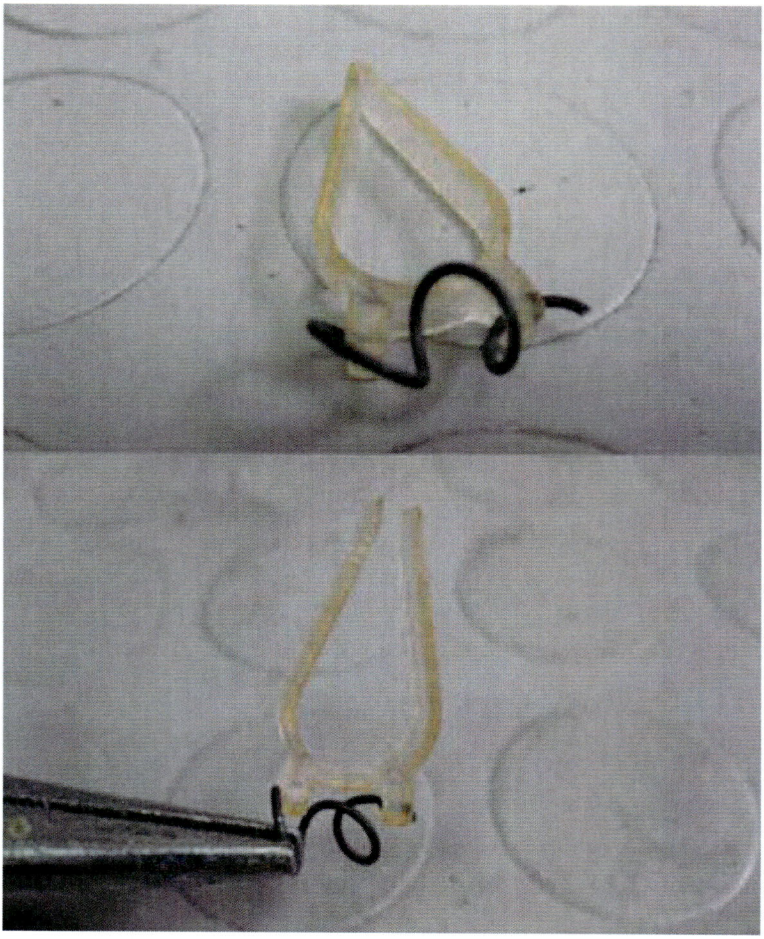

Figure 4.14 Example of tweezer activation as a possible end for an active catheter, activated by a linear shape-memory alloy actuator.

By precisely adjusting the dimensions of the actuator, devices can be obtained that can be activated many times over where heating causes them to go from deformed martensite to austenite. When heating is stopped, the part's own elasticity is again able to induce the passage from austenite to deformed martensite in the actuator, and so it returns to its original condition.

In whichever case, depending on the final purpose of the device, either conventional memory effect or dual memory effect, alloys can be used according to whether activation is required on one or more occasions and according to other design constraints.

To help fix the "muscle wires" and other linear actuators in place, particularly in devices or on more complex test benches, rapid connectors are usually used, like those in Fig. 4.15, that are able to withstand the mechanical stress generated by the actuator during the activation process. They are also of help for performing characterisation tests on raw materials as well as the associated devices.

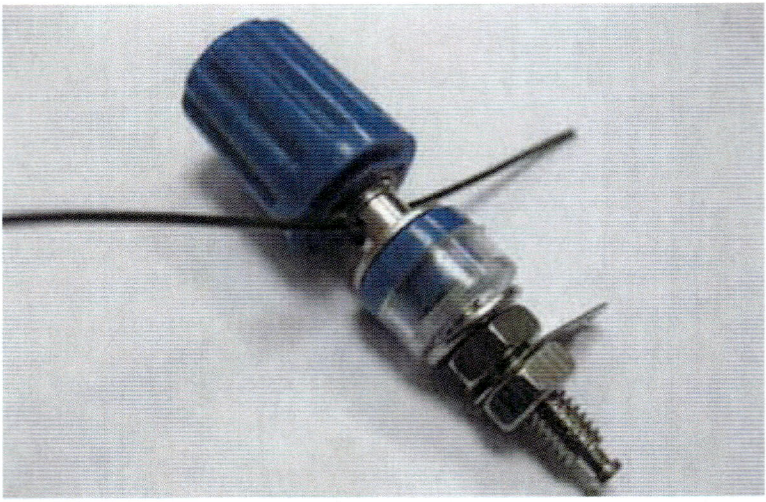

Figure 4.15 Rapid connectors to facilitate the testing and integration of more complex devices.

Before any kind of *in vivo* testing, it must be remembered that the devices must be thoroughly validated *in vivo*. Sometimes, to supplement these tests, particularly when the actuators are intended for use on body tissues, it may be a good idea to use synthetic tissues with mechanical properties similar to those of body tissues (e.g., the "Pericardial Patch" from Edwards Lifesciences), for producing more suitable samples than would probably be obtained by more customary solutions that use offal.

As an additional recommendation for testing, it is important to mention the benefits of using infrared thermography tools to help characterise thermoactive materials (alloys and shape-memory polymers, among others) and for evaluating the effects of their activation on other components of the device into which they are integrated, as well as any possible effects on surrounding tissues.

More detailed examples of the uses of this technique for evaluating the behaviour of active materials is provided in the following Chapter 5, although the conclusions are the same for shape-memory alloy-based devices.

4.4 Main Challenges

4.4.1 Enhancing Mechanical Response

Much research into the use of intelligent materials, such as actuators, is connected with the development of new materials or new actuator designs that can exert greater force and displacements during the activation process, if possible with actuators that gradually consume less (and generally lower applied voltages and current intensities for better end device safety).

In the case of shape-memory alloys, multiple active fibre or "muscle wire" actuators are being developed that help increase the attainable forces, and which in combination with movement multiplying mechanisms also increase the attainable displacements during the activation process (Lafont *et al.*, 2007). With a view to optimising consumption, research still needs to continue into the control mechanisms of activation, as described in the following sub-section.

The behaviour under fatigue of these kinds of actuators should also be examined, regarding the feasibility of performing a large number of activation cycles to compare how the different alloys gradually deteriorate, as a way of assisting the choice of materials for device design. For single activation devices, behaviour under fatigue is not especially relevant. However, for designs required to withstand hundreds or thousands of cycles the effects of the appearance and propagation of cracks associated with the load and unload procedure can be critical in certain compositions. We must once again mention the importance of structuring, and if possible of normalising the characterisation procedures of these alloys in order to obtain more relevant information for design work.

Research is also being conducted to optimising the response speed of these actuators to attempt to attain the frequencies of ceramic actuators. For this purpose, emphasis is being placed on producing smaller actuators (Lai *et al.*, 2004), particularly microactuators based on thin film manufacturing processes (see Chapter 13 for more detailed information on these processes).

In fact, for MEMS (micro-electromechanical systems) applications, SMA thin films, especially Ti-Ni systems, have very desirable properties, like high energy density, the ability to withstand considerable forces, and in principle, good biocompatibility. Recent studies have resulted in the manufacture of prototypes that demonstrate the advantages of what we are proposing as well as their potential for microvalve and micromanipulator design for biomedical applications (Krulevitch *et al.*, 1996; Fu *et al.*, 2009).

A recent alternative with a promising future consists in using ferromagnetic shape-memory alloys that are activated through variations in the magnetic field, more rapid and with less hysteresis than conventional memory alloys. Some of these materials are alloys such as Ni-Mn-Ga, Ni-Fe-Ga and Co-Ni-Ga, although their major limitation is the intensity of the magnetic fields needed to activate them, in addition to which they are sometimes excessively fragile. Research is currently being conducted into improving these aspects due to the advantages to be had from their greater speed (thermal activations are usually slower in comparison with electromagnetic activations) and their lower thermal hysteresis.

However, it is important to compare the potential of these ferromagnetic shape-memory alloys with the potential of other "intelligent" materials like those detailed in the chapter (Chapter 10).

4.4.2 Optimising Activation Power and Control Systems

Shape-memory alloys present some non-linearities and hysteresis effects that make it difficult to implement high level control systems, especially in devices having a large number of actuators. To model these extremely complex systems in real time and manage their control systems, artificial neural networks (ANN) have proved to be effective in some devices and microdevices, provided that these ANN have been properly trained with the results from tests (Ikuo *et al.*, 2003; Asua *et al.*, 2008; Ahola *et al.*, 2009).

As an example of these tools' potential for modelling intelligent materials with marked non-linear behaviour, the handbook includes a detailed example, further on, regarding the modelling of quantum tunnelling composites, in Chapter 15.

As a way of controlling the activation of shape-memory materials the focus is moving towards obtaining step-by-step or progressive activations. Let us consider, for a moment, a step-by-step activation of a shape-memory alloy device with conventional heating by Joule effect by applying a voltage between the ends of the alloy filament or "muscle wire".

When the activation has begun (after exceeding the activation temperature), the only way of "freezing" the structure again is to cut off the power supply, which cools the material and stops the geometry change.

However, after cutting off the power supply when the activation temperature has been exceeded, it does not cool immediately but continues to have a higher temperature than activation temperature for sometime, which on occasions is quite considerable. During this time the geometry continues to change from "temporary geometry" to "permanent geometry", with the result that the permanent shape can be attained before the device temperature cools to below activation temperature.

For a more exact control over the activation of these devices, thermoelectric heating-cooling devices can be used based on the Peltier effect as they have proven their usefulness in various developments that have led to devices that can activate "step-by-step" (Luo *et al.*, 2000; Abadie *et al.*, 2002; Wakasa *et al.*, 2008).

If Peltier cells can be inserted into an active device together with shape-memory alloy actuators and an electronic control, they can be used as a heating/cooling system. This will ensure a more precise control over the geometry changes produced by activating the shape-memory effect by facilitating step-by-step, progressive activations. On enabling current to pass through the Peltier cell, one of the surfaces of this cell and the adjacent SMA actuator increases the temperature (up to actuator activation), while the other surface of the Peltier and the adjacent zone of the device undergo a drop in temperature.

In order to stop the geometry recovery process there are two main alternatives; the first consists in cutting off the current to the Peltier, and the second consists in reversing the direction of the current. This second alternative can stop the recovery process much more quickly than other shape-memory material activation systems, which is one of the advantages of the system described. This control over the current intensity flowing through the different Peltier devices can be achieved by associated control electronics.

The same concept can be used to control geometric changes in any device made of shape-memory material, like shape-memory polymers. These will be examined in Chapter 5. In fact, the main advantages of step-by-step activation by Peltier devices have a more marked effect when dealing with polymers since their low conductivity means activations can be performed in different zones of the device which multiplies the number of attainable geometries.

They are even more suitable for obtaining shape-memory polymer actuators that are able to undergo more than one geometry change (more than one activation), which helps overcome some of the limitations of these polymers as active materials compared to other families (like shape-memory alloys and electroactive polymers) that can intrinsically activate many times (Díaz Lantada *et al.*, 2010).

4.4.3 Enhancing the Synthesis and Manufacturing Processes

Very recent works are focused on a detailed study of the use of new alloying materials to produce increasingly more complex alloys with ever more controllable properties (in the same way that additives have strengthened the use of polymers in every type of application providing greater control over their properties).

Apart from alloying materials, using different thermal processing gives rise to a practically unlimited number of combinations for adjusting the end properties, and contributes a wider range of materials from which to choose depending on the initial requirements of the device under development.

Many centres are conducting research into the production of more affordable alloys to enable researchers and companies to "embark on" trying out rapidly manufactured cheap prototypes that could bring improvements to their products or conventional processes.

However, from a biomedical standpoint, including new alloying materials can turn out to be negative. This is because the different synthetic alloys also need to be studied from a biological standpoint, evaluating their effects on surrounding biological tissues in addition to verifying their long-term stability, in order to prevent rejection by the body and encourage their use.

Regarding the development of more complex geometry medical devices, the gradual advances in laser micromachining are beginning to show results. A wide range of mesh models and self-expanding stents have been developed with geometries that aid the attainable deformations while their enhanced surface finish helps prevent the formation of thrombi. Processes like micro-abrasive blasting are also helping achieve surface finishes that are more suitable for contact with body tissues, which contributes to optimising the final biocompatibility of the devices.

The use of micro waterjet machining is also being promoted. This has already been shown to be a faster technology than other alternatives like EDM (electrical discharge machining) and possesses a similar precision to laser micromachining (MicroManufacturing, 2010).

Micro waterjet machining compared to laser micromachining has the advantage of preventing the appearance of zones affected by heat ("HAZ") which sometimes limits the mechanical properties of the end devices. However, not all alloys are suitable for this kind of waterjet machining as some of the effects of oxidation and corrosion can be reinforced.

4.4.4 Complex Geometries for New Applications

It is also a good idea to continue studying these device manufacturing processes in depth, not only by using machining technologies (subtractive), but also considering the potential to be gained from changing the approach to layer manufacturing technologies and other rapid manufacturing technologies like selective laser sintering or selective laser fusion by which particularly complex geometries could be rapidly produced in combination with CAD-CAM approaches (computer-aided design and manufacturing). Positive results are beginning to appear, especially in the micro-electromechanical system (MEMS) industry (Clare *et al.*, 2007).

These rapid manufacturing approaches have already been used to develop components and parts for complex medical devices activated by SMA muscle wires, as previously described in the chapter as well as by other researches (De Laurentis and Mavroidis, 2002). However, it could be highly positive to produce a whole range of SMA structures to assist specific activations and not have to only rely on intelligent or "muscle wires".

4.4.5 Commercial Materials and Devices

One of the factors restricting the large-scale use of "intelligent" alloys is their high price, especially when compared to the other intelligent materials dealt with in the following chapters (mostly polymers), as both the base materials and the alloying materials are expensive. When manufacturing prototypes for concept validation the difference in price may not be particularly significant, but for mass production it can mark the difference between a product that is viable and one that is not.

Moreover, the geometries usually supplied are very simple (wires, sheets, tubes), which means suppliers sometimes have to be consulted or have to customise these geometries. This increases the final cost of the devices (even when the final actuators do not have excessively complex geometries, such as rings, springs and the like).

A close examination of how to normalise or standardise the synthesis procedures, and the processing, testing and characterisation of these shape-memory alloys is important if more companies are to be encouraged to develop these materials, so that as the supply increases prices will fall. This will lead to these materials having a greater impact on industry.

Work to publicise the properties and applications of these "intelligent" alloys, above all in the area of university teaching could lead to their being used in many fields. For this reason it is important for teaching resources to be prepared on these materials and for these subjects to be gradually included in the syllabuses of the different Science and Technology degrees and even health science-related degrees. For example, some practical handbooks could help understand the properties of SMAs in a few brief sessions (Case *et al.*, 2004; Boohan, 2006)

Setting up collaborative online groups, whose web pages are incorporated into data bases, to connect the demand to solve specific problems concerning the use of shape-memory alloys (or other intelligent materials) with technology supply, could be an excellent tool to promote collaboration among different universities, research centres and companies and achieve a marked expansion of these materials throughout the industry.

4.5 Enhancing Outcomes and Main Conclusions

This chapter has focused on the study of the properties and applications of shape-memory alloys as thermomechanical actuators, specifically oriented towards encouraging their use in the biomedical sector.

In general, these applications correspond to minimally invasive implantable medical devices due to their properties of superelasticity or to active implantable medical devices designed to bring about shape-memory property-based geometry changes in surrounding body tissues or structures (either simple or two-way effect). The two-way effect is also particularly suited to the development of surgical devices that can repeatedly act on specific tissues during an operation.

Aspects linked to the synthesis, processing, characterisation, simulation and integration of these materials into more complex materials have been described in detail, the chapter being completed by highlighting the main lines of action and the possibilities for enhancement, as a way of encouraging the use of these alloys in industry.

One of the priorities for study is different research into the development of new formulas with enhanced thermomechanical response for producing more complex geometries capable of being integrated even into micro-electro-mechanical systems. Another priority is to obtain information from thorough characterisation tests for more accurate modelling of these materials.

In order to develop active implantable medical devices, it is again important to point out the need to form teams comprising engineers who are experts in many branches of technology, professionals from the different areas of health sciences and the fortunately increasing number of biomedical engineers. Their members should work in close collaboration to encourage communication among the experts in the teams and lead these kinds of research projects.

If this is to become a reality, it is important to gradually include shape-memory alloy-related matters (and "intelligent" materials in general) in the various Master's and PhD programs, in faculties of technology and biotechnology as well as in faculties of medicine and biology.

Additional information can be found in the following list of references as well as in the websites of the different suppliers included in the annexes of the handbook. We hope this will be of use to researchers interested in these materials and their applications, as well as for establishing future contacts among research centres.

References

Abadie, J.; Chaillet N.; Lexcellent, C. "An integrated shape memory alloy micro-actuator controlled by thermoelectric effect". Sensors and Actuators A: Physical A, 99(3), 297–303, 2002.

Ahola, J.; Makkonnen, T.; Nevala, K.; *et al.* "Model-based control of SMA actuators with a recurrent neural network in the shape control of an airfoil". Solid State Phenomena (147–149), Mechatronic Systems and Materials, 278–283, 2009.

Asua, E.; Etxebarria, V.; García-Arribas, A. "Neural network-based micropositioning control of smart shape memory alloy actuators". Engineering Applications of Artificial Intelligence, 21(5), 796–804, 2008.

Asao, F.; Suzumori, K.; Kanda, T.; Yamada, Y. "Development of an SMA micro valve (2nd report : Design, prototype and characteristics evaluation)". Nippon Robotto Gakkai Gakujutsu Koenkai Yokoshu, 23, 1–15, 2005.

Besseghini, S.; Villa, E. "DMA characterization of shape memory alloys". E-MRS Fall Meeting, 2005.

Boohan, R..- "Innovations in practical work: Metals and smart alloys". Gatsby Science Enhancement Programme, 2006.

Buehler, W.J.; Wiley, R.C. "Nitinols are nonmagnetic, corrosion resistant, hardeneable". Materials in Design – Engineering, 82–93, February, 1962.

Calvo, F.; Gómez de Salazar, J.M.; Ureña, A.; Méndez, F.J.; Guilemany, J.M. "Aleaciones base Cu (Cu-Al-Mn y Cu-Al-Zn), con efecto de memoria de forma soldadas por difusión: Estudio microestructural de la unión". XVI Reunión bienal de la SEME. Universidad de Cádiz. Cadiz, 1990.

Case, L.; Kreiner, Z.; Redmond, J.; Trease, B. "Shape memory alloy shape training tutorial - A teacher's guide to teaching shape memory alloy shape training". ME559 - Smart Materials and Structures, University of Michigan, 2004.

Clare, A.T.; Chalker, P.R.; Davies, S.; Sutcliffe, C.J.; Tsopanos, S. "Selective laser melting of high aspect ratio 3D nickel-titanium structures two way trained for MEMS applications". International Journal of Mechanics and Materials in Design, 4(2), 181–187, 2007.

De la Flor, S. "Simulación numérica y correlación experimental de las propiedades mecánicas en las aleaciones con memoria de forma". PhD Thesis, Universidad Politécnica de Cataluña, 2005.

De la Flor López, S.; Urbina Pons, C.; Ferrando Piera, F. "Caracterización de la evolución de las transformaciones de fase con el tratamiento térmico previo en aleaciones NiTi con memoria de forma". 9° Congreso Iberoamericano de Ingeniería Mecánica, Las Palmas de Gran Canaria, 2009.

De Laurentis, K.J.; Mavroidis C. "Mechanical design of a shape memory alloy actuated prosthetic hand". Technology and Health Care 10, 91–106, 2002.

Díaz Lantada, A.; Lafont Morgado, P.; Muñoz García, J.; *et al.*- "". Smart Materials and Structures, 19(5), 055022, 2010.

Duerig, T.; Pelton, A.; Stöckel, D..- "Superelastic nitinol for medical devices". Medical Plastics and Biomaterials Magazine. March, 30–43, 1997.

Fu, Y.Q.; Luo, J.K.; Flewitt, A.J.; *et al.* "Thin film shape memory alloys and microactuators". International Journal of Computational Materials Science and Surface Engineering, 2(3-4), 208–256, 2009.

Gad-el-Hak, M. "The MEMS Handbook". CRC Press. Florida, 2002.

Greninger, A.B.; Mooradian, V.G. "Strain transformation in meta stable copper-zinc and beta copper-tin alloys". AIME Transactions, 138, 337–368, 1938.

Ha, C.D.; Calagnano, D. "Amplatzer Vascular Plug to occlude the internal iliac arteries in patients undergoing aortoiliac aneurysm repair". Journal of Vascular Surgery, 42(6), 1058–1062, 2005.

Ikuo, S.; Masaru, F.; Hirohsi, Y.; Yukinori, K. "Control of SMA-net robot using distributed chaotic neural networks". Nippon Robotto Gakkai Gakujutsu Koenkai Yokoshu, 21, 3B26, 2003.

Krulevitch, P.; Lee, A.P.; Ramsey, P.B.; *et al.* "Thin film shape memory alloy microactuators". Journal of Microelectromechanical Systems, 5(4), 270–282, 1996.

Lafont Morgado, P.; Díaz Lantada, A. "Self-contained mechanical window -opening and -closing system". World Intellectual Property Organization (WIPO) - International Bureau - Patent Document WO/2008/071818 - PCT/ES2007/000720.

Lagoudas, D. "Shape memory alloys: Modelling and engineering applications". Springer Science + Business Media LLC, New York, 2008.

Lai, B.K.; Kahn, H.; Phillips, S.M.; Heuer, A.H. "A comparison of PZT-based and TiNi shape memory alloy-based MEMS microactuators". 306(1), 221–226, 2004.

Luo, Y.; Takagi, T.; Yamada, M. "A shape memory alloy actuator using Peltier modules and R-Phase transition". Journal of Intelligent Material Systems and Structures, 11 (7), 503–511, 2000.

Mineta, T.; Mitsui, T.; Watanabe, Y.; *et al.* "An active guide wire with shape memory alloy bending actuator fabricated by room temperature process". Sensors and Actuators A: Physical, 97, 632–637, 2002.

Olander, A. "An electrochemical investigation on solid cadmium-gold alloys". Journal of the American Chemical Society, 56, 3819–3833, 1932.

Rapp, B. "Nitinol for stents". Materials Today, May, 13–13, 2004.

Sánchez Pérez-Grueso, J. "De la hemivectebrectomía en escoliosis infantil a la aplicación de materiales con memoria". Noticias Médicas, Noticias del Siglo XXI, XLIV, n 3951, 20–24, 2010.

Schwartz, M. "New Materials, Processes, and Methods Technology". CRC Press, Taylor & Francis Group, 2006.

Smith, W.; Sung, G.; Saver, J.; *et al.* "Mechanical thrombectomy for acute ischemic stroke: Final results of the Multi MERCI Trial". Stroke, 39(4), 1205–1212, 2008.

Suzumori, K.; Asao, F.; Kanda, T.; Yamada, Y. "Development of a three-directions switching micro valve with SMA-wire (1st Report: Design, prototype and characteristics evaluation)". Electromagnetics Symposium Proceedings, 17, 351–352, 2005.

Wakasa, Y.; Watanabe, Y.; Yoshida, A.; Tanaka, T.; Ashaki, T. "Response improvement of shape memory alloy actuators with Peltier elements". Proceedings of 2008 IEEE International Conference on Mechatronics and Automation, 587–592, 2008.

Chapter 5

Shape-Memory Polymers for Biodevices

Andrés Díaz Lantada and Pilar Lafont Morgado
Mechanical Engineering Department, E.T.S.I. Industriales,
Universidad Politécnica de Madrid, c/ José Gutiérrez Abascal 2,
28006 Madrid, Spain
adiaz@etsii.upm.es, plafont@etsii.upm.es

5.1 Brief Introduction to Shape-Memory Polymers

Shape-memory polymers (SMPs), as previously introduced (see Chapter 3), are materials that show a mechanical response to external stimuli, usually to changes of temperature. When these materials are heated above their "activation" temperature, there is a radical change from rigid polymer to an elastic state that will allow deformations of up to 400%.

If the material is cooled down after manipulation it retains the shape imposed; the said structure is "frozen" and returns to a rigid but "non-equilibrium" state. If the material is again heated above its vitreous transition temperature (T_{act}) or "activation temperature" it recovers its initial non-deformed state.

The cycle can be repeated numerous times without degrading the polymer and most suppliers can formulate different materials with activation temperatures ranging from −30 to 260°C, depending on the application required.

Of all the polymers developed that show shape-memory properties, those most worthy of mention due to their applicability

---

Handbook of Active Materials for Medical Devices: Advances and Applications
Edited by Andrés Díaz Lantada

www.panstanford.com

are epoxy resins, polyurethane resins, cross-linked polyethylene, styrene-butadiene copolymers and other formulations (Lendlein and Kelch, 2002; Liu *et al.*, 2007).

They are therefore active materials with thermomechanical coupling and a high capability for recovery from deformation (much greater than that shown by shape-memory metal alloys), which when combined with their lower density and cost has favoured the appearance of numerous applications.

Their properties allow applications for manufacturing sensing devices or actuators, especially for the aeronautics, automobile and medical industry, some of which have already been explained.

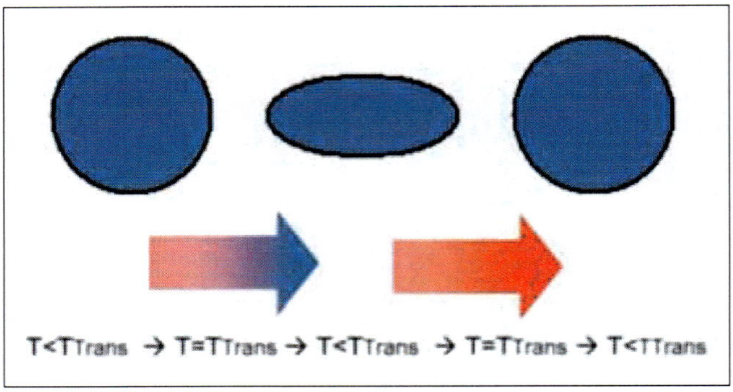

Figure 5.1 Training process of the shape-memory effect and recovery of permanent form.

5.2 Potential for Biodevices

5.2.1 Some Advantages

As polymers, SMPs can be easily conformed into different complex shapes and their properties designed or adapted to specific applications and can also be integrated with other microelectromechanical sensors ("MEMS") to produce "intelligent" bioactuators and biodevices.

Compared to other shape-memory alloys used in numerous medical devices, SMPs show a far greater capability for changing their geometry during activation.

They are also much cheaper to synthesise and their large scale mass production costs are reduced by using technologies such as injection moulding or extrusion. At the same time the use of additives provides possibilities of tailoring their properties for improving and adapting their properties to final applications.

All this makes them very versatile active materials with a high potential for industry, provided they overcome some of the limitations set out in the following sections.

5.2.2 Proposed Devices

Shape-memory polymers can be used as active materials in medical devices for two main proposals or for solving two different kinds of medical problems:

- **Minimally invasive surgery.** Capabilities of SMPs can be employed for obtaining reduced temporary forms that make surgical tasks or implantation easier. In this way a device can be conduced, in its temporary small size, to the desired location, where activation leads to the implantable geometry.
- **Actuation on tissues and organs.** SMP-based devices can be implanted with a temporary form and, after the patient has recovered from intervention or when the related pathology has reached a limit level, activation can be promoted in order to modify the surrounding tissue geometry.

Below are explained some specific proposals for developing medical devices based on the use of shape-memory polymers, most of which have undergone *in vitro* laboratory testing. After undergoing *in vitro* testing and meeting the requirements for official approval, in some cases their commercialisation is subject to their attaining the goals described at the end of this chapter.

Self-expanding stents

Like the one designed by Boston Scientific Corporation using the polymer from CRG Industries known as "Veriflex" under its trade-name, to treat the problems arising when the arteries become narrow or obstructed and also for removing obstructions from other "tube-shaped" body parts, like the ureter and the bronchial tubes. The stent is inserted in its temporary form (reduced) and the body's own heat causes it to dilate and become attached to the artery.

They may be used to replace stents based on shape-memory alloys such as Nitinol, once the appropriate biocompatibility studies have been carried out. Developments of self-expanding stents have also been carried out by using injected polyurethane (Wache *et al.*, 2003).

Intelligent sutures

Like those developed at the Forschungszentrum in Karlsruhe by Lendlein's team and at the M.I.T. by Langer's team, which have a temporary linear shape and a permanent shape in the form of a knot, with the change in geometry being activated by the body's own temperature. They have numerous applications in minimally invasive surgery and, as they are biodegradable, they have additional advantages over the use of textile sutures and metal clips (Lendlein *et al.*, 2002, 2005).

Thrombectomy devices

With the recent discovery that the thermal effect of shape memory can be activated by a laser, part of whose energy is absorbed by the polymer, devices with special geometries have been proposed for removing clots (Wilson *et al.*, 2006). The polymer is shaped in a spiral mould and then heated and stretched to give it its temporary shape. When the laser light passes through the polymer, the shape-memory effect is activated and the device recovers its spiral shape trapping the clot which can then be removed.

Active catheters

By using shape-memory polymers for the distal point of catheters together with a subsequent activation of the memory effect by laser light or body heat, different drugs and antitumoural agents can be released. The presence of an active catheter point can also help reach zones that are difficult to access in minimally invasive surgery tasks (Yakacki, 2007).

Drug release devices

If biodegradable shape-memory polymers are used for implantable medical devices, drug supply reservoirs can be incorporated into the device itself. After implant, the polymer begins to be absorbed by the organism and the drug is released. Patents have been taken out in this respect for self-expanding coronary stents or intra-urethral stents (Boston Scientific Co. and Surmodics Inc.). The possibility of obtaining temporary geometries with micro-reservoirs for drug storage has also been studied. The drugs would then be released on activation of the shape-memory effect by body heat (Gall, 2004).

Active annuloplasty rings

Aimed at obtaining a progressive postoperative treatment of mitral insufficiency, they are based on the use of a polymeric ring with heating resistances distributed around the inside to activate the shape-memory effect by Joule effect. This activation must allow the cross-section of the mitral ring to be gradually reduced and, therefore, the mitral insufficiency improved.

Figure 5.2 shows a schematic design of such a device. Prototypes of these rings, with different geometries and materials, have been developed and tested *in vitro* in pig's hearts (Díaz Lantada *et al.*, 2008).

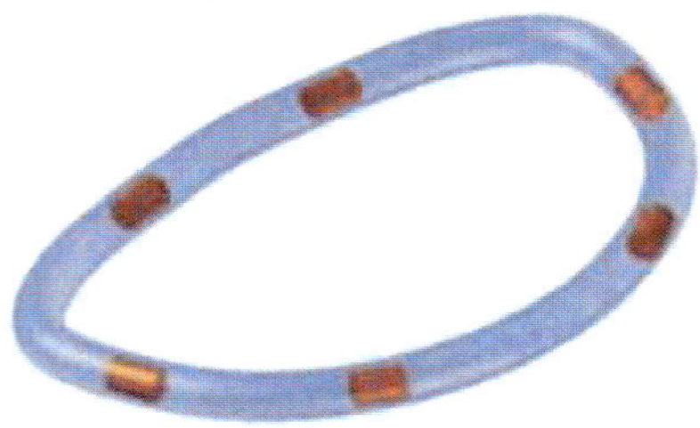

Figure 5.2 Active annuloplasty ring design. SMP with internal heating resistances (Biodevices, 2008).

The different devices explained will provide considerable therapeutic benefits compared to conventional devices, due to their capability to act inside the body, thanks to the use of shape-memory polymers.

5.3 Current Capabilities and Recent Advances

Set out below are some of the main advances achieved in the last decade concerning shape-memory polymers and the technologies associated with their use.

5.3.1 Synthesis

In recent years particular emphasis has been placed on obtaining new formulations of polymers with shape-memory properties, by changing the proportions of monomers, including additives, and inducing multiple crosslinkings and working on previously known formulations whose shape-memory properties have been boosted (Lendlein and Kelch, 2002; Liu *et al.*, 2007).

Different prestigious laboratories have conducted exhaustive work on synthesis and subsequent classification in accordance with the molecular structure of the polymers.

The recent synthesis of polymers capable of remembering two pre-set shapes using two programming stages (triple shape effect) has brought new possibilities for future medical devices, due to the fact that two postoperative changes can be made to the geometry (Bellin *et al.*, 2006).

In spite of the numerous formulations for the shape-memory polymers that have been synthesised recently, the main problems for obtaining commercial biodevices based on these materials are the small number of commercial formulations, the toxicity of many of them and problems regarding thermomechanical properties, as will be explained in the following sections.

5.3.2 Characterisation

During the last decade most experiments linked to characterising different shape-memory polymer properties have attempted to compare the thermomechanical response of different formulations.

At the Langley Research Centre the results of tests using thermomechanical analysers (TMA) has been compared with those obtained by using differential scan calorimeters (DSC) to obtain precisely the vitreous transition temperature in shape-memory polymers (Volk and Whitley, 2005). This research also explains deformation recovery tests conducted by heating under constant deformation and under constant stress, for which MTS Alliance RT1 traction machines and a heating chamber are used (Fig. 5.3).

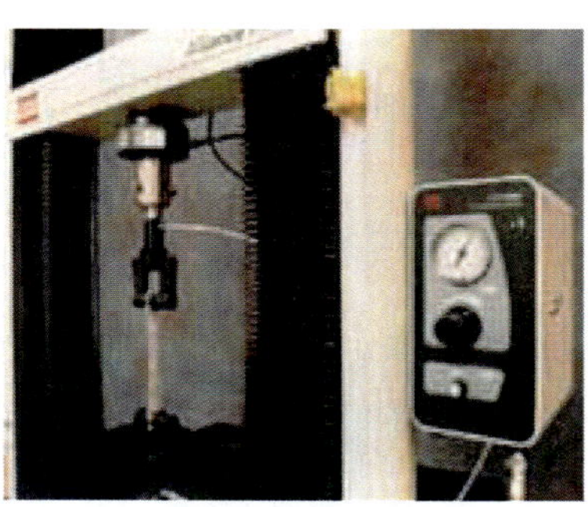

Figure 5.3 MTS Alliance machine for characterization (www.mts.com).

Three-point bending tests have also been used in heated chambers in order to evaluate the geometric recovery capability of these materials subjected to different levels of stress and deformation (Lendlein and Kelch, 2002; Tobushi, 2008).

Dynamic mechanical analyses (DMTA) have been used basically to evaluate the elastic modulus of these materials according to temperature. They also enable the vitreous transition temperatures of the materials to be found (Mather and Liu, 2002; Liu *et al.*, 2003, 2006; Huang and Lee, 2006; Yakacki, 2007). This is a supplementary technique to DSC tests (which are usually used for the study of vitreous transitions, polymorphisms, crystallisations and aging).

All these experiments and many others have helped to provide basic knowledge concerning the thermomechanical behaviour of these materials, which is decisive for future developments.

5.3.3 Processing Technologies

CAD-CAE-CAM tools

Computer-aided design, calculation and manufacturing technologies (CAD-CAE-CAM) have become essential tools for product development. They let 3D geometries and alternative designs to be obtained rapidly. Calculations on stress, deformations, ergonomics, dynamic response and other aspects including material comparison and design can also be performed for design optimization.

The numerous benefits of these technologies for developing conventional products can also be applied to the development of shape-memory polymer–based medical devices.

The recent use of programs such as MIMICS for processing medical image technique files (TAC, NMR and others) enables biodevices to be made-to-measure (Harrysson *et al.*, 2007). With these programs three-dimensional geometries of parts of the human body can be obtained and exported to other CAD-CAE-CAM programs to perform the customised designs and obtain prototypes by using techniques that we will now explain. They also contribute new possibilities to the design of customised implants that benefit from the use of SMPs.

Rapid prototyping technologies

A new set of manufacturing techniques and technologies has appeared in the last two decades to address market requirements in an ever more customised way and to provide support for research work where physical models are needed for tests and trials that are optimised in terms of time and cost.

These new techniques and technologies go by the name of *Rapid Prototyping and Manufacturing* technologies. They are usually based on manufacturing processes that add layers or "Layer Manufacturing Technologies" (like "laser stereography" or selective laser sintering) in rapid shape-copying processes, or in manufacturing processes through the elimination of materials (such as in high speed numerical control machining). The different technologies available allow prototypes to be obtained in a wide range of metallic, ceramic or polymeric materials with remarkable precision (Freitag and Wohlers, 2003; Kuklick, 2006; Lafont *et al.* 2007, 2008).

These technologies enable physical parts to be had in a short time (hours or a few days) directly from the designs made with the help of computer-aided design, calculation and manufacturing programs or "CAD-CAE-CAM technologies". They greatly help to optimise design iterations, contribute to early error detection and speed up production start-up.

In spite of their being rapidly incorporated into product development methodologies, these new types of technologies are still in their initial stages of development. Up to present, with most of these new technologies, prototypes or short production runs of a part can be obtained, in most cases by using materials different from those of the end product but very often with mechanical properties that are inferior to those of the end parts.

The direction in which these new techniques have been heading in recent years is towards obtaining the end parts as quickly and precisely as possible. To this end, one possibility is material innovation that will enable this goal to be attained by applying these new techniques.

Another option, linked to the former, is to develop new techniques and technologies that did not exist until now. A third way is to seek out new combinations from among existing manufacturing techniques and technologies, including traditional ones like rapid prototyping, in order to make the best use of the benefits provided by each of them.

To this end, the technologies set out below under the name of "rapid tooling technologies" are particularly relevant and intimately linked to the mentioned "rapid prototyping technologies".

So-called "rapid tooling" technologies seek to manufacture different tools (moulds, matrices, inserts, tools and equipment) with these new manufacturing and rapid prototyping techniques in combination with other traditional manufacturing techniques.

The manufactured tools can then be used with traditional production techniques (injection, extrusion, moulding) and obtain the required parts in end materials or with properties much more in line with those stipulated in the design. Depending on the life of the parts and the number that can be produced using the tools resulting from these technologies, "rapid tooling" processes are usually classified as

- **Soft tooling.** A term referring to equipment built from materials that are easy to process, shape and machine (silicones, resins, aluminium, wood and others) designed for short production runs and with a very limited useful life.
- **Hard tooling.** A term referring to equipment designed for large production runs or mass production end runs. This equipment is usually obtained in very hard and highly resistant materials that usually have a very long useful life.
- **Bridge tooling.** This term refers to the techniques for obtaining a finite production run of "prototype parts" from equipment that has a longer life than those considered as "soft tooling", but less than those classified as "hard tooling". They are normally obtained by rapid prototyping technologies.

Choice basically depends on the size of production required, on the available budget and the schedule to be met. "Soft tooling" technologies provide a faster, cheaper solution for customers requiring short production runs (around 50–100 parts). However, for longer runs, bridge or hard tooling technologies must be resorted to, but these also require greater investment.

Of all the possible applications of these technologies for supporting research work, one that is becoming particularly relevant is their use in obtaining demonstration prototypes, both conceptual and end ones, using active or "intelligent" materials.

This sub-chapter helps to explain some of the remarkable benefits of using different "rapid prototyping" and "rapid tooling" technologies as a supplement to tasks for developing devices based on shape-memory polymers.

The applications and examples explained are linked to the development of medical devices, as this is the sector that can mostly benefit from the use of these active materials. However the conclusions of this study, on the advantages of using rapid prototyping technologies as a support for development works related to devices based on active materials, may be extended to other fields of science and engineering.

Normal procedure for the following examples includes the following stages:

- Designing the 3D geometry of the device and obtaining a CAD file.
- Manufacturing the first prototype by rapid prototyping, in our case using Laser Stereolithography, which enables the use of epoxy resin as a material with acceptable shape-memory properties.
- Using the initial prototype for obtaining a rapid mould through "form coping". In our examples we use a "soft tooling" process for manufacturing silicone moulds.
- Manufacturing a second prototype by vacuum casting within the silicone mould, in which materials with enhanced shape-memory properties, such as polyurethane resins, can be used.

Figure 5.4 shows how a pincer-shaped end for an active catheter can be obtained from its 3D geometry in a CAD file. An SLA-350 machine was used to polymerise a 3D Systems epoxy resin sold under the trade name of Accura® 60.

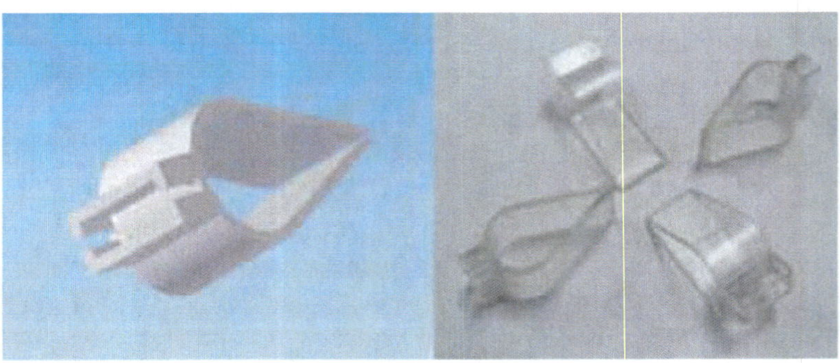

Figure 5.4 Active pincer design and prototypes (Biodevices, 2009).

The pincer can be forced to open by hot deformation during the shape-memory "training" process ($T_{training} = T_g + 20°C$), so as to obtain the "temporary form". Afterwards by reheating it with the help of an incorporated heating resistance, the pincer closes, as Figs. 5.5 and 5.6 show schematically. This ability can be used in similar devices, with different geometries and materials, to extract foreign bodies and in minimally invasive surgery. The help of infrared "IR" thermography, as in Fig. 5.6, proves to be valuable for measuring temperatures within the devices and for controlling when activation temperature is reached (Díaz Lantada, 2009).

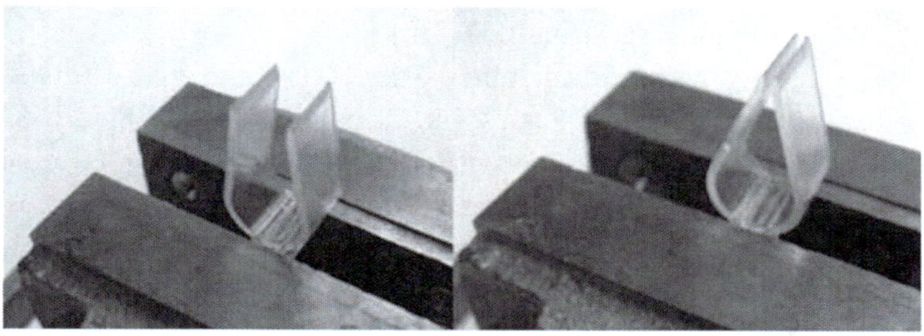

Figure 5.5 Geometric activation in an epoxy resin pincer.

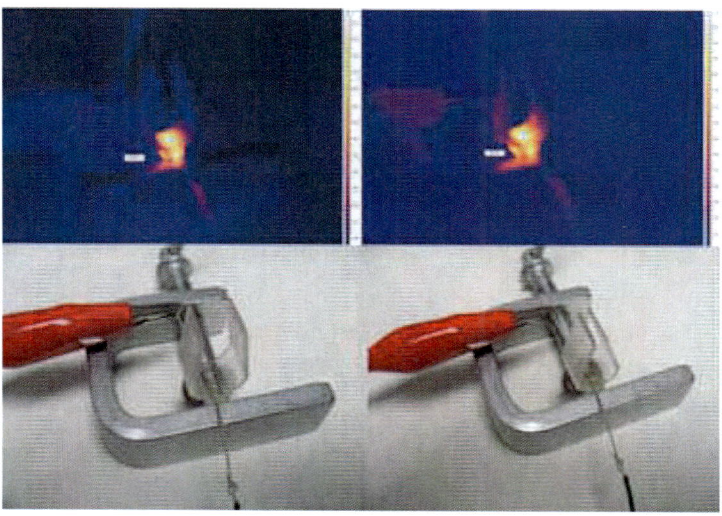

Figure 5.6 Illustrative example: active catheter extreme for minimally invasive surgery. Temporary form before activation (left) and permanent form recovery through heating above T_g for activation and closing (right) (Biodevices, 2009).

The parts obtained by laser stereolithography are especially useful for dimensional and visual checks, as well as for carrying out conceptual tests of the shape-memory effect. They can be used as models for obtaining silicone moulds that can then be used for obtaining replicas in other polymers that are more resistant and more suited to functional tests and which, in addition, possess more remarkable shape-memory properties than the epoxy resin of the first models. Vacuum casting procedure allows different types of dual component resins to be used, with modifiable properties, and the resulting prototypes reproduce the mould cavities with great precision (roughnesses around 50 μm).

Using silicone mould vacuum casting, polyurethane prototypes with shape-memory properties can also be obtained. Figure 5.7 shows a ring device obtained with this technology using a type of polyurethane sold under the trade name MCP Iberia 3115, whose capability for recovering shape through heating is also remarkable. Similar devices can be used to change soft tissue geometry (annuloplasty, sutures, cerclages and others).

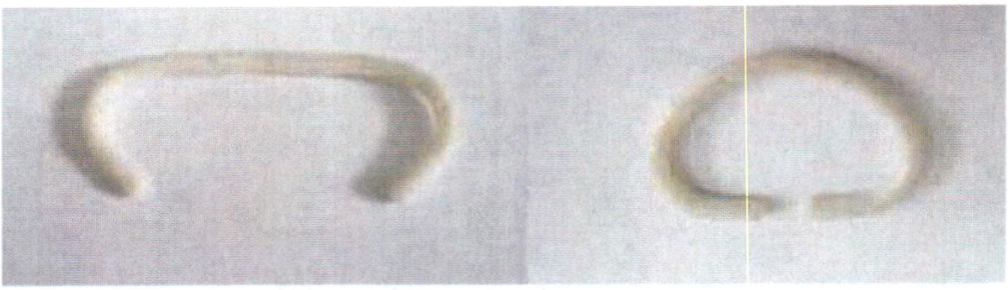

Figure 5.7 PU geometric cerclage activation (Biodevices, 2009).

The main benefits of these technologies are that designs and functionalities can be efficiently compared and that the associated products can be more rapidly developed. Being able to apply these technologies to SMP-based devices is of great importance to their becoming widespread in industry. Additional examples of conceptual trials linked to different medical devices manufactured using SMPs with shape-memory properties are shown in Fig. 5.8.

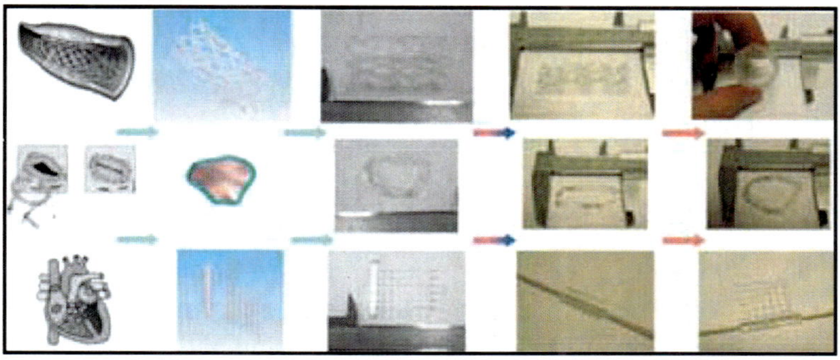

Figure 5.8 Global processes of design, manufacture, shape-memory training and recovery for different biodevices.
(A) Expandable stent for thoracic aortic diseases. (B) Annuloplasty ring for mitral valve insufficiency.
(C) Net-shaped structure for septal defects. All of them, due to reduced temporal shape, allow minimally invasive surgery approaches.

Microfabrication

Being able to use microfabrication technologies with SMPs provides a new line of use for these materials inside the medical device industry, particularly in lab-on-a-chip and controlled drug delivery systems.

Typical devices for these applications require surface channels and microtextures with micrometric geometries that can be obtained in polymeric materials by using technologies such as "hot-embossing", "micro injection moulding" or "LIGA".

To be precise, by applying hot-embossing to SMPs, surface microtextures and microreservoirs with temporary geometry can be achieved (Gall, 2004).

The possible use of physical or chemical vapour deposition technologies, combined with the ability to produce protective masks by applying UV photolithography, enables surface embossing to be performed on very different materials (metals, alloys and ceramics) using shape-memory polymers as substrate (Paumier *et al.*, 2008).

Thus, by making connection microtracks, these can be used to send an order to certain parts of a device to activate a geometric change by heating an adjacent resistance. In some cases, the connection track itself can be used as a heating element if its cross section is sufficiently small and its electrical resistance, therefore, high enough.

This ability to manufacture by layers and combine different materials enormously strengthens the capability to integrate certain SMP-based active parts into complex systems (such as implantable medical devices).

5.3.4 Shape-Memory Effect Training

The shape-memory effect training process is usually conducted through heat deformation of the device manufactured in SMP and subsequent cooling to maintain the deformation, thereby obtaining the temporary shape.

To increase the length of the temporary shaped devices traction machines with heated chambers are used. To produce temporary surface marking hot compression moulding presses are used.

Recently, the use of cone-shaped counter shapes, for hot-embossing, has been proposed to obtain SMP ring devices with a temporarily enlarged diameter (Díaz Lantada, Lafont Morgado, 2008, Fig. 5.9).

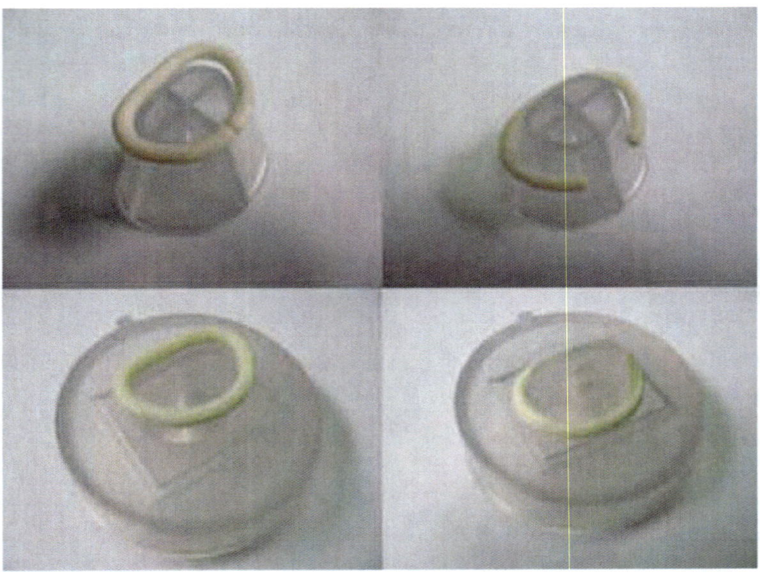

Figure 5.9 Different rapid prototyped counter shapes for obtaining temporary forms of medical bands (above) and rings (below), through hot pressing and cooling down.

5.3.5 Activation

Another aspect where most progress has been made is the activation of the memory effect by various methods, described in detail below, especially

Joule effect activation

Based on distributing heating resistances at the core of the polymer where the passing of an electric current generates the necessary heat. The Fig. 5.10 shows as example a prototype of annuloplasty ring aimed at inducing geometrical changes to the mitral valve, thus treating mitral insufficiency. The trial was controlled using a thermographic "IR" camera marketed under the name of "Flyr Systems Thermacam E300" with its accompanying "Thermacam Reporter 8.0" analytical software, which enables the thermographs taken to be more exactly and thoroughly analysed.

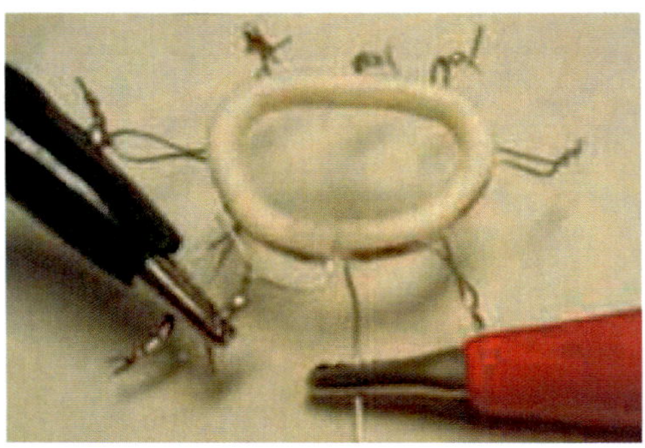

Figure 5.10 Shape-memory polymer polyurethane annuloplasty rings. Concept prototype with eight heating resistances (SMART 09, 2009).

As heating system for the annuloplasty rings a set of six or eight resistances was used with a nominal value of 4.7 Ω fed in series using a variable voltage transformer. The tests performed with a prototype including eight heating resistances are shown in Fig. 5.11 (Díaz Lantada, SMART09, 2009).

The image shows that, for reaching the glass transition temperature throughout the ring (around 70°C), certain zones need to reach up to 91°C, which means that heating is not homogeneous (and neither are the mechanical properties of the whole implant during the activation process).

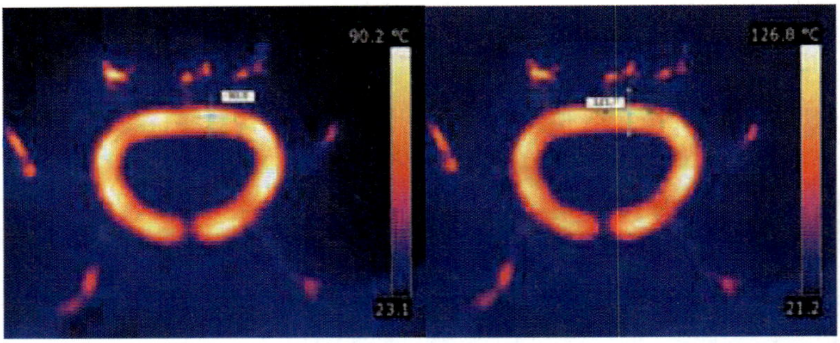

Figure 5.11 Thermograms associated with the ring heating tests (eight resistances).
0.63 W (left image) and 0.97 (right image) heating power per resistance (SMART 09, 2009).

On the other hand, the size of the resistances and their need to be integrated into the body of the polymer brings about a reduction in the mechanical resistance of these implants.

It has to be noted that final device should be manufactured using SMPs with lower activation temperature, so as not to damage surrounding tissues. The polyurethane resin MCP3115 of these trials has been used as a proof of concept, due to its processing facilities.

One of the main problems of using Joule effect activation lies in the fact that distributing punctual heating resistances among the polymer leads usually to a decrease of mechanical resistance and to important temperature differences along the structure during activation.

We propose and explain below some improvements for SMP activation, obtained by substituting punctual heating resistances by silver-cloth thread knitted along the structure and used as single Joule effect heating element.

Figure 5.12 shows the prototype of a net-shaped SMP structure with the heating silver-cloth thread already knitted to it. Such thread was acquired from the MUTR (www.mutr.co.uk) special materials facilities.

For manufacturing the prototypes (directly from 3D CAD files with part geometry) a laser stereolithography "SLA-350" machine was used to polymerise a 3D system epoxy resin sold under the trade name of Accura® 60.

A total electrical resistance of around 40 Ω was measured between ends of the thread, which proves to be an acceptable value for activating the whole structure through Joule effect heating, as Figs. 5.14 and 5.15 show. Such values can be modified and adjusted for final implantable or surgical devices, so as to comply with the acceptable values described in regulations related to maximal current through such devices.

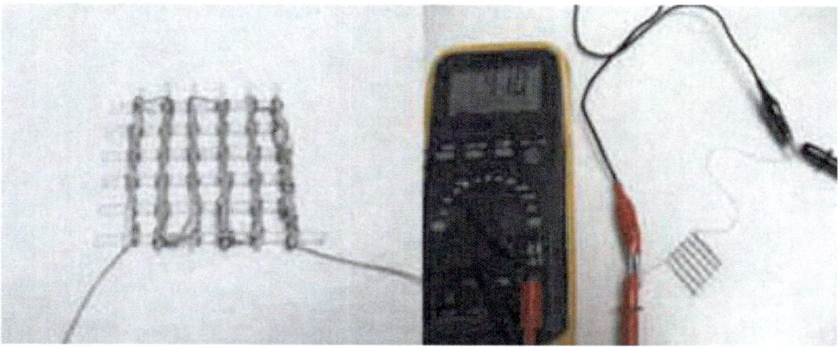

Figure 5.12 Prototype of net-shaped SMP structure with knitted silver-cloth thread for improving activation (resistance around 40 Ω).

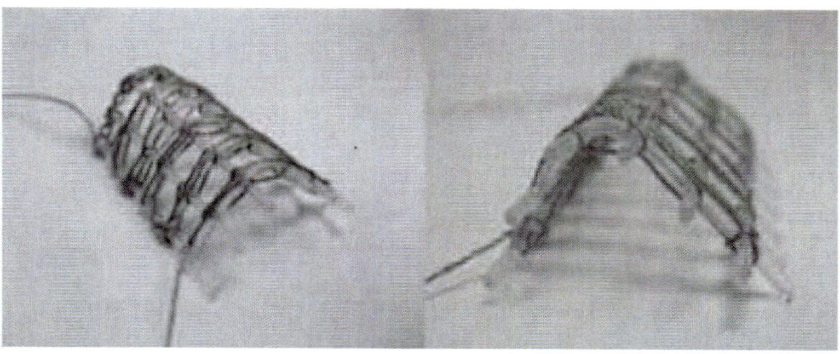

Figure 5.13 Temporary form obtained through heating, imposing a 90° deformation between extremes of the structure and finally cooling down.

Once the prototypes had been fabricated and the heating thread knitted to the structure, temporary form was obtained through heating, imposing deformation and cooling down.

Afterwards the *in vitro* heating was carried out to verify the designed heating system and to show that it is possible to exceed the glass transition temperature that leads to the "shape-memory effect" being activated (Fig. 5.14).

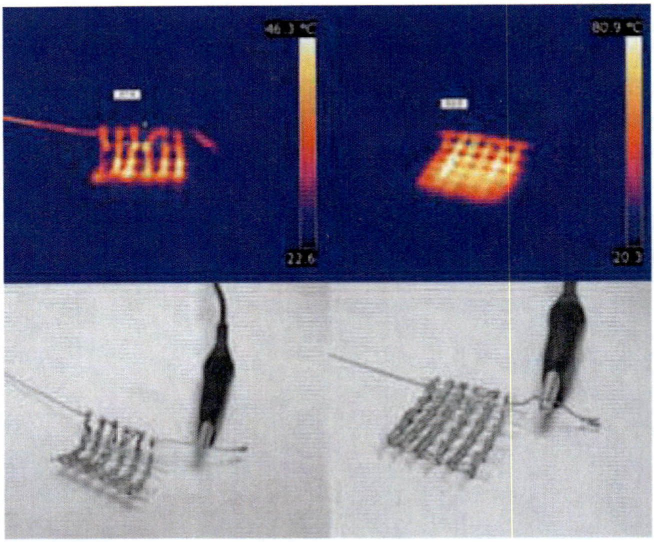

Figure 5.14 Recovery process by distributed heating (view using IR thermography). Total recovery time, 20 s. Images taken every 5 s (image corresponding to $t = 0$ not included).

The activation process, including temperature evolution and shape recovery, is represented in Fig. 5.15. Similar graphics help to appreciate the response of active devices and to compare performance and time response between different possible active materials used as transducers.

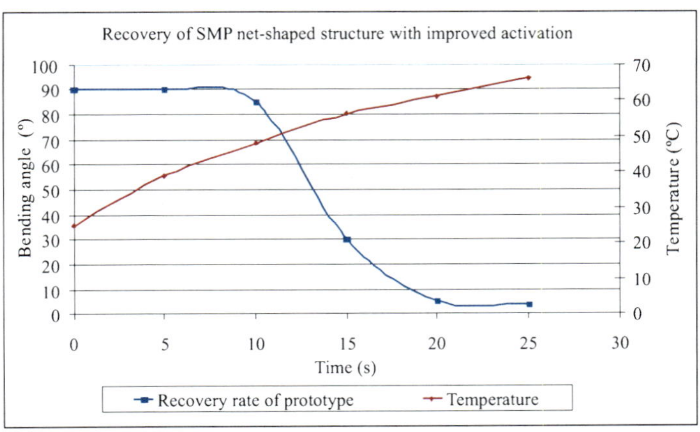

Figure 5.15 Recovery process, from 90° to 0°, as a function of time and temperature.

SMP-based devices normally have a response time ranging from around 5 to 20 s, which limits some applications, where other actuators such as piezoceramics, piezopolymers or shape-memory alloys can be used, because of their faster activation.

A remarkable fact for the trials is to verify that no short-circuit appears during the training process, which limits the attainable size reduction. When bending and reducing structure size during training, the heating thread can separate slightly from the polymeric material and promote such problems.

Therefore, fixing points for the heating element have to be taken into account from the design stage, so as to improve final performance. Another option consists of totally embedding the heating element within the polymeric structure during manufacture, but that leads to additional problems when casting or injecting into the moulds.

Light or laser activation

This kind of activation is based on projecting a laser through a shape-memory material with a similar absorption frequency to that of the laser used, which produces heating (Lendlein and Kelch, 2005; Wilson *et al.*, 2006).

Such activation usually reduces the problems related to designing an internal heating system with additional elements within the polymeric structure. On the other hand, "light/laser activation" is normally limited to tubular/linear structures, which limits applications.

Magnetic activation

This sort of activation is based on heating by induction of magnetic or metallic microparticles, distributed at the core of the polymer while it is being conformed to its shape (Buckley *et al.*, 2006). However, the biocompatibility of the associated devices needs to be further optimised.

New prototypes of annuloplasty rings have been manufactured using composite shape-memory polymers with electrically conductive materials within to test the feasibility of a heating system based on the effect explained. To do this, a copper thread rolled into a coil and soldered at its ends was used, as the Fig. 5.16 shows.

This thread was fitted into the cavities of some silicone moulds that reproduced the geometry of the rings to be manufactured by vacuum casting (see Fig. 5.16).

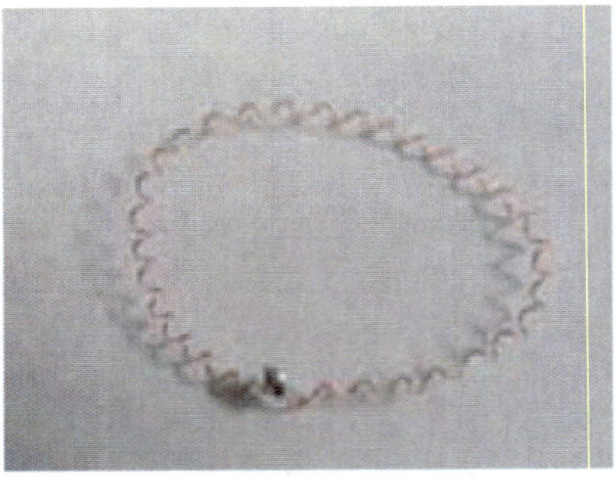

Figure 5.16 Obtaining the coil for homogeneous induction heating from a rolled and soldered copper thread.

After performing the vacuum casting using MCP Iberia 3115 polyurethane resin and subsequent oven ageing at 70°C for 25 min, the prototype annuloplasty rings can be extracted. The different geometries are similar to some of the most common rings in industry. The circular-shaped ring was obtained to show the validity of the process, not only for annuloplasty rings designed for treating mitral insufficiency, but also for other tubular-shaped body structures that can benefit from the use of changeable-geometry prosthetic rings (Fig. 5.18.

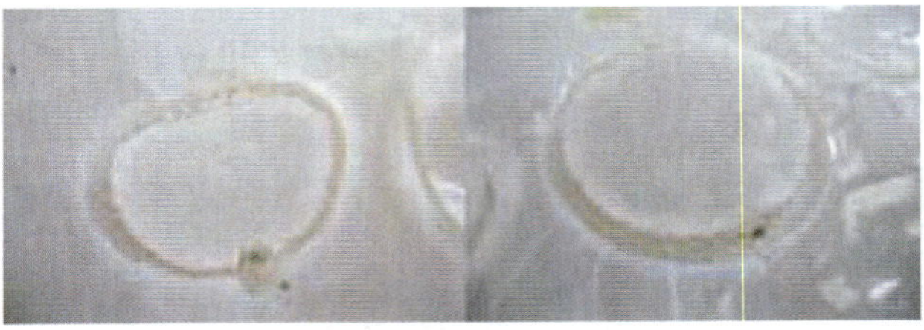

Figure 5.17 Copper coils for induction placed in various silicone mould cavities to obtain the rings by vacuum casting.

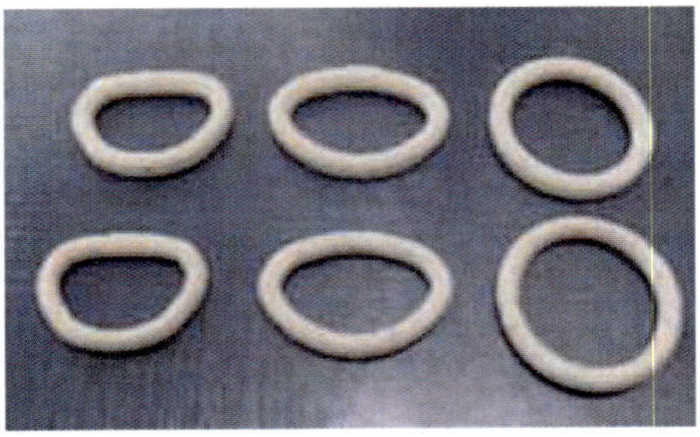

Figure 5.18 Shape-memory polymer rings with coils for induction heating.

After manufacturing the prototypes, they were subjected to induction heating to verify it was possible to activate the shape-memory effect based on this heating principle. For this, a set of copper coils was used connected to a power supply of variable intensity and frequency. It was thus possible to control the intensity of the magnetic field and study how the heating of the rings responded to this intensity. The tests were performed with a 10 kHz frequency power supply with the intensity of the magnetic field being made to vary around the annuloplasty rings from 20×10^{-4} to $80 \cdot\times 10^{-4}$ T so as to be able to evaluate the temperature that could be reached according to the intensity of the magnetic field, as can be seen in the images and graphs of Figs. 5.19 and 5.20, respectively.

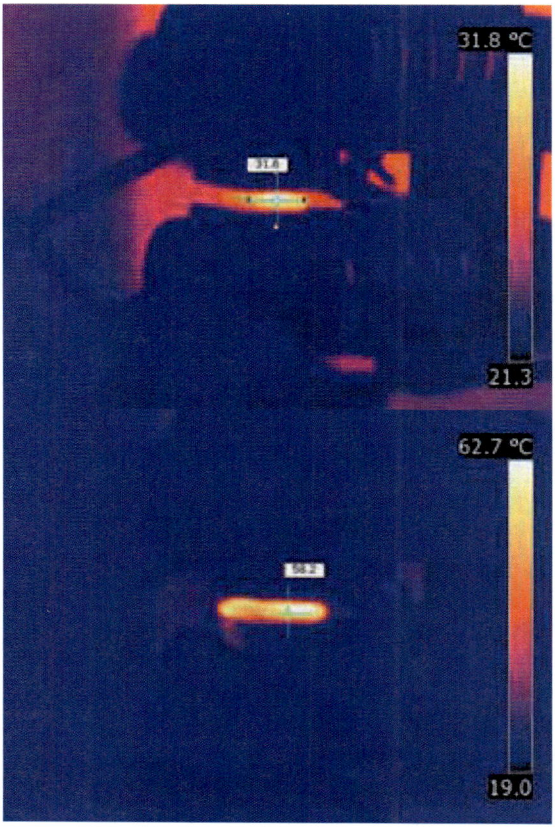

Figure 5.19 Thermograms of the induction heating tests performed. Annuloplasty SMP ring prototypes at the centre of a variable magnetic field.

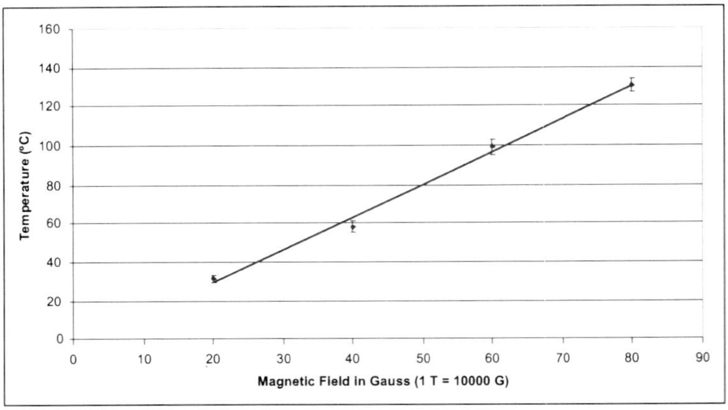

Figure 5.20 Temperature reached according to the intensity of the magnetic field applied (10 kHz frequency power supply).

The results show a remarkable homogeneous heating of the annuloplasty rings (especially when compared with previous trials using Joule effect as exposed in Fig. 5.21) and the possibility of going beyond the glass transition temperature, T_g, so as to activate the "shape-memory effect" and the subsequent geometrical changes.

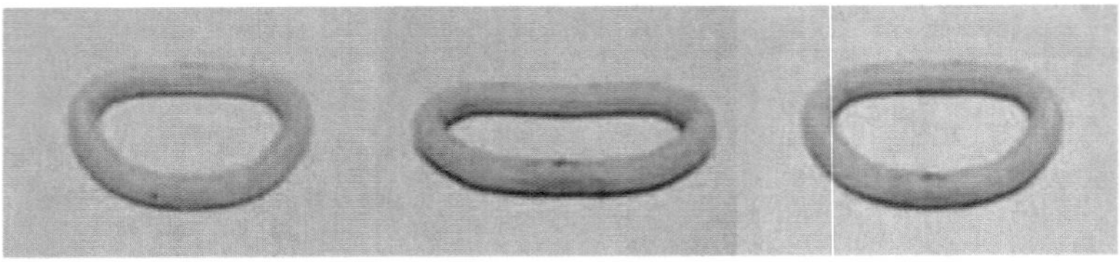

Figure 5.21 Shape-memory effect training process: Hot deformation of the original ring (left image) to obtain the temporary shape (centre image) and recovery of the original geometry through subsequent heating (right image).

In fact, the high deformations that can be attained (and subsequently recovered) not only let us contemplate possible postoperative activations for a progressive treatment of mitral insufficiency but also new percutaneous approaches for minimally invasive annuloplasty ring implants (and other therapeutic devices).

Direct activation of conductive polymers

Recent studies (Leng *et al.*, 2007; Liu *et al.*, 2009) have clearly shown the possibility of obtaining shape-memory polymers that are electrical conductors, based on the incorporation of micro and nanoparticles (NPs) into the body of the polymer during its processing.

Prototypes can then be produced that can be heated by directly applying a voltage between different zones or ends of the device in question. However, the inclusion of these particles can negatively affect the body's response to the polymers used and their thermomechanical properties.

Among the particles studied for obtaining conductive SMPs, good results have been found when using carbon nanotubes (specially multi-walled nanotubes "MWNT"), pure metals and metal oxide nanopowders (some manufactures, such as NanoAmor.Inc., have already started selling such dispersions in polymeric solvents).

The importance of using NPs lies in the fact that percolation threshold decreases together with particle size for obtaining conductive polymers and, with a lower proportion of particles needed, negative influence on other polymer properties is reduced.

Support technologies for activation

Progress in the field of wireless communications means that devices can now be remotely activated, which is promoting the appearance of new active implantable biodevices.

Such wireless applications have already been studied for other medical devices with sensing capabilities (González Bris and Díaz Lantada, 2009), based not only on the use of Bluetooth/radio links, but also on the use of magnetic near-field communications for energizing semi-passive devices inside the body from an outer source.

Similar proposals can be adapted for actuators based on the use of SMPs, always taking into account the regulations on admissible frequencies and other requirements for communication links surrounding the human body.

Such possibilities can promote the development of several multipurpose medical applications, especially when combining sensing capabilities (for detecting some kind of pathology or problem) together with actuation means (for solving the problem).

5.3.6. Combining Simulations and *in vitro* Trials

Development of medical devices entails important responsibilities; as such devices must be tested in living systems (*in vivo* testing) in order to be approved by the competent administrations for clinical pre-market trials.

A medical device designer must always be mindful that working with live animals is a privilege that should never be taken lightly, due to moral and economic reasons (Kuklick, 2006). Therefore, recent theories related to the development of medical devices have highlighted the great importance of exhaustive *in vitro* trials, which together with results from simulations can provide enough confidence for undertaking *in vivo* studies.

The important advances in CAD-CAE-CAM programs, which now provide great capabilities for carrying out precise FEM simulations, have proven to be valuable for optimising developments and reducing the number of design iterations. Several researchers have concentrated on modelling living tissue behaviour and contact phenomena between implants and tissues, which gives additional information for developing SMP-based devices.

At the same time, the possibilities for *in vitro* testing have greatly increased in the last decade, as several companies are focussing their efforts at developing artificial tissues (normally based on hidrogels and other polymeric materials), which are slowly substituting the traditional *in vitro* trials on explanted tissues. Sometimes an artificial circulatory system is needed, which can be supplied by several independent model makers (mainly plastic or glass models that work well enough).

As an application example, Fig. 5.22 shows FEM. simulations of SMP annuloplasty ring actuating for promoting mitral valve cross-section reduction, together with results from *in vitro* testing with a SMP prototype implanted on porcine mitral valve; showing temporary shape and recovery of permanent shape, before and after activation (Díaz Lantada, 2009, Munich World Congress on Biophysics and Biomedical Engineering).

5.3.7 Commercial Formulations

The promising applications of these materials, particularly in the field of medicine, together with a growing industrial demand, has led to departments dedicated to the synthesis of shape-memory polymers being set up in large companies and the appearance of some spin-off. The major companies are:

- Mitsubishi Heavy Industries Ltd.
- DIAPLEX
- mNemoscience GmbH

- CRG Industries LLC

Most of these recently set up companies and departments offer "a la carte" design work and prototyping applications using SMP. They also commercialise their developments, both synthesised materials and products based on those materials.

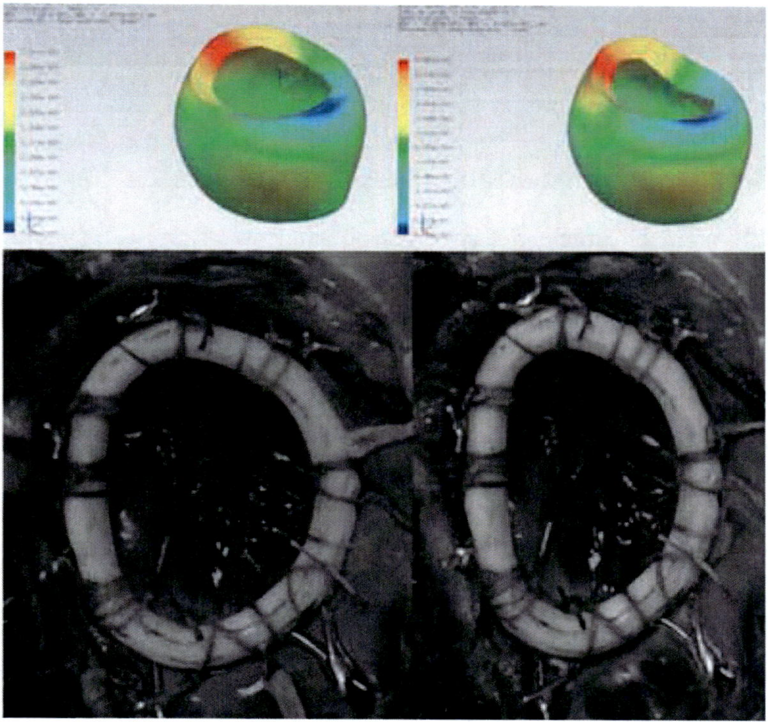

Figure 5.22 Above: FEM simulations of SMP ring actuating for mitral valve cross-section reduction (in order to treat mitral insufficiency). Below: *In vitro* trial of SMP ring, implanted on porcine mitral valve, actuating for mitral valve cross-section reduction.

Recently, some SMPs are beginning to be commercialized in "pellets" form for part manufacture by injection moulding, therefore aiming at the promotion of mass fabrication of related devices. Until now most parts with shape-memory properties should be obtained after mixing of two components (a base one and a polymerizing agent) and subsequent curing inside a mould. The process of obtaining an SMP-based part following such process uses to last from 30 min to 36 h. Because of this, availability of SMPs for injection moulding will be of great importance for promoting its application and reducing the price of end devices.

5.4 Main Challenges

This section deals with the main fields where more in-depth study is particularly important, in order to facilitate the industrial expansion of shape-memory polymers as an integral part of active implantable medical devices or as surgical tools.

5.4.1 Thermomechanical Response

Unfortunately, the shape-memory polymer materials developed up to now only let forces of approximately 3 MPa be withstood during activation, which is insufficient for certain medical applications intended for use as actuators, especially when wishing to change the geometries of biological tissues.

Enhancing the activation forces requires greater understanding of the basic physical-chemical principles of these phenomena. To this end, computational models can be used that help apply a combined knowledge of materials science, thermodynamics, mechanics and heat transmission (Conti *et al.*, 2007).

5.4.2 Modelling and Simulation

Using the data obtained from the characterization tests (of materials and specific applications) behaviour models can be obtained that facilitate the development of new applications with the same material or similar applications with other polymers.

The possibility of combining models developed ad hoc, together with the multivariable simulations that allow finite element calculation programs, will help to simplify the design of training systems and the heat activation of SMP-based devices. Some promising results of using stress-strain simulations for estimating device's capabilities have already been explained (see sub-section 5.3.6). The Figs. 5.23 and 5.24 show additional examples, now linked to the design of the activation system of several devices, in which thermal simulations are used to estimate the *in vitro* trial results also included (Díaz Lantada, SMART09, 2009).

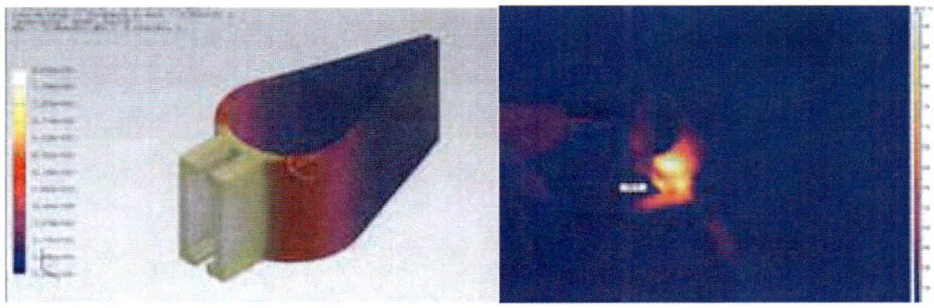

Figure 5.23 Simulation and trial of heating system for activating a SMP-based pincer with applications as active catheter extreme (SMART 09, 2009).

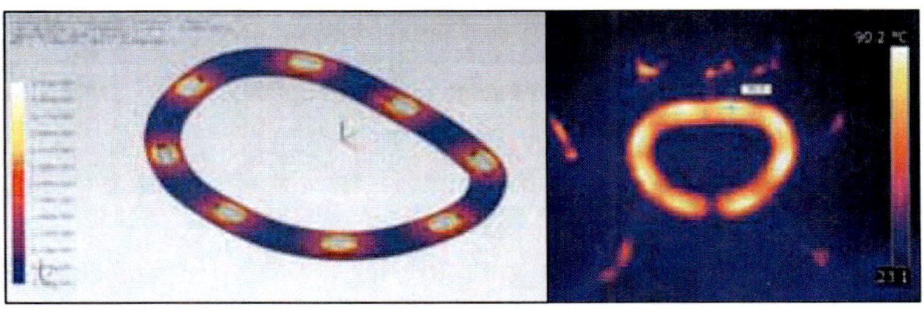

Figure 5.24 Simulation and trial of heating system for activating a SMP-based annuloplasty ring. FEM results and IR thermogram (SMART 09, 2009).

5.4.3 Stability of Properties

In general, the variation in the properties of polymeric materials through aging has major economic implications as it affects the in-service performance. Particularly in the case of shape-memory implants, any change in the vitreous transition temperature (or activation temperature) can cause problems when activating the necessary geometric changes.

Physical ageing has been reported as a cause of notable changes in the vitreous transition temperature or activation temperature of shape-memory polymers and studied by means of digital scanning calorimetry (DSC), as Fig. 5.25 shows (Lorenzo and Díaz Lantada, 2009). Additional structural changes of the polymer, due to secondary polymerisations, UV exposure and other environmental factors, can also increase activation temperature of SMPs and related devices, thus affecting performance either *in vitro* or *in vivo*.

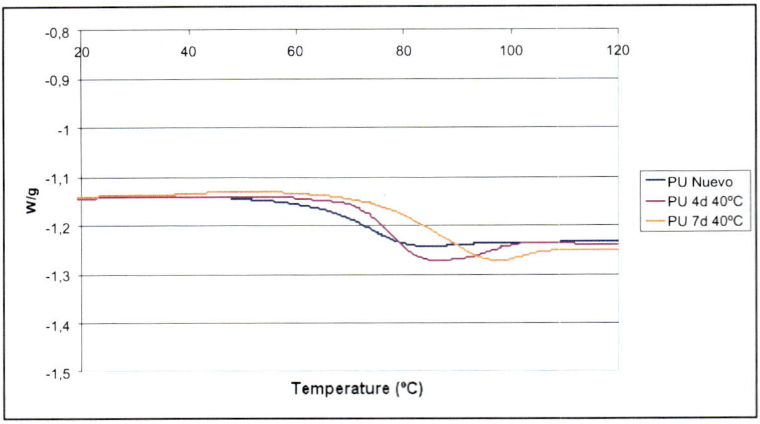

Figure 5.25 Evolution of glass transition temperature *T*" (activation temperature) due to physical ageing in a shape-memory polyurethane - MCP Iberia 3115. DSC measurements for ageing times of 1 h (blue), 4 h (pink) and 7 days (orange).

It is also necessary to study the changes to the mechanical properties of these polymers (elasticity modulus, hardness, and resilience), due to their being implanted in the human body. Figure 5.26 shows an example how the (micro)hardness of a shape-memory polyurethane evolves at 40°C for a total ageing time of 80 days. A Vickers microhardness tester was used with a 0.98 N load and a 15 s contact time.

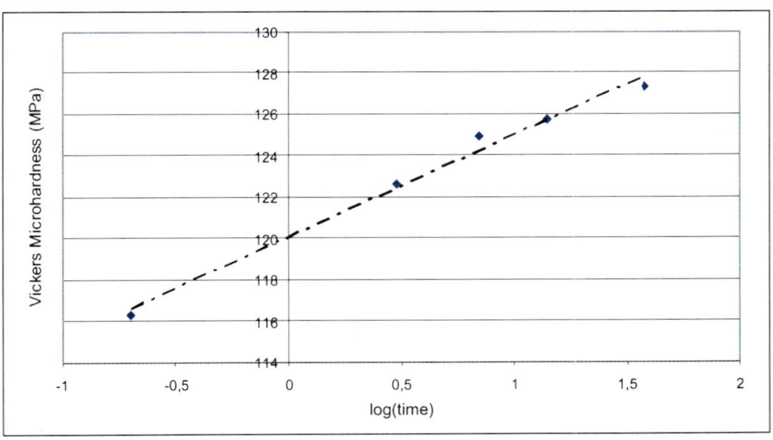

Figure 5.26 Evolution of hardness in a shape-memory polyurethane. (Ageing time expressed in h) (Biodevices, 2009).

Changes in the thermo-mechanical properties, like that shown in Fig. 5.26, can considerably affect the applicability of devices based on these materials. The use of additives and the synthesis of new formulations that help minimise the changes to properties with the passage of time will be highly useful for optimising device performance.

However, the effects of moisture on changes in the properties of SMPs may be determining factors for making an application invalid. This effect has been studied on shape-memory polyurethanes by conducting DMTA and DSC tests with samples submerged in water for different lengths of time to age them (Yang, 2004).

5.4.4 Activation Temperature

Only on rare occasions, in the polymeric products industry, have materials with vitreous transitions of between 0 and 50°C been used, as in-service changes to properties are not usually desirable. For this reason, it is difficult to find commercial formulations for polymers with T_g in the 25 to 45°C range.

However, for the development of shape-memory polymer–based active implantable medical devices, it is precisely temperatures near to the 37°C of body heat that are sought. SMPs with a T_g of around 30°C may give rise to devices that change their geometry on contact with the patient's body. SMPs with a T_g of around 45°C can be used to develop implants intended for postoperative activation through heating to induce geometric changes.

Some laboratories and companies achieve noticeable changes in the T_g of dual component SMPs by modifying the proportion of monomers and additives for cross-linking that are used to synthesise them. Most formulations still have activation temperatures that are too high to be used in implantable devices without causing damage to surrounding tissues.

Fortunately, in the last 5 years new SMPs with a T_g closer to body temperature have been synthesised and could be used in conjunction with appropriate protective coatings to develop percutaneous implants. Table 5.1 shows some prime examples.

Table 5.1 Materials and Acceptable T_g for Biodevices

Material	Vitreous transition temperature	Reference
tBA-co-PEGDMA	40–52°C (according to % of cross linking)	(Yakacki, 2008)
Polynorbornene (Norsorex ®)	Around 40°C	(Liu and Mather, 2003, 2007)
Polyurethane	Room Temp. ±50°C	(Tobushi, 2008)
Polyurethane Diaplex MM5520	55°C	DIAPLEX Ltd. (Small, 2005)
Poly(ε-caprolactone)	40–59°C	(Lendlein and Kelch, 2002)
Epoxy-based	35–105°C	CRG Industries
Styrene-based	45–95°C	CRG Industries

Very recently CRG Industries has developed *two new formulations* under trade name "Esssemplex" with shape-memory properties and activation (T_g) temperatures of around 34°C and 43°C, thus leaving normal body temperature (37°C) between them, hopefully for promoting different medical applications once biocompatibility is verified or improved.

However, additional considerations, which are set out below, must be taken into account concerning the feasibility of using these materials for the development of medical devices.

5.4.5 Security Issues

Biocompatibility improvements

Starting up production of shape-memory–based polymers is closer than ever as more emphasis is being placed on improving the biocompatibility of these devices.

Many SMP formulations are toxic; however, some of them have been shown to be compatible with human tissues (Cabanlit *et al.*, 2007; Sokolowsky *et al.*, 2007), which results hopeful for future developments.

In whatever case, the use of protecting coatings (using "PVD" or "CVD" technologies) may be of considerable help in improving this aspect (particularly when using the new DLC "diamond like carbon", Salgueiredo *et al.*, 2007) of coatings, as well as textile coatings to ensure biocompatibility.

Perhaps the best starting point for understanding biocompatibility requirements is standard ISO 10993 "Biological evaluation of medical devices", which includes guidelines for specific test procedures and related issues, many of them tightly linked to the use of polymeric materials, which can provide useful information when developing and assessing effectiveness of SMP-based actuators.

Sterilisation

Before *in vivo* implantation the devices need to be sterilised using some of the methods that are usually applied to polymers (steam, ethylene oxide, gamma radiation, low temperature plasma "LTP" or the Noxilizer process).

In spite of the numerous methods that can be used, it is preferable to choose low-temperature sterilisation (LTP, ethylene oxide or the Noxilizer method) to avoid activating the memory effect before implanting the devices.

The influence of these methods on toxicity and thermomechanical response of these materials has recently begun to be studied with promising results (Yakacki, 2008).

Regulations

In order to optimise the safety of devices based on these materials they must be in compliance with the guidelines of the "European Directive on Medical Devices – 93/42/EEC" and the "European Directive on Active Implantable Medical Devices – 90/385/EEC".

It is also advisable to follow the recommendations of Standard ISO 13485 on quality in medical devices as well as specific legislation concerning materials characterization tests (ISO and ASTM Standards especially).

5.4.6 Structured Development Process

If the development of commercial medical applications based on these devices is to be promoted, it is important to increase the connection between all the actors taking part in the different development stages.

In this way, they could collaborate to establish a structured design process to combine the tasks of synthesis, materials characterization and processing, mechanical design, prototype manufacture, *in vitro* and *in vivo* trials, official approval and subsequent production start-up.

Similar proposals are being successfully applied to promote developments based on other active materials for different industries, such as electroactive polymers (EAPs) (Bar-Cohen, 2002, 2006). Final chapter of this handbook covers in-depth a global proposal of structured systematic methodology for the development medical devices based on active or "intelligent" materials.

5.5 Improving Results and Conclusions

Shape-memory polymers have emerged with enormous potential allowing the development of medical devices with special features and capabilities for activation hitherto unachievable.

The development of bioactuators based on these materials at present requires progress in various scientific-technological aspects to optimise their possibilities. It will then be possible to obtain marketable medical devices (diagnostic and therapeutic) that fulfil all the mechanical, therapeutic, stability and safety requirements.

Recent advances in issues of international co-operation concerning active materials with the setting up of specific forums like Scientific.net, Biomat.net and others, are helping to disseminate results and exchange opinions. However, it would be of great interest to create a specific forum on shape-memory polymers and their applications, where researchers, universities and enterprises could make contact in order to fit technological supply with market requirements, which is of particular importance for the Medical Industry.

While the new capabilities brought by these materials give rise to expectations that many medical devices will become more effective, considerably more effort still needs to be put into research and development, so as to obtain robust and effective actuators based on these materials.

References

Bar-Cohen, Y. "Electroactive polymer actuators as artificial muscles: Reality, potential and challenges". SPIE Press. Washington, 2002.

Bar-Cohen, Y. "Electroactive polymer (EAP) actuators as artificial muscles: Reality, potential and challenges". SPIE Press, 2nd Edition. Washington, 2006.

Bellin, I.; Kelch, S.; Langer, R.; Lendlein, A. "Polymeric triple-shape materials". Proceedings of the National Academy of Sciences, 103(48), 18043–18047, 2006.

Buckley, C.P.; Prisacariu, C.; Caraculacu, A. "Novel triol-crosslinked polyurethanes and their thermorheological characterization as shape-memory materials". Polymer, 48, 1388–1396, 2007.

Buckley, P.R.; Mc Kinley, G.H.; Wilson, T.S.; *et al.* "Inductively heated shape memory polymer for the magnetic actuation of medical devices". IEEE Transactions on Biomedical Engineering, 53(10), 2075–2083, 2006.

Cabanlit, M.; Maitland, D.; Wilson, T.; *et al.* "Polyurethane shape-memory polymers demonstrate functional biocompatibility in vitro". Macromolecular Bioscience, 7(1), 48–55, 2007.

Conti, S.; Lenz, M.; Rumpf, M. "Modelling and simulation of magnetic shape-memory polymer composites". Journal of Mechanics and Physics of Solids, 55(7), 1462–1486, 2007.

Díaz Lantada, A.; Lafont Morgado, P.; Lorenzo Yustos, H.; *et al.* "Treatment of mitral valve insufficiency by shape memory polymer based active annuloplasty". International Conference on Biomedical Electronics and Devices Biostec 2008 – Biodevices, 1, 17–22. IEEE Engineering in Medicine and Biology Society. 28–31 January 2008 in Madeira. INSTICC Press, 2008. I.S.B.N.: 978-989-8111-19-7.

Díaz Lantada, A.; Lafont Morgado, P.; Lorenzo Yustos, H.; *et al.* "Biodevices based on shape-memory polymers: Current capabilities and challenges". Biodevices 2009 – International Conference on Biomedical Electronics and Devices. IEEE Engineering in Medicine and Biology Society. 14–17 January 2009 in Porto. I.S.B.N.: 978-989-8111-64-7.

Díaz Lantada, A.; Lafont Morgado, P.; Lorenzo Yustos, H.; *et al.* "Rapid prototyping and rapid tooling technologies for developing shape-memory polymer based devices". IV ECCOMAS Thematic Conference, Smart Structures and Materials (SMART'09). 13–15 July 2009 in Porto. I.S.B.N.: 978-972-752-113-5.

Díaz Lantada, A.; Lafont, P.; Muñoz-García, J.; *et al.* "Stress-strain simulations for optimising the design of shape-memory polymer based annuloplasty rings". "World Congress on Medical Physics and Biomedical Engineering 2009". 7–12 September, 2009 in Munich.

Freitag, D.; Wohlers, T. "Rapid prototyping: State of the Art". Manufacturing technology information analysis centre. Chicago Illinois, 2003.

Gall, K.; Kreiner, P.; Turner, D.; Hulse, M. "Shape memory polymers for MEMS systems". Journal of Microelechtromechanical Systems, 13(3), 472-483, 2004.

González Bris, C.; Díaz Lantada, A. "A wearable passive force sensor/active interrogator intended for intra-splint use for the detection and recording of bruxism". 3rd International Conference on Pervasive Computing Technologies for Healthcare 2009. 1–3 April 2009 in London. I.S.B.N.: 978-963-9799-42-4.

Harrysson, O.; Hosni, Y.A.; Nayfeh, J. "Custom-designed orthopaedic implants evaluated using FEM analysis of patient computed tomography data". BMC Musculoskelet Disorders, 8, 91–91, 2007.

Huang, W.; Lee, C. "Thermomechanical behaviour of a polyurethane shape memory polymer foam". Journal of Intelligent Material Systems and Structures, 12(4), 283–287, 2006.

Kuklick, T.R. "The medical device R&D handbook". CRC Press, Taylor and Francis Group. Florida, 2006.

Lafont Morgado, P.; Díaz Lantada, A.; Martínez Álvarez, A.; *et al.* "Instrumented splint for the diagnosis of bruxism". International Conference on Biomedical Electronics and Devices Biostec 2008 – Biodevices, 2, 216-222. IEEE Engineering in Medicine and Biology Society. 28–31 January 2008 in Madeira. INSTICC Press, 2008. I.S.B.N.: 978-989-8111-19-7.

Lafont Morgado, P.; Lorenzo Yustos, H.; Suarez García, D. *et al.* "Rapid tooling: Moldes rápidos a partir de estereolitografía". Revista de plásticos modernos, 524, 150–157, 2000.

Lendlein, A.; Hiang, H.; Jünger, O.; Langer, R. "Light-induced shape-memory polymers". Nature, 434, 879–882, 2005.

Lendlein, A; Kelch, S. "Shape-memory polymers". Angewandte Chemie International, 41(12), 2034–2057, 2002.

Lendlein, A.; Kelch, S. "Shape-memory polymers as stimuli-sensitive implant materials". Clinical Hemorheology and Microcirculation, 32, 105–116, 2005.

Lendlein, A; Langer, R. "Biodegradable, elastic shape-memory polymers for potential biomedical applications". Science, 296(5573), 1673–1676, 2002.

Leng, J.; Lv. H.B.; Liu, Y.J. Du, S.Y. "Electroactive shape-memory polymer filled with nanocarbon particles and short carbon fibers". Applied Physics Letters, 91, 144105, 2007.

Liu, C.; Mather, P.T. "Thermomechanical characterization of a tailored series of shape memory polymers". Journal of Applied Medical Polymers, 6(2), 47–52, 2002.

Liu, C., Qin, H.; Mather, P.T. "Review of progress in shape-memory polymers". Journal of Materials Chemistry. 17, 1553–1558, 2007.

Liu, Y.; Gall, K.; Dunn, M.L.; Greenberg, A.R.; Diani, J. "Thermomechanics of shape memory polymers: Uniaxial experiments and constitutive modelling". International Journal of Plasticity, 22(2), 279–313, 2006.

Liu, Y.; Gall, K.; Dunn, M.L.; Mc Cluskey, P. "Thermomechanical recovery couplings of shape memory polymers in flexure". Smart Materials and Structures, 12, 947–954, 2003.

Liu, Y.; Lv, H.; Lan, X.; Leng, J.; Du, S. "Review of electroactive shape memory polymer composite". Composites Science and Technology (in press), 2009.

Lorenzo, V.; Díaz Lantada, A.; Lafont Morgado, P.; *et al.* "Physical ageing of a PU based shape memory polymer: influence on their applicability to the development of medical devices". Materials and Design, 30(7), 2431–2437, 2009.

Paumier, G.; Siv, S.; Bancaud, A.; Sudor, J.; Gué, A.M. "Thermoresponsive polymer-based microdevice for nano-liquid chromatography". International Conference on Biomedical Electronics and Devices Biostec 2008 – Biodevices, 1, 178–181. IEEE Engineering in Medicine and Biology Society. INSTICC Press, 2008.

Salgueiredo, E.; Vila, M.; Silva, M.A.; *et al.* "Biocompatibility Evaluation of DLC-coated Si3N4 Substrates for Biomedical Applications". Diamond and Related Materials. 17(4), 878–881, 2008.

Sokolowsky, W.; Metcalfe, A.; Hayashi, S.; Yahia, L.; Raymond, J. "Medical applications of shape memory polymers". Biomedical Materials, 2, 23–27, 2007.

Volk, B.; Whitley, K. "Characterization of shape memory polymers". NASA Langley Research Centre. Texas A&M University, 2005.

Wache, H.; Tartakowska, D.J.; Hentrich, A.; Wagner, M.H. "Development of a polymer stent with shape memory effect as a drug delivery system". Journal of Materials Science–Materials in Medicine, 14(2), 109–112, 2003.

Wilson, T.; Small IV, W.; William, B. J.; Bearinger, J.P.; Maitland D.J. "Shape memory polymer therapeutic devices for stroke". Smart Medical and Biomedical Sensor Technology III. Proceedings of the SPIE, 6007, 157–164, 2005.

Yakacki, C.M.; Shandas, R.; Lanning, C.; Rech, B.; Eckstein, A.; Gall, K. "Unconstrained recovery of shape-memory polymers networks for cardiovascular applications". Biomaterials, 28(14), 2255–2263, 2007.

Chapter 6

Electroactive Polymers as Actuators for Biodevices

Andrés Díaz Lantada
Mechanical Engineering Department, E.T.S.I. Industriales,
Universidad Politécnica de Madrid, c/ José Gutiérrez Abascal 2,
28006 Madrid, Spain
adiaz@etsii.upm.es

6.1 Brief Introduction to Electroactive Polymers

The synthetic polymer industry emerged in the second half of the 19th century, although its expansion and use in practically every sphere of daily life did not occur until the last decades of the 20th century. This was a consequence of the gradual appearance of new formulas and the improvements in mass production manufacturing processes, mainly injection and extrusion moulding and the use of additives, especially reinforcement fibres to obtain composite materials.

All this has made synthetic polymers very versatile materials that possess mechanical, thermal, chemical, optical, electrical and even aesthetic properties that can be adapted to most of the standard requirements of device development. They are often materials that have mechanical characteristics that are similar to those of body tissues. This, combined with their resistance to corrosion, makes them excellent candidates for materials in implantable medical devices.

Handbook of Active Materials for Medical Devices: Advances and Applications
Edited by Andrés Díaz Lantada

www.panstanford.com

On the other hand, advances in microfabrication technologies since the 1970s and their gradual application (and adaptation) to polymer materials, particularly since the 1980s, have sought to combine the benefits of speed and low cost of mass produced polymer parts with the intrinsic capabilities of micro-electromechanical systems (MEMS), which stand out for their low consumption of materials and energy resources and a greater sensitivity and response speed.

This has helped boost the impact of polymer materials on the development of devices for different health science work (medicine, biology, biochemistry and others). Moreover, since the final decade of the 20th century special attention has been paid to integrating functionalities (couplings between different properties) into a wide range of polymers in order to obtain active or "intelligent" properties that can be used as transducers to develop sensors and actuators. Various chapters of the handbook focus on analysing the fundamental properties of these intelligent polymers and their potential for active medical device development.

In the previous chapter, we saw how shape-memory polymers (SMPs) present thermo-mechanical coupling that capacitates them as thermoactive or thermosensitive actuators. The concept of electroactive polymer could be equally applied to all polymers that can change their geometry or their mechanical, optical or chemical properties, among others, in response to electrical stimuli. But it could also be applied to all polymers that can generate an electrical response to changes in environmental variables, like pressure, temperature, pH, and light intensity among others.

However, the term "electroactive polymer" is usually used, above all, for polymers with a coupling of mechanical and electrical properties. When electroactive polymers receive electrical stimuli they can change their geometry and transmit mechanical forces and can be used as actuators. It is on this behaviour that we are going to focus this chapter, beginning in the following section with an analysis of the most recent proposals for their application.

On the other hand, when electroactive polymers are subjected to deformations or mechanical forces, they are capable of displacing charges (and generating potential differences) at their core, enabling them to be used as force or pressure sensors. These will be dealt with in Chapter 7.

Further on, the handbook will also deal with other kinds of polymers with specific elctroactivity, like pyroelectric polymers (with thermo-electrical coupling) in Chapter 9, electro-optical polymers in Chapter 11 and some hydropolymers in Chapter 12, with different responses to electrical stimuli. In Chapter 10 special emphasis will be placed on electro/magnetorheological elastomers, to which the addition of ferrofluids, during the polymerisation process, enables flexible actuators to be obtained that are sensitive to changes in the magnetic field around them.

6.2 Applications in Medical Devices

As already introduced, since the beginning of the 1990s, new polymers have been obtained that respond to electrical stimuli with considerable changes in shape or size, which has been a big step forward in the use of polymeric materials.

They are called electroactive polymers (EAPs), although they also go by the name of "Artificial Muscles" due to the similarity of their behaviour with animal muscles (electric impulse-based mechanical activation).

The large differences in properties between the different kinds of electroactive polymers enable them to be used as sensors and actuators contributing versatility to device development. As previously stated in this chapter, we will focus on its applications as actuators within biodevices. The main designs proposed for medical device development will now be explained (Ashley, 2003; Herr and Kornbluh, 2004).

Micropumps for drug delivery

Based on existing designs of piezoelectric micropumps or diffusers or diaphragm micropumps, by replacing the traditional ceramic activator component (usually PZT, zirconate-titanate or lead zirconate) by dielectric electroactive polymers, micropumps can be had that can be used to deliver drugs. They have also been proposed for use in the treatment of glaucoma and hydrocephaly. Such micropumps have been developed by Medipump LLC Inc. and Ophthalmotronics Co. and utilise a dielectric electroactive polymer laminate as activation element.

Microanastomosis devices

Anastomosis is an operation for reconnecting communication between vessels, ducts and nerves. The smaller the diameter of the vessel, the more difficult is the operation. Micromuscle AB enterprise has designed a cylindrical device made of electroactive polymer on the outside and biocompatible material on the inside. This means an operation can be done simply as the cylinder can be made to dilate or contract by applying a voltage.

Devices for minimally invasive surgery

Electroactive polymers can be used as guides for active catheters; by applying opposite voltages the catheter bends in one direction or the other thereby allowing access to more inaccessible areas.

Once the catheter is in position, drugs can be supplied through it or optic fibre inserted to perform an inspection. They can also be used in other minimally invasive surgery work such as removing intravenous (IV) clots or to help in positioning stents.

Fluid system microdevices

The development of electroactive polymer-based active microvalves and microchannels is being used to design controlled drug delivery devices. They can also be used in lab-on-a-chip devices, and microsystems that integrate various laboratory functions in a few square centimetres. They can be used for blood analysis, DNA sample extraction, perform antigen-antibody reactions and others; all of this in the fastest, most controlled, cheapest way. In these designs the polymer generally acts as an agitator to speed up the chemical analysis process (Lanceros-Méndez *et al.*, 2008).

Haptic devices

Teleoperators are those that control tools remotely and in these cases the contact resistance forces need to return to the teleoperator. This is called "haptic teleoperation". When these devices are user-operated by means of computer-guided simulation, it is important to provide the return force that could be felt in real operations. As the objects being handled do not exist in reality, the haptic forces generated (by the computer) as return force must be such that they give a feeling as to the surroundings.

Haptic simulators are currently widely used for training in surgical operations. They are useful when attempting to minimise damage caused by the use of invasive procedures (invasive laparoscopy/radiology) and let operations be performed remotely.

Electroactive polymers have been used as the active part that generates the return force in these devices in various research centres such as the Jet Propulsion Laboratory NASA (Bar-Cohen, 2004) or the Research Centre of EAP Devices in Switzerland.

Heartbeat aid devices

There are various patents that propose using electroactive polymer bands located around the heart wall that are electronically synchronised with the heart beat to aid pumping, particularly in cases of insufficiency (US Patents 6464655, 2002, US Patent 7198592, 2007, Shahinpoor and Kim, 2004). In fact, firms like Environmental Robots Inc. put their services out for hire to carry out research projects that culminate with the *in vivo* validation of these proposals.

Devices to correct eye problems

Other patents propose using electroactive polymer actuators as an aid to correcting different eye problems. Patent US6511508 developed through collaboration between Environmental Robots Inc. and Ophthalmotronics Corp. describes the use of bands placed next to the eyeball to correct refractive errors.

Other patents like US6168575, US6589198 and US6682500 detail the possible development of micropumps with an active polymer diaphragm to help treat glaucoma, although they also have some applications for drug delivery or the treatment of hydrocephaly. They are being developed in collaboration between Environmental Robots Inc. and Medipump LLC Inc.

6.3 Current Capabilities and Recent Advances

6.3.1 Main Kinds of Electroactive Polymers

Polymers that undergo dimensional changes in response to an electrical stimulus can be divided into two basic families: electronic (electronic EAP, with activation as a result of applying an electric field or Coulomb forces) and ionic (ionic EAP, with shape changes due to movement or ion diffusion).

This section deals with the different kinds of polymers in each of the two families, in line with the usual terminology, especially after the publication of the handbook *Electroactive Polymer Actuators as Artificial Muscles* by Dr. Yoseph Bar-Cohen, a world reference in the development of electroactive polymer-based devices, who continuously publicises the principle scientific advances concerning these materials through his web page (http://eap.jpl.nasa.gov).

Electronic electroactive polymers

They usually comprise an elastic or elastomeric polymer core with metallic electrodes deposited on the opposing surfaces of the material. Activation is usually produced by electrostatic forces between the electrodes, which compress or expand the middle polymer layer. Their main limitation is that they require high activation voltages.

Of all the types of electronic electroactive polymers the following families should be mentioned:

- **Ferroelectric polymers.** Their non-centrosymmetric structure causes the application of mechanical forces to lead to charge displacements and the appearance of potential differences between different zones of the material. The poly(vinylidene fluoride) or PVDF -(CH2-CF2)-n and its copolymers, like poly(vinylidene trifluoride-ethylene) or P(VDF-TrFE), are the polymers of this type that are most used in industry. They possess partial crystallinity, with an inactive and an elastic modulus between 1 and 10 GPa. Their use as actuators is limited by the need to apply strong electric fields (around 20 V/μm for 3% deformations), but they are replacing traditionally used piezoelectric ceramics as pressure sensors. They will be examined in detail in Chapter 7.
- **Dielectric EAP.** These are laminated polymer materials (mainly acrylics and silicons) with a very low mechanical stiffness and high dielectric constants that can be used as actuators by applying a strong electric field between the electrodes deposited on their sides (Gisby *et al.*, 2008). For deformations of between 10% and 200%, they require around 100 V/μm, which is close to the material's dielectric breaking point. For the present, this is limiting their applications outside I+D+I tasks. One of the major commercial products is VHB 4910 from 3M Company.
- **Electrostrictive graft elastomers.** This type of electrostrictive material comprises a flexible macromolecule which acts as a skeleton and grafted polymer chains that are able to form a crystalline structure. These chains respond to electrical stimuli and attain deformations of 4% when strong electric fields are applied (NASA development, 1998). If they are combined with piezoelectric copolymers, systems can be obtained that can be operated as pressure sensors and electrostrictive actuators, thereby combining detection and activation capabilities.

- **Electrovisco-elastic elastomers.** These are a family of composites comprising silicon and a polar phase, which before polymer chain bonding, behave as electrorheological fluids. During curing, an electric field is applied to orient and fix the position of the polar phase in the elastomer silicon matrix. In this way, composites are obtained whose shear modulus changes with the electric field (values lower than 6 V/μm).

  Electrorheological fluids in active suspensions can be used as an alternative for the automobile industry as well as for precision control of robot arms in a closed loop. However, at present their uses are limited compared to the increasing use of electro/magnetorheological fluids and magnetorheological elastomers (analysed in Chapter 10).
- **Liquid-crystal elastomer "LCE".** A particular kind of thermotropic liquid crystal has been recently developed that presents a nemetic to isotropic phase transformation when heated above its transition temperature. This phase change (with a change in the structure of its network and associated volume) can be achieved through the Joule effect, which means they can be used to produce electroactive actuators or rather, with electro-thermomechanical coupling, as is also the case with some of the shape memory polymers already examined. Those most studied are aromatic polyesters like HBA and its copolymers (Vectra A9000 from Hoechst - Celanese). In less than 1 s, the transition from the nematic to the isotropic phase can be achieved. However, the opposite process requires around 10 s of cooling, which limits its response speed and applications.

Ionic electroactive polymers

Activation is produced by ion movement at the core of the polymer. Their main limitation is that they usually need to function when wet and the developable mechanical forces are usually small. The following families of ionic electroactive polymers need to be mentioned:

- **Ionic polymer gels "IPGs".** Polymer gels for producing actuators can be synthesised that will be able to attain the force and energy density of biological muscles. These (like polyacrylonitrile) are usually activated by a chemical reaction, changing from an acidic environment to a basic one that causes the gel to become less dense. When an electrical stimulation is applied, a multilayer structure ionic polymer gel bends since the cathode becomes more alkaline and the anode more acid. However, the response speed is relatively slow as it requires the diffusion of the ions through the gel (around 20 min). Resistance to fatigue is also critical (around 3 cycles) because the large deformations damage the electrodes. Current work is focused on discovering better deposition technologies to obtain thinner metallic layers that are adapted to the mechanical properties of the substrate.

- **Ionomeric polymer-metal composites "IPMCs".** These are polymer-metal composites that bend in response to an electrical stimulus which, in turn, is a response to ion movement through the polymer network (Shahinpoor and Kim, 2004, 2005). A typical IPMC consists of an approximately 200 μm thick polymer film or membrane with approximately 10 μm thick electrodes deposited on the opposite sides of the polymer film.

  Nafion from Du Pont and Flemion from Asashi Glass are usually used as base membrane. We should also mention the development kits supplied by Environmental Robots Inc. which integrate control electronics for teaching activities and preliminary concept tests.

  They require a relatively low voltage to activate them (1–10 V) which produces bendings of around 90° with frequencies and responses below 1 Hz. The main drawback is their low output power (and associated activation force) of around 10 W/kg, compared to around 1000 W/kg in biological muscles. On the other hand, their having to activate in the presence of water, (submerged or wet), to enable the migration of cations also limits their applications. Recent developments are using solid coatings with dissolved electrolyte for dry operation.
- **Conductive polymers (CPs).** These consist of a two-electrode conductive polymer sandwich structure (like polypyrrole or polyaniline or PAN doped with HCl), with an electrolyte layer between them. When a voltage is applied between the electrodes, oxidation is produced in the anode and reduction in the cathode. The ions (H+) migrate between the electrolytes and the electrodes to balance the electric charge. This causes

an increase in the volume of the polymer receiving the ions and a narrowing of the polymer releasing them. As a result, the sandwich bends. They usually require voltages of around 5 V and response speeds of 40 Hz for thin films (around 100 μm). Current research is being channelled towards activation in dry environments, for which quasi-solid electrolytes are being used. Neither should we forget the artificial muscle fibres from EAMEX Co. that work in this way, which are managing to reach developable forces close to those of biological muscles.

Other materials sometimes included in these classifications, like magnetorheological fluids or carbon nanotubes (and associated actuators), will be dealt with further on in the handbook in more specific chapters, due to the recent surge in interest in them and because they behave very differently from the polymers mentioned above.

We should also mention an additional member of the pneumatic muscles family, sometimes called "Mc Kibben artificial muscles", which are only made up of tubular polymer structures (very flexible) which respond to compressed air power which causes them to swell and shorten. Pneumatic power can be controlled by electrovalves, which means there is a certain electromechanical coupling that makes these materials part of the electroactive polymer family.

Some firms, like Festo Didactic, have a wide range of models and control systems for these kinds of actuators. This allows test benches to be quickly and effectively set up for characterising a range of medical applications like those shown in Chapter 7, that use Mc Kibben muscles as actuators on a test bench for simulating human bite.

When using this kind of actuator for design and calculation work the characteristic sheets of the different manufacturers will prove helpful as they usually include the ratios between activation force, attainable deformation and power pressure.

Finite elements simulation tools can also be used in the same way that a balloon-mounted catheter was simulated in Chapter 4 (which is used as the front cover picture of the handbook).

Other electroactive polymer actuators, like those based on carbon nanotubes integrated into the material core or microstructured actuators that combine various families of active materials will be dealt with further on in Chapter 14.

6.3.2 Synthesis and Processing

In this introduction to electroactive polymers it is quite impossible to include a detailed description of all the different ways of synthesising these materials as each family has its individual method. These are explained in numerous patents and scientific articles, many of which involve complex chemical reactions that are outside the scope of this handbook. A lot of information on the subject can be had by consulting patent data bases, some of which are online, like www.espacenet.com, ISI Web of Knowledge, and www.wipo.int among others.

When the materials required for developing practical applications, particularly in the biomedical field, have been synthesised, the transformation methods that allow processing the materials until the right geometries for activation have been obtained, become particularly important. The standard processing technologies for conventional polymers will produce more affordable actuators in less time at a lower cost. This may well be a determining factor if these "intelligent" materials are to enter into general use in industry.

Some of the processes that can be used are injection moulding for complex geometries, calendering and laminating for the production of flat actuators, stretching to produce linear actuators and fibres, hot-embossing and injection micro-moulding to produce micro-components. These are just some of the many standard processes which can also be used in the field of electroactive polymers.

Developing practical applications for EAPs requires the aid of other effective processing technologies so that actuators with the right-shape connective electrodes can be produced ready to be integrated into more complex systems. Other requirements are to maximise activation or detection capabilities, ensure that the durability and strength of the material is suited to the use it will be put to and bear in mind how it can be integrated with other electromechanical components.

Special emphasis is being placed on deposition processes for electrodes so that the voltages required to activate these polymers can be applied (or voltages generated when they are used as sensors), as is described in Chapter 13 when dealing with CVD and PVD deposition technologies, sol-gel, spin-coating, dip-coating processes and other more specific processes.

6.3.3 Characterisation and Modelling

One way of embarking on a study of electroactive polymers and the devices that are based on these materials is to purchase some of the so-called "kits or development packages" that are sold by various firms that specialise in the synthesis and use of EAPs.

These kits usually come with various samples of different EAPs, complete with power and control electronics for managing activation as well as short handbooks full of useful tips and practical teaching activities. Worth mentioning are the development kits supplied by Environmental Robots Inc., some of which include (together with standard linear samples) specific toys or mini-robots with active moving parts, due to EAP bands being integrated into the devices.

These "plug and play" packages are an ideal first approach to the essentials of characterising electroactive polymers and then modelling their behaviour according to the information resulting from the characterisation tests. They are ideal for setting up more complete test benches for testing different electroactive polymers that allow studying the attainable deformations, developable forces and the response speed according to the voltages and current intensities applied.

They can also be directly used in practical teaching sessions in Universities to supplement standard subjects in Master's or PhD programmes in "Biomedical Engineering", "Biomechanics" or "Biomaterials" and other more innovative subjects such as "Intelligent Materials" or "Active Implants".

Below, we include an example of the characterisation process performed with the aid of one of the development kits supplied by Environmental Robots Inc. that includes IPMC samples, as well as electronics for generating a square wave to control the applied voltage (mainly responsible for the deformation obtained) and the frequency of the signal (which marks the response speed).

Different examples of characterisation tests are shown in the Figs. 6.1 to 6.3 and are summarised in by the graphs in Fig. 6.4, showing the outcomes of a specific study on the influence of moisture on the way these ionic polymers function. As we have stated, most of these polymers have to work in the presence of water or be recently hydrated so that the water can enable the ions to move that cause the polymer to bend. It can be seen how after 1 h out of the water, the polymer has partially dried and the attainable deformations are around 40% smaller than in the initial hydrated state.

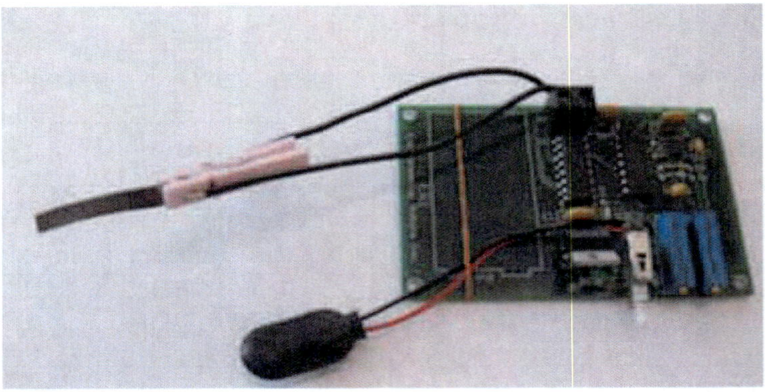

Figure 6.1 Teaching kit for ionic electroactive polymer study. Supplied by Environmental Robots Inc.

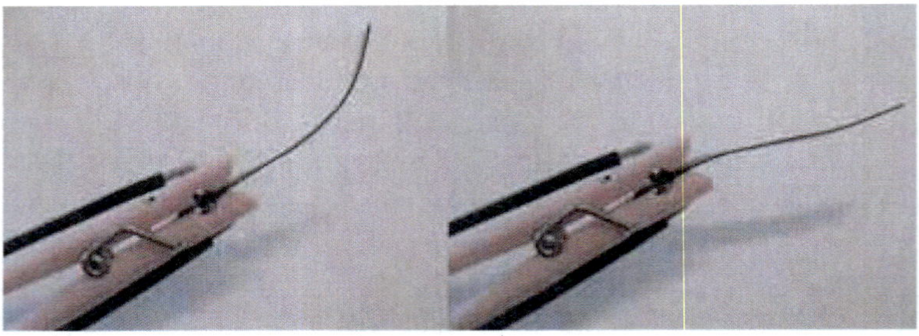

Figure 6.2 Free activation of IPMC film. Supplied by Environmental Robots Inc.

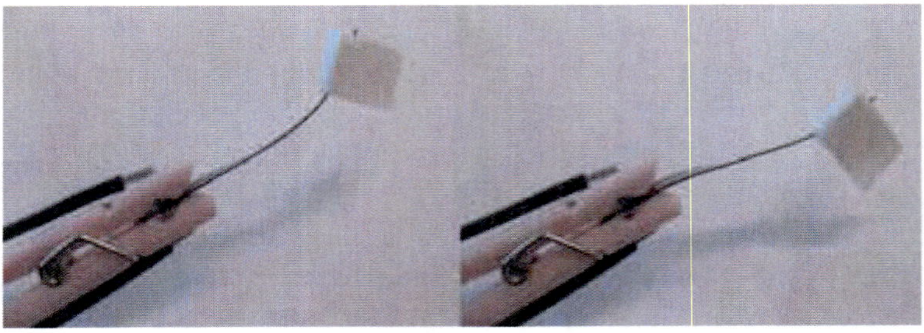

Figure 6.3 Free activation of IPMC film with a mass of 5 g attached to its end. Supplied by Environmental Robots Inc.

These are some of the issues that need to be borne in mind right from the design stage so that when the prototypes have been obtained for a specific device, they will work as designed, thereby avoiding design iterations having to be performed with the ensuing impact on time scales and costs. We will again underline the importance of thorough characterisation tests in order to discover the response of the active candidate materials for the development of a device, since the innovative nature of these materials often leads to design uncertainties.

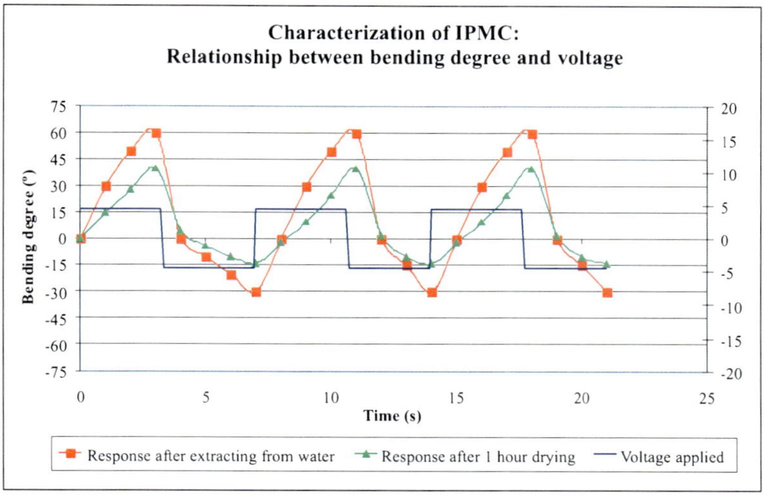

Figure 6.4 Standard IPMC film response to a variable power voltage. Influence of moisture loss which limits ion movement and activation.

Signal generators with voltage, current and frequency that can be controlled to suit the kind of polymer used are usually required. It is a good idea to have two different models for one laboratory; one for electronic electroactive polymers and another for ionic electroactive polymers.

Video cameras are usually used to aid characterisation tasks, and on occasions, high speed cameras, as well as other optical or electromechanical systems used to measure displacements, such as laser measurement systems, LVDTs or optical position sensors depending on the degree of accuracy sought and the speed of the system to be monitored.

6.3.4 Simulation Tools to Aid Device Development

By using the information from the characterisation tests, it is a simple matter to simulate the behaviour of an electroactive polymer that is part of a complex device and analyse what impact the actuator and device geometry will have on the final system response. Finite elements calculation programs are an invaluable aid to simulation, as was seen in Chapter 4.

Depending on the voltage-deformation-developable force ratio found from the characterisation tests on the electroactive actuator (usually with linear geometry similar to the "muscle wires" dealt with in Chapter 4), the deformation of the actuator can be known, as well as the activation force and the voltage required for the actuator to respond in a specific way (opening or closing tweezers, movement of an active catheter end, closing a valve, relative motion between two system components etc.).

When the actuator has a more complex geometry or when activation is by resonant effects produced by applying periodic voltages, finite elements programs for calculating vibration frequency and modes become even more valuable, given the additional difficulties of calculating even more problems. These resonant effects are being used in many multiple systems and microsystems to design sensors with optimised sensitivity (especially microcantilevers), as well as to produce sensors that can develop greater forces and achieve more marked deformations.

Numerous microfluid devices like diaphragm pumps, diffusion pumps and other volumetric pumps use resonant membranes to pump the fluid from aspiration to impulsion. In these cases it is more complicated to characterise electroactive actuators without any help, so we suggest using FEM simulations that help with these decisions and provide solutions concerning the best geometries and the power systems required before embarking on prototype manufacture for validating the designs through functional tests.

Two case studies are presented below; one of a circular membrane and another of a rectangular membrane. Both are electroactive polymers that are able to resonate at different frequencies and give rise to activations for different fluid device geometries. It is interesting to compare these examples with those described in Chapter 9, where passive membranes are activated by piezoelectric ceramic actuators.

It is advisable to revise the differential equations for finding the vibration frequencies and modes of membranes and plates (Santamarina Pol, 1998), in order to then be able to compare the theoretical predictions from the data found by applying the finite elements method as part of the design validation procedure.

To analyse transverse vibrations in membranes that are considered as perfectly flexible, very thin films that are uniformly stretched in all directions, the following differential equation is usually solved:

$$T \cdot \left(\frac{\partial^2 w}{\partial x^2} + \frac{\partial^2 w}{\partial y^2} \right) - \sigma \cdot \frac{\partial^2 w}{\partial t^2} = 0$$

where T is the uniform stress per unit of length of the boundary; w is the displacement of any point of the membrane, at a right angle to the xy plane restraining the membrane; and σ is the specific surface mass.

On the other hand, to analyse the vibrations of flat thin plates, with bending stiffness, the following differential equation must be solved:

$$\Delta\Delta w + \frac{\sigma}{D} \cdot \frac{\partial^2 w}{\partial t^2} = 0$$ $\Delta\Delta$ is the double Laplacian operator

$$\Delta\Delta = \frac{\partial^4}{\partial x^4} + 2 \cdot \frac{\partial^4}{\partial x^2 \partial y^2} + \frac{\partial^4}{\partial y^4}$$

where w is the displacement of any point of the membrane, at a right angle to the xy plane restraining the membrane; σ is the specific surface mass and D is the bending stiffness of the plate according to the expression:

$$D = \frac{E \cdot h^3}{12 \cdot (1 - \upsilon^2)}$$

where E is the Young modulus of the plate material, h is the thickness and v is the Poisson coefficient of the plate material.

The case under study, which is the use of an electroactive dielectric thin film elastomer attached to the casing of a fluidic device inside which the film acts as an actuator (pumping or supplying some liquid), corresponds to an intermediate situation that can be modelled in an approximate manner by using both approaches.

But it is also a good idea to conduct a parallel simulation of these systems using a finite elements model. When the FEM models in the Figures had to be implemented, the NX-7 system was used ("Siemens - PLM Solutions") in which the standard properties of dielectric elastomers were applied to the active membrane zone. The data on the geometries designed, meshing and properties of the materials are detailed below.

In order to simulate the polymer membrane, in the first case a 20 mm diameter, 0.2 mm thick circular membrane was designed. In the second case a 20 mm × 10 mm rectangular membrane was used that was also 0.2 mm thick.

Standard plate elements were used in the finite elements models for the membranes[1] with 2D meshes with 0.5 mm side squares. The characteristics taken for the electroactive polymer material were the standard ones for dielectric elastomers used in some fluid device prototypes. The following were used as mechanical properties:

Young modulus: 0.5 MPa

Poisson ratio: 0.4

Density: 900 kg/m^3

We should point out that to simulate these effects and other non-linearities there are calculation programs like ANSYS or Abaqus, which are currently the most effective for adding increasing complexities to the models. The results shown here are useful for design work, as an initial approximation, due to the similarities existing between boundary-fixed membrane models (with stress-stiffening effects) and boundary-supported thin plate models, regarding that deformations are controlled and with low values (Blevins, 1979).

Figures 6.6 and 6.7 reflect the outcomes of the dynamic simulation performed, showing the initial vibration modes for the different active membrane settings. The frequencies at which these modes appear can be seen in Fig. 6.8 and help predict the power frequencies that must be applied to the electroactive membranes to achieve the different activation modes.

It is important to state that, in general, the fit between the calculations or simulations of vibration frequencies (of the different modes) and the test results with actual devices is usually more suitable for the initial modes, since for the modes that appear at higher frequencies any slight modification in the boundary conditions can have a determining influence on the associated frequency.

[1]The models prepared for the simulations are depicted in Figs. 6.5 and 6.7 (top left corner), in which supported edges were used as boundary conditions so that standard very thin plate elements could be used to approximate thin membrane behaviour through simulations. By considering sufficiently small deformations in these simulations we did not need to do calculations under the hypothesis of "large deformations" and neither were stress stiffness effects included.

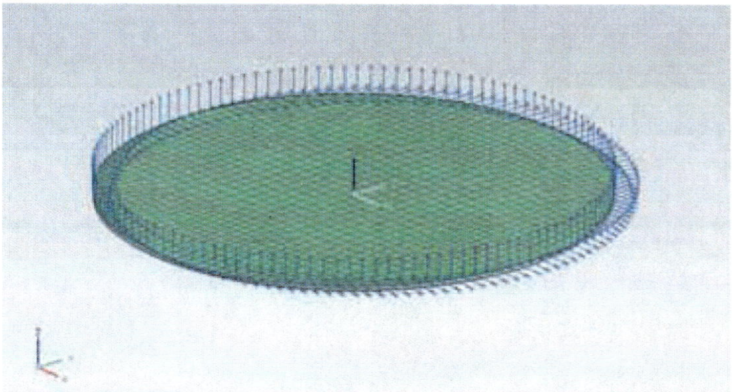

Figure 6.5 Finite-elements model for simulating the response of a dielectric elastomer membrane. Thin plate supported on its boundary as an approximation.

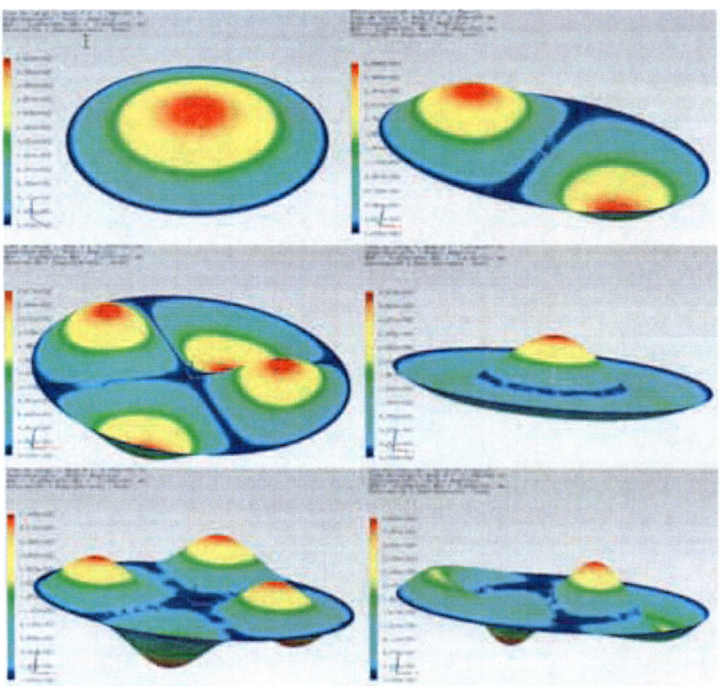

Figure 6.6 Vibration modes of a circular dielectric elastomer membrane used as an actuator in a fluidic device. Ordered by rows: modes 1 to 6.

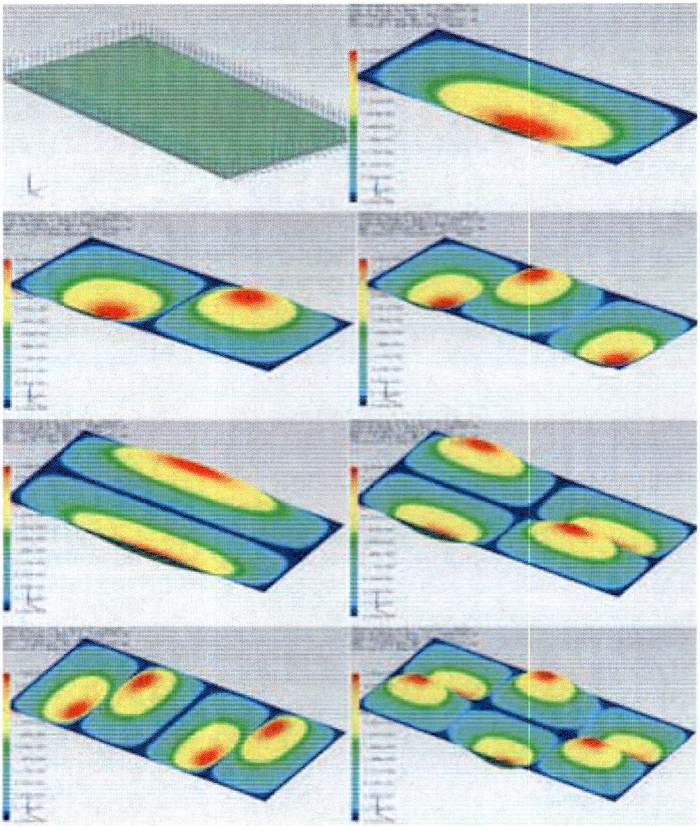

Figure 6.7 Vibration modes of a dielectric rectangular elastomer membrane used as an actuator in a fluidic device. Ordered by rows: modes 1 to 7.

It should be underlined that the geometry of the different modes helps design the casing geometry, which, together with electroactive polymer film (and the power supply system), make up the active device under development.

For example, as the mission of the film is to aspire and propel the fluid, it is reasonable to locate the aspiration and propulsion in antinodes (zones of maximum amplitude during vibration) separated by a node (zones of minimum amplitude during vibration); so that there is suction in one area of the pump and propulsion in the other. The use of the right diffusers in the input and output channels will do positive pumping in the required direction, as described in some handbooks on Microsystems (Koch *et al.*, 2000; Maluf, 2000; Gad-el-Hak, 2002).

Since the boundary conditions of the polymer film have a determining influence on the natural frequency vibration values and are difficult to simulate, it is important to remember that prototypes can be used to help validate or correct the initial design estimates made with the aid of theoretical or simulation models. These boundary conditions include the bond with the protective casing, and the bonding of the power supply wires to the electroactive membrane and the surrounding fluids in the case of a fluidic device. It is now that rapid manufacturing and prototyping tools can be of tremendous help, as we have shown in other chapters.

In whatever circumstances, simulations performed with FEM tools are excellent for displaying the geometry of each mode and the design questions of the device depending on the way it will be excited for activation. On the other hand, if we are dealing with complex geometries, the theoretical models combined with the FEM simulations are enormously useful for estimating the principle dimensions of the various components. Comparing the results of the analytical and simulation models serves as an additional tool for verifying that the calculations are being performed correctly.

As an example, we have included a comparative study of the values found for the vibration frequencies at the different settings (associated with the different modes), either analytically or using simulation tools.

Solving the differential equation representing the behaviour of circular plates subjected to bending vibrations (described at the beginning of the sub-section), leads to the following expression for calculating the natural frequencies of a circular plate supported on its boundary, an expression that helps model the system under study:

$$f_{ij} = \frac{\lambda_{ij}^{2}}{2\pi \cdot a^{2}} \left[\frac{E \cdot h^{3}}{12 \cdot \sigma \cdot (1 - \upsilon^{2})} \right]^{1/2}$$

where

- *i* is the number of nodal diameters;
- *j*, the number of nodal circumferences;
- *a*, the plate radius, in the example 20×10^{-3} mm;
- *h*, the plate thickness, in the example 0.2×10^{-3} mm;
- *E*, the Young modulus of the plate material, in the example 0.5×10^{6} Pa;

ν, the Poisson coefficient of the plate material, in the example 0.4; and

σ, the mass per unit of plate surface, in the example 0.18 kg/m^{2}.

Although the applicable theoretical model should be closer to a membrane model than a thin-plate model, if we consider that the displacements are small, the behaviour of a membrane can be based on a thin-plate model bisupported on its entire boundary.

For a deeper understanding of this analogy some excellent references can be consulted (Blevins, 1979), a text from which the values of λ_{ij} were taken for the previous expression.

For rectangular plate geometry the same previous expression can be used to calculate the natural frequencies, although the values of λ_{ij} depend on the a/b ratio, where in this example, a is the length of the long side of the rectangle, b is the length of the short side, and i and j are the number of nodal lines in perpendicular directions. They are also well-tabulated in "Formulas for Natural Frequency and Mode Shape" (Blevins, 1979).

According to the tabulated data of λ_{ij} for geometries that are "circular bisupported on the boundary" and "rectangular bisupported on the boundary", natural frequency values were calculated that were associated with different modes. These can be found in Fig. 6.8 together with the FEM simulation results shown before, so that they can be compared.

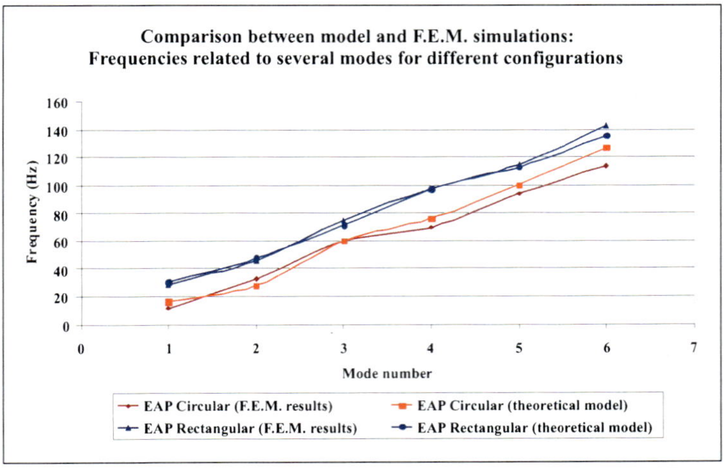

Figure 6.8 Relative frequencies of different vibration modes. Comparison for the two settings (circular and rectangular membrane) of the theoretical model and the simulations.

Figure 6.8 shows an acceptable fit between the values found for each of the settings ("Circular EAP" and "Rectangular EAP"), using the theoretical model and the finite elements simulations. However, tests still need to be conducted with pre-prototypes and prototypes to make the calculations performed for these types of design more reliable.

We have used these examples to demonstrate the effectiveness of using a structured design methodology and the equations from theoretical models to pre-select concepts, materials and working principles and simulations for evaluating, purchasing and improving geometries.

It is also important carry out tests to verify, adjust and optimise the designs in a controlled manner.

Additional simulation tools can be adopted, such as Matlab–Simulink programs for evaluating the response of an electromechanical system, even under non-linear conditions, just as will be shown in the following chapter for designing an electroactive polymer-based system as sensors. Taking this example, applying the specific simulator for activation tasks is direct. The simulator only needs to be constructed in reverse (since the input is mechanical in the sensor and the output electrical and in the actuator the input is electrical and the response mechanical).

Simulink will prove to be a valuable tool throughout the handbook on many occasions. Its ability to simulate complex systems by combining simpler sub-systems is especially suited to designing "intelligent" or multifunctional-based devices.

6.3.5 Device Integration: *In vitro and in vivo* Tests

To supplement calculation and simulation tools it is essential to use prototypes for validating the designs produced (both *in vitro* and *in vivo*). For this reason, "rapid prototyping & manufacturing" technologies are becoming more important in industry, particularly in research work connected with product development.

As an example of their use, Fig. 6.9 shows a prototype of some tweezers fabricated by laser stereolithography. In this technology a laser beam photopolymerises an epoxy resin and constructs the parts layer by layer, following the CAD design guidelines programmed in the computer to guide the laser movement.

They are extremely versatile technologies that can be used to produce a wide range of complex geometry parts quickly and cheaply (at a prototype level) as a way of not only producing devices but also the casings and fittings required to test the device or to build test benches.

When the prototypes have been obtained, the electroactive polymer actuator is inserted into the zone designed for such. In this example, that zone is the tiny "legs" designed at the end opposite the pincer so that the *in vitro* tests can be conducted to verify the capabilities of the actuator as a movement guidance system, as Fig. 6.9 shows.

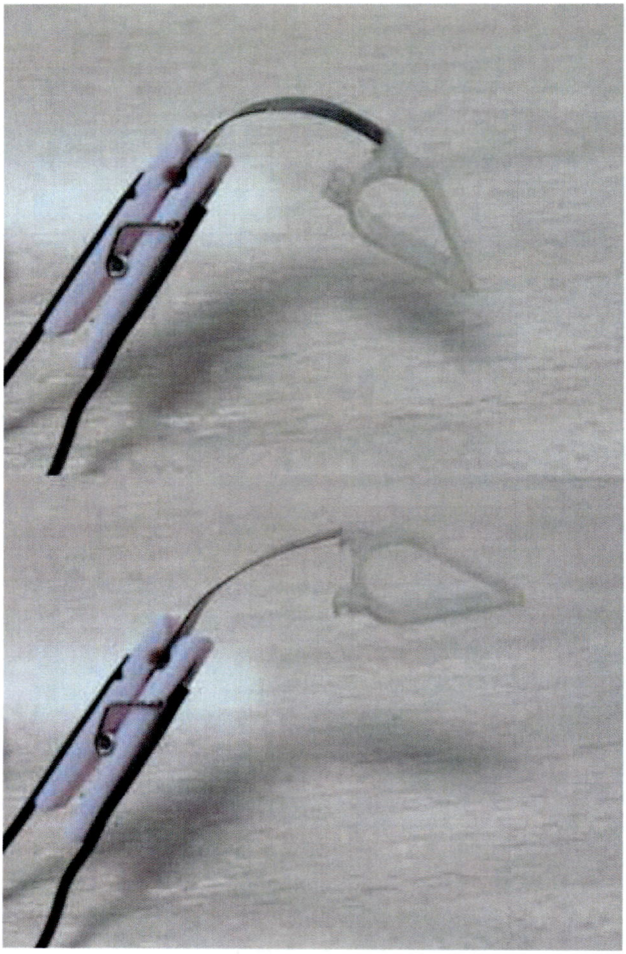

Figure 6.9 IPMC as an aid for active catheter development: Microtweezer guidance.

Once again, an "ionic polymer-metal composite" actuator was used supplied by Environmental Robots Inc., as part of one of its development kits. It can also be used for teaching as an introduction to research into these materials.

If active polymers are to be used as actuators or sensors on structures or metallic, ceramic, polymer or composite parts, it is advisable to use carefully chosen adhesives in accordance with the materials to be bonded and look for biocompatible adhesives, particularly for implantable devices.

The catalogues and online selectors of the leading manufacturers will be sufficient to make a good choice (Loctite, Henkel among others) whose web pages often offer manuals and examples of guided calculation to aid the choice of material and even parts design, especially in the bonding zone.

Should the actuators be for fluidic devices, the right insulation is important in order to prevent leakage. The connection zone on the electroactive polymer sides must be specially protected to avoid short-circuits when they come into contact with fluids, which could lead to impaired function.

To this end, elastomer coatings with pressure additives have proved to be effective, as can be seen from the various examples described in Chapters 7 and 8.

On the other hand, in order to strengthen the activation capabilities of devices like that shown in Fig. 6.9, antagonist actuators are often used (in the same way that the biological muscles of animals act), with one of them usually made to produce movement in a specific direction.

Automatic spring-based return systems can also be used as well as combining different actuators that are able to respond to different stimuli in order to produce multifunctional systems. When ionic electroactive polymers are used, automated drip or spray systems can be adopted to keep these polymers moist (e.g., IPMCs), especially for extracorporeal work where they will operate in a dry environment, which with the passage of time, may limit the forces generated or the attainable deformations.

6.4 Main Challenges and Research Trends

6.4.1 Enhancing Mechanical Response

For EAPs used as actuators

Although EAPs can be easily shaped, their properties can be acted on by using additives and can be integrated with other Microsystems to produce "intelligent actuators", there are many unsolved problems that limit their use.

Firstly, we will list the drawbacks related to the low activation force obtained and/or the small attainable deformations:

- Most electronic electroactive polymers need the application of strong electrical fields (around 100 V/μm for 5% deformations) which limits their use. With such high voltages, prototypes have been achieved that can lift up to hundreds of grams.
- Most ionic electroactive polymers reach much larger deformations than electronic polymers (90° bending with around 5–10 V power), but they can only lift a few grams. Their response speed is also slower, usually just a few Hz, compared to the kHz reached by some electronic polymers. They normally require "wet" activation, which prevents them from being used, although recent developments use electrolytes embedded in solid-paper supports.

Like all polymers, EAPs present ageing problems connected with the formation of new links between chains, which causes them to become stiff, thus restricting their use as actuators. Exposure to UV light and environmental conditions can also be a determining factor in the degradation of polymers (dissociation of bonds and fragility), so they have to be taken into account as well as an estimate made of the useful life of the device. The use of absorbent pigments and antioxidants may help solve these problems.

Behaviour under fatigue is also decisive to obtain devices subject to continuous and prolonged activation. Characterising the behaviour under fatigue of the different components of EAP families is one of the priority lines of research in the universities, companies and technology centres that develop applications for these materials.

The synthesis and transformation processes used need to be optimised if more robust materials are to be found with a greater activation capability. It can be useful to use chemical models and simulations for processing to predict the end properties according to the process parameters. More reliable and standardised methods for characterisation must also be used so that a data base can be created that documents the properties of EAPs to aid designers.

For EAPs used as sensors (additional information in the next chapter)

As for actuators, the use of EAPs in sensors presents ageing problems as the polymer gradually becomes stiffer and loses sensitivity. To prolong the life of the device some kind of behaviour model can be included in the microcontroller to regulate the system thresholds. Whatever the case, the useful life of the sensor must be estimated and the material to be used chosen as a result, but without losing sight of basic requirements like sensitivity and response speed.

The behaviour of the materials under fatigue is also decisive here and must be borne in mind in the behaviour models right from the design stage, taking test data to obtain long-lasting sensors. The environmental conditions the actuator will be operating in also need to be considered as metallic electrodes are easily oxidisable. Using Cr and Al or Pt and Au helps delay the process, but the films must be kept clean. Contact with the hands may dirty and slightly oxidise the electrodes, producing changes in resistance. However, the encapsulations limit the harmful effects of the external conditions and protect the devices.

Another important question concerning aging and behaviour under fatigue of EAP-based devices are the problems deriving from using metallic electrodes. As explained in the section on electrode deposition technologies (Section 6.3.2 and Chapter 13), the different coefficients of expansion between the base polymer and the deposited metal lead to the appearance of unwanted in-service stresses that accelerate the peeling and breaking of the deposited layer. On the other hand, the additional stiffness passed on to the polymers by the metallic electrodes restricts the movement of EAP-based actuators. Technologies such as ion implementation and the use of electrical point contacts may solve these problems.

In the specific case of piezoelectric polymers (PVDF and copolymers) used as pressure transducers, it must be borne in mind that these materials are also pyroelectric (charge displacement associated with temperature change), which means the repeated action of charges that leads to heating by hysteresis can affect measurements. Pyroelectricity, therefore, which is an interesting property for use in infrared detection sensors can be harmful for some applications and must be included in the behaviour models so that predictions can be made before developing the sensor. More thorough data bases of EAP properties, their standardised characterisation and the use of models that simulate the behaviour of different settings is crucial for the successful development of sensors based on these materials (as was the case for actuators).

6.4.2 Optimising the Power and Control Systems for Activation

Numerous types of electroactive polymers present some non-linearities and hysteresis effects that make it difficult to implement control systems that attain high precision, particularly in devices with a large number of actuators. In order to model these markedly complex systems in real time and manage their control systems, the use of artificial neural networks (ANN) has proved to be effective in some devices and microdevices, providing those ANN have been properly trained using test results (Arena *et al.*, 2002; Biddiss and Chau, 2006; Kim *et al.*, 2007). Proper, precise, real-time control is especially recommended for medical devices due to their enormous responsibility, since most of the research referred to is linked to biomedical developments.

As an example of the potential of these tools for modelling intelligent materials with high non-linear behaviour, the handbook includes a detailed example further on of quantum tunnelling composites modelling in Chapter 15.

6.4.3 Enhancing Synthesis and Manufacturing Processes

Since innovative materials are being dealt with (Nobel Prize for Chemistry in 2000 shared by Alan G. Mac Diarmid, Alan J. Heeger and Hideki Shirakawa), efforts are being made to adapt the conventional processes used for polymer material mass production to electroactive polymer production.

Software packages are also being produced that can predict properties according to the chemical structure of the polymers and simulation programs. These are similar to the programs used for the parts production of plastic materials that are used to make prior predictions about processing and speed up the development process of electroactive polymer-based systems.

This will lead to more affordable electroactive polymers to enable researchers and companies to "embark on" trying out rapidly manufactured cheap prototypes that could bring improvements to their products or conventional processes.

Attention is focusing on the use of microfabrication technologies that can be applied to polymer materials to produce smaller and smaller active components that can interact directly, even with isolated cells and microorganisms. Further information on some of the more marked processes is included in the references of the chapter (Ward and Bashir, 2001; Díaz Lantada, 2006).

6.4.4 Commercial Formulations

The interest aroused in the last decade by these kinds of polymer materials possessing special activation and detection capabilities is giving rise to the appearance of numerous companies, often spin-offs of universities. They are beginning to commercialise electroactive polymer formulations developed during research. The processes of synthesis and transformation are often clearly described in recent patents.

They are therefore subject to the restrictions of intellectual property as they are recent materials, but their use in specific devices can be sufficiently innovative to generate new product patents, the results of which can benefit not only the inventor of the material but also the inventor of the application.

So, when trying to solve a specific medical problem using a device that can activate through an electroactive polymer, it can be profitable to work in collaboration with material manufacturers. This can lead to a better final results quality, optimise time and costs and encourage the new system to be taken up by industry. However, the delivery time of the suppliers of these kinds of intelligent polymers must be taken into account, as sometimes the synthesis process is still done semi-manually and the fabrication of a few samples can often take a week or up to a month. This should be taken into account if the time frames of complex development projects are to be adhered to that involve a large amount of mutually dependent work.

Some researchers have proposed using very common polymer materials that have certain piezoelectric properties, like cellophane, to develop biodegradable prototypes (Je and Kim, 2004). This may be effective for preliminary conceptual prototypes with especially affordable materials (and quickly obtainable).

6.4.5 Biomimesis as a Source of Inspiration: Biological and Artificial Muscles

Biomimesis or Biomimetics is the application of natural systems and methods to solve the problems of seeking effective solutions to problems of Engineering and Technological Sciences. During its evolution Nature has designed a number of innovations far superior to what the human mind alone would have conceived, due to the fact that Nature has been contributing effective solutions to real-world problems over millions of years of trial and error (Dawkins, 2006, 2009).

Some of the main areas of research strategies for Biomimesis-related solutions are

- The imitation of structures and natural mechanisms
- The imitation of fabrication processes and biological recycling
- The imitation of energy management systems in Nature
- The imitations of the principles of organisation of organisms and micro-organisms

The observation of Nature (animal and vegetable) is a source of inspiration for a range of devices that use active materials as sensors or actuators. This is particularly so in the case of devices that use electroactive polymers, since their behaviour is similar in many ways to that of human muscles.

So, it is becoming habitual to design devices whose parts are bonded by at least two electroactive polymers that can achieve movements in opposite directions, as is the case with the animal joints that are the basis of these designs.

It is also recommendable to study the mechanical behaviour models of biological muscles, as these models can be suitable for analysing artificial muscle behaviour (based on the use of electroactive polymers), as with slight modifications these models can be used to adjust the behaviour of many synthetic formulations.

As an example, we will now describe a typical mechanical model frequently used to simulate biological muscle behaviour, Hill's model (Peterson and Bronzino, 2008), which is shown schematically in Fig. 6.10 and the equations of which are shown further on. It basically corresponds to a Kelvin-Maxwell model completed in parallel with an actuator that introduces the mechanical stress generated by the muscle, in accordance with time and the length of the muscle fibres.

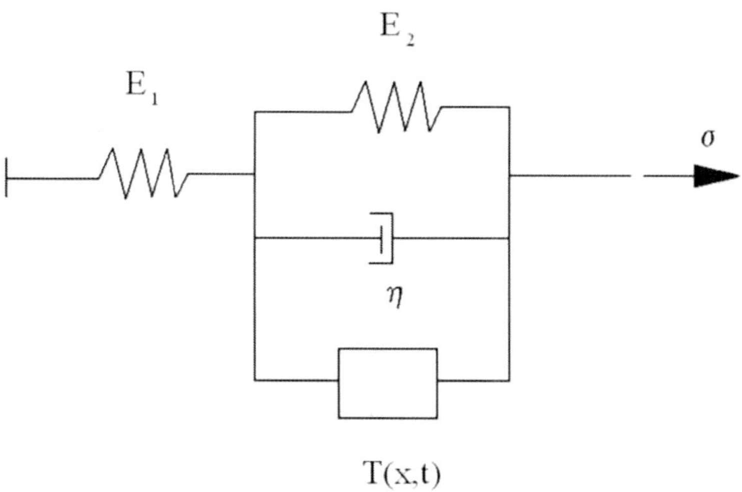

Figure 6.10 Typical human skeletal muscle model.

The deformation of the muscle subjected to a stress σ [N/m^2] and able to generate, in turn, a force T, is given, according to the model by the sum of two deformations ε_1 and ε_2, in which the elasticity moduli of the different muscle fibres E_1 and E_2 [N/m^2] play a special role, in addition to the parameter η [Pa· s] which marks the ease of displacement between fibres (essentially a dynamic viscosity). The set of ratios is shown below and has also been modelled with the aid of Simulink, in line with the outline in Fig. 6.11.

$$\begin{cases} \varepsilon(t) = \varepsilon_1(t) + \varepsilon_2(t) \\ \varepsilon_1 = \dfrac{\sigma_1}{E_1} \\ \sigma_2 = \sigma_1 = \sigma = \eta \dfrac{d\varepsilon_2}{dt} + E_2\varepsilon_2 + T_{musc}(\Delta l, t) \end{cases}$$

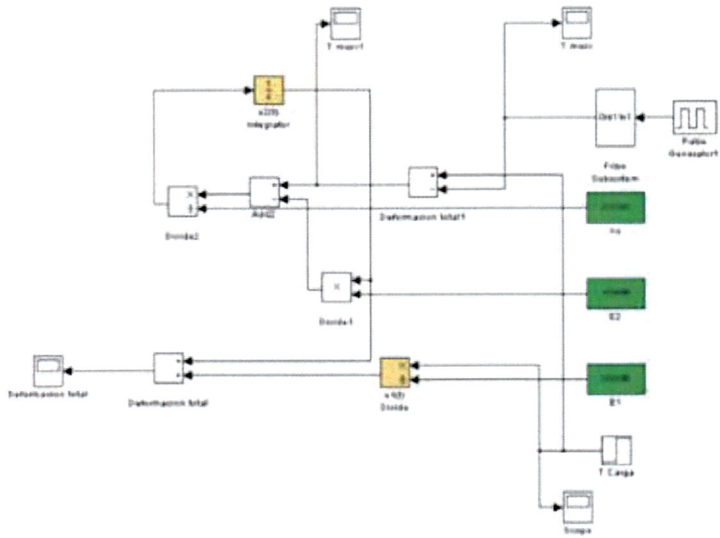

Figure 6.11 Simulink model in line with the preceding equations.

The two load models shown in Fig. 6.12, were simulated using the model, the first (upper image) associated with a muscle at rest subjected to a mechanical force and the second (lower image) associated with the contraction and relaxation of a muscle subjected to a mechanical force. The figure reveals some similarities with the behaviour of electroactive IPMCs, whose characterisation has been shown in preceding sections.

Similar models could possibly be applied to many synthetic active polymers and Simulink is a very apt tool for the gradual addition of aging effects, progressive stiffness, electro-mechanical couplings and other effects that complicate the analytical solving of the differential equations involved. In biological muscles some relationships are known between the developable forces and the attainable activation speed, as the following relation shows, but which can also be applied to some basic electroactive-based polymer actuators (and to other intelligent materials).

$$(T + a)\ v = b\ (T_0 - T)$$

where T is the generated mechanical stress, v is the activation speed and T_0, a and b, the fitting parameters according to muscle type.

Their inclusion in already implemented Simulink models is practically immediate, while their inclusion in differential equation systems increases the non-linearities and the complexity of the system, often resulting in changes to the analytical solution strategy or even the need to use numerical methods.

We think this is a parallel way of trying to reach a deeper understanding of the way biological and synthetic materials behave so as to be able to benefit from the progress in these fields in a combined manner.

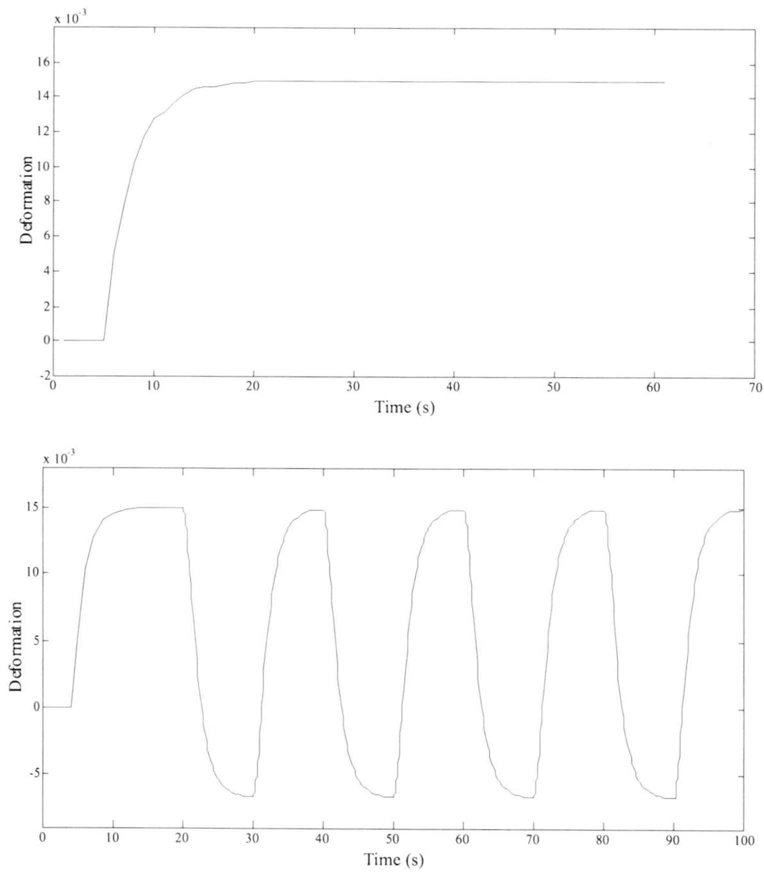

Figure 6.12 Results of simulating muscular fibre deformation over time: (A) Muscle at rest subjected to a mechanical force (person holding a weight). (B) Contraction and relaxation of a muscle subjected to a mechanical force (person doing weight-lifting).

Setting up online collaborative groups whose web pages gradually include data bases that help connect the demands for solutions to specific problems with technological supply, to solve these problems by using electroactive polymers (or other intelligent materials), could be an excellent tool to encourage collaboration between different universities, research centres and companies as a way of spreading the use of these materials in industry.

Major work has been done in this respect by Prof. Bar-Cohen through his web page (http://eap.jpl.nasa.go), although it can be complemented by other new sites devoted to more specific areas of application.

We must once again insist on the need to set up teams for device development where engineers who are experts in numerous branches of technology work in close collaboration, as well as professionals from various areas of health sciences and the fortunately ever increasing numbers of biomedical engineers, in order to strengthen the communication between team experts and lead these kinds of research projects.

If this is to become reality, it is important to gradually include electroactive polymer-related subjects (and "intelligent" materials in general) in the various Master's and PhD programs, in faculties of technology and biotechnology as well as in faculties of medicine and biology.

6.5 Improving Results and Conclusions

This chapter has focused on the main families of electroactive polymers and their specific applications as components in actuators for active medical devices, although the following chapter will continue with their applications as sensors.

The transformation processes that can be applied to EAPs have been detailed, dividing them into conventional processes and specific electrode deposition technologies, highlighting the benefits of using rapid prototyping technologies in combination with the information from using simulation tools for optimising the development of the associated devices and boosting the impact of these materials on industry.

After having closely examined the main problems of integrating electroactive polymers into "intelligent devices", it is clear that the improvement in most current processes combined with the progressive application of mass production processes for traditional electroactive polymers is key work for achieving an infrastructure that will enable the potential of these materials to be harnessed.

The current lines of research of the major technology centres, firms and universities related with the world of electroactive polymers is focused on the following aspects, all of which are complementary:

- The development of chemical models to predict material properties after synthesis.
- The development of models that simulate transformation processes, possibly by adapting the already existing programs for conventional materials (Moldflow, Magma Soft or Solidworks).
- The development of electromechanical models to predict the behaviour of EAP-based sensors and actuators.
- To enhance the transformation processes, including shaping, deposition, integration and miniaturisation techniques.
- To improve and standardise the testing and characterisation methods for these materials in order to find their properties and classify them better.
- To develop more complete data bases (and freely accessible) that include all the previous results to enable designers to select materials more simply and reliably.
- To search for new applications that will make the most of the unique benefits of these materials, in spite of their limitations.

Worldwide collaboration among researchers to spread the word (through web pages, handbooks and specialised journals, the organisation of monographic congresses and the gradual inclusion of these topics in technical university syllabuses) will prove essential in the coming years to encourage the use of these intelligent materials, and particularly electroactive polymers for their outstanding novelty.

Additional information can be found in the following list of references as well as in the websites of the different suppliers included in the annexes of the handbook. We hope this will be of use to researchers interested in these materials and their applications, as well as for establishing future contacts among research centres.

References

Arena, P.; Bonomo, C.; Fortuna, L.; Frasca, M. "Electro-active polymers as CNN actuators for locomotion control". IEEE International Symposium on Circuits and Systems, 4, 281–284, 2002.

Ashley, S. "Artificial muscles". Scientific American, 53–59, October, 2003.

Bar-Cohen, Y. "Electroactive polymers (EAP) characterization methods". Proceedings of SPIE's 7th Annual International Symposium on Smart Structures and Materials, 2000.

Bar-Cohen, Y. "Electroactive polymer (EAP) actuators as artificial muscles: Reality, potential and challenges". SPIE Press, 2nd Edition. Washington, 2004.

Biddiss, E.; Chau, T. "Electroactive polymeric sensors in hand prostheses: Bending response of an ionic polymer metal composite". Medical Engineering & Physics, 28(6), 568–578, 2006.

Blevins, R.D. "Formulas for natural frequency and mode shape". Litton Educational Publishing, 1979.

Cardoso, V.F.; Rocha, J.G.; Soares, F.O.; *et al.* "Lab-on-a-chip fluid acoustic microagitation: Piezoelectric polymer beta-PVDF used as ultrasonic transducer". International Conference on Biomedical Electronics and Devices Biostec 2008 – Biodevices, 2, 262–267.

Dawkins, R.- "The blind watchmaker". Penguin Books, 1986, reissue 2006.

Dawkins, R.- "The greatest show on earth, the evidence for Evolution". Spanish Edition, Espasa Calpe, S.A., 2009.

Díaz Lantada, A. "Procesos de transformación para polímeros electroactivos". Universidad Politécnica de Madrid, 2006.

Gad-el-Hak, M. "The MEMS Handbook". CRC Press. Florida, 2002.

Gisby, T.A.; Anderson, I.A.; Calius, E.P.; Xie, S. "Smart dielectric elastomers and their potential for biodevices". International Conference on Biomedical Electronics and Devices Biostec 2008 – Biodevices, 2, 285–290. IEEE Engineering in Medicine and Biology Society. 28th–31st January in Madeira. INSTICC Press, 2008.

Herr, H.; Kornbluh, R. "New horizons for orthotic and prosthetic technology: Artificial muscle for ambulation". Smart Structures and Materials 2004: Electroactive Polymer Actuators and Devices (EAPAD). Proceedings of the SPIE, 5385, 1–9, 2004.

Je, C.H.; Kim, K.J. "Cellophane as a biodegradable electroactive polymer actuator". Sensors and Actuators A: Physical, 112(1), 107–115, 2004.

Kim, H.J.; Shin, J.; Kang, S.; *et al.*- "Ionic electroactive polymer control using co-evolutionary optimisation". Electronic Letters, 43(16), 859860, 2007.

Koch, M.; Evans, A.; Brunnschweiler, A. "Microfluidic technology and applications". Research Studies Press Ltd., Philadelphia, 2000.

Kofold, G. "Dielectric Elastomer Actuators". Ph. D. Thesis 2001. The Technical University of Denmark.

Lafont Morgado, P.; Díaz Lantada, A.; Martínez Álvarez, A.; *et al.* "Dispositivos médicos basados en el empleo de polímeros electroactivos". 8° Congreso Iberoamericano de Ingeniería Mecánica. Pontificia Universidad Católica del Perú. 23–25 October in Cuzco, 2007.

Lafont Morgado, P.; Díaz Lantada, A.; Martínez Álvarez, A.; *et al.* "Instrumented splint for the diagnosis of bruxism". International Conference on Biomedical Electronics and Devices Biostec 2008 – Biodevices, 2, 216–222. IEEE Engineering in Medicine and Biology Society. 28–31 January in Madeira. INSTICC Press, 2008.

Maluf, N. "An introduction to microelectromechanical systems engineering". Artech House Inc., 2000.

Nye, J.F. "Physical properties of crystals: Their representation by tensors and matrices". Oxford University Press. Oxford, 1957, 1985, 2006.

Peterson, D.R.; Bronzino, J.D. "Biomechanics: Principles and applications". CRC Press, Taylor & Francis Group, 2008.

Santamarina Pol, P.; Santamarina Siruana, M.C. "Vibraciones Mecánicas en Ingeniería". Universidad Politécnica de Valencia, 1998.

Shahinpoor, M.; Kim, K. "Ionic polymer-metal composites: III. Modeling and simulation as biomimetic sensors, actuators, transducers and artificial muscles". Smart Materials and Structures, 13, 1362–1388, 2004.

Shahinpoor, M.; Kim, K. "Ionic polymer-metal composites: IV. Industrial and medical applications". Smart Materials and Structures, 14, 197–214, 2005.

Ward, J.; Bashir, R. "Micropatterning of biomedical polymer surfaces by novel UV polymerization techniques". Journal of Biomedical Materials Research, 56(3), 351–360, 2001.

Wong, J.Y.; Bronzino, J.D. "Biomaterials". CRC Press, Taylor & Francis Group, 2007.

Chapter 7

Electroactive Polymers as Sensors for Biodevices

Andrés Díaz Lantada and Pilar Lafont Morgado
Mechanical Engineering Department, E.T.S.I. Industriales, Universidad Politécnica de Madrid, c/ José Gutiérrez Abascal 2, 28006 Madrid, Spain
adiaz@etsii.upm.es, plafont@etsii.upm.es

7.1 Brief Introduction to Electroactive Polymers as Sensors

There are various types of polymers that can be called electroactive (depending on the type of stimulus received, either thermal, mechanical, chemical, optical or other). However, the concept of "electroactive" usually refers to materials with electro-mechanical coupling. We are therefore dealing with materials where the application of forces gives rise to the displacement of charges at their core. This enables them to be used as sensors where applying a voltage between the ends of the material leads to the appearance of deformations, which means they can be used as actuators.

This chapter will deal with the use of electroactive polymers as sensors, looking particularly carefully at how they can be used in the development of medical devices with enhanced diagnostic capabilities. Piezoelectric polymers will be analysed in greater detail due to their remarkably increasing number of applications as substitutes for

Handbook of Active Materials for Medical Devices: Advances and Applications
Edited by Andrés Díaz Lantada

www.panstanford.com

active ceramics. Mention will also be made of the potential possessed by piezoresistive polymers for certain tasks as well as the novel cellular ferroelectrets. The main operating principles of these types of sensors will be compared and comparisons of properties will be included to help in the process of selecting materials for devices and designing them.

In spite of their recent appearance, these electroactive polymers (especially piezoresistive ones) are replacing piezoelectric ceramics in many applications as sensors. The main reasons behind this interest in promoting the use of polymers as sensors are

- Their greater flexibility favours larger charge displacements at the core of the material than those achieved using piezoceramics.
- This flexibility and their ability to be shaped into very fine film makes it easy to integrate them into the end device as well as their easy adaptation to the surface over which the measurements will be taken.
- They possess a low dielectric constant, low density and a high resistance to impact, which makes them ideal as sensors.
- They are easier to process than ceramics as large areas can be obtained that can then be again cut and shaped to obtain complex forms.
- Their high resistance to high dielectric breakdown lets them withstand higher activation fields than ceramics. This is also positive for applications as actuators (based on the inverse piezoelectric effect).
- An absence of toxic components such as lead and rare earths in their composition is a plus for their use in the development of medical devices of a diagnostic nature.
- The recent appearance of suppliers that mass produce sensors based on this type of material, like those shown in Figs. 7.1 and 7.2, whose remarkable features and repeatability favour their use in responsibility devices.

The chapter contains a comparison of piezoelectric material properties (Table 7.1), ceramics as well as polymers, although ceramics are examined in more detail in Chapter 9, with an explanation of their capabilities, mainly as actuators but also as sensors.

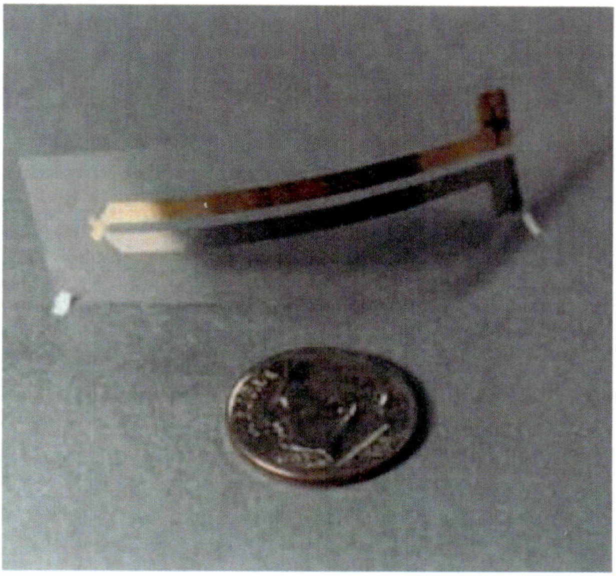

Figure 7.1 Example of EAP-based sensor. Ktech Corp. (ktech.com).

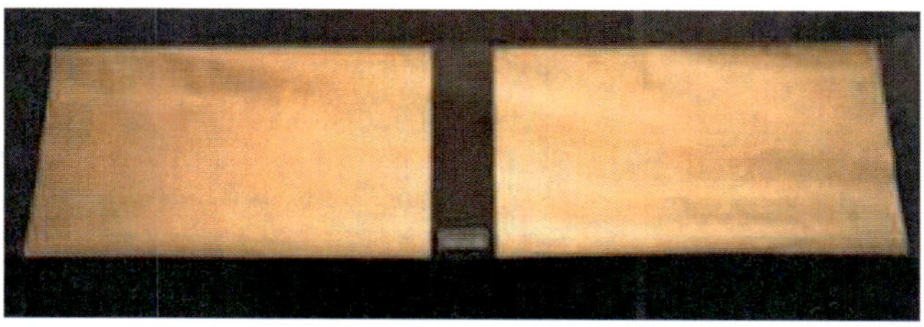

Figure 7.2 Metallised PVDF film. Piezotech S.A. (www.piezotech.fr).

As an aid to the development work for medical devices integrating these materials as sensors, we will show a detailed case study concerning the development of an intraoral device for measuring pressure. With the help of this case study different basic issues are explained that are connected with modelling, simulation, design, processing, material and device characterisation, *in vitro* and *in vivo* tests and pre-commercial validation.

We hope the methodology shown will be of interest to researchers working on these issues. The references included at the end of the chapter provide very detailed information on the different aspects of the development process set out. The characteristics sheets provided by the suppliers mentioned in the chapter and the annexes to the handbook must be very carefully borne in mind when comparing alternatives and selecting candidate materials for a specific application.

The following section begins with a review of the main applications of these polymers as sensors in medical or health-oriented devices, many of which have passed the *in vivo* test stage and have reached the pre-marketing stage or are already on the market.

7.2 Potential for Biodevices

Biomedical applications of these kinds of materials are mainly related to their being used as pressure/force sensors. Below are explained some specific proposals for developing medical devices based on the use of electroactive polymers (normally piezoelectric polymers) as sensors, most of which have undergone *in vitro* laboratory testing. After undergoing *in vitro* and animal *in vivo* testing and meeting the requirements for official approval, in some cases their commercialisation is subject to their attaining the goals described at the end of this chapter.

Pressure sensors for dentistry

As part of the "FEMAB" project of Madrid Polytechnic University, a pressure sensor has been developed with applications in dentistry for diagnosing and treating bruxism (Lafont Morgado and Díaz Lantada, 2008, 2009), based on the use of PVDF piezoelectric film. This film is marketed with the electrodes already in position, usually Au or Pt, by companies like "Piezotech S.A." or "KTech Corp.".

Pressure sensors for monitoring lesions

On occasions, it is advisable to integrate sensors, normally pressure sensors, into orthetic or prosthetic devices to study the evolution of different lesions that change the normal movement patterns of patients. These systems help to verify when a balanced state is reached that shows the damaged organ has recovered.

Piezoelectric polymers are also used inside special footwear to enable the user's footsteps to be analysed to detect any problems and check improvements using orthopaedic apparatus or prostheses (Aguado and González, 1995; Brady *et al.*, 2006).

Sensor gloves

In many tasks involving orthopaedic surgery and physiotherapy, particularly in the area of paediatrics, the availability of sensor gloves

means the specialist can know the intensity of the massages applied at any instant as well as receive a warning in cases where there is a potential harm for the patient. When dealing with the newborn or babies they are especially useful during examinations. The small size of polymer piezoelectric sensors together with their remarkable flexibility has opened up the way to their being integrated into textiles to develop this kind of device and also as an aid to the blind (Bailey–Van Kuren, 2005; Wagner, 2006).

Cochlear implants

These are high-precision, high-tech active implantable health products that help bring back hearing to persons whose cilia cells of the cochlea are damaged -whose mission is to send coded information to the brain- by stimulating the ganglionar cells (of the auditory nerve). The capability of piezoelectric materials to generate charges in response to mechanical stimuli, such as pressure waves, makes them clear candidates for transducers for this type of device, combined with their small size when incorporating the typical functionalities of the active materials already mentioned.

Electroactive polymers have recently been used as parts of cochlear implants with promising results for enhancing sensitivity, durability and the body's response as well as the quality/price ratio of those already available (Mukherjee, 2003).

Haptic devices

Teleoperators are used to control tools remotely. In these cases, the resistant contact forces need to return to the teleoperator. This is called "haptic teleoperation". When these devices are used with a user by means of computer guided simulation, it is important to provide the return force that could be felt in real operations. As the objects to be handled do not actually exist in these cases, the haptic forces generated as user return force must provide a sensation of the environment.

Haptic simulators have a wide application in training for surgical operations. They are useful for attempting to minimise the damage caused by the use of invasive procedures (laparoscopy/intervention radiology) and allow operations to be performed remotely. Electroactive polymers have been used for the sensor part that detects contact with the object being manipulated as well as for the active part that generates the return force of these devices, in various research centres like NASA's Jet Propulsion Laboratory (Bar-Cohen, 2006) or the Research Centre of EAP Devices in Switzerland.

"Haptic" scalpels have also been developed intended for enhancing precision in surgical tasks (not remote in this case but conventional), as described in other documents (Schena, 2008) and which are currently being marketed by Inmersion Corp.

The different devices explained will provide (and some are already providing) considerable diagnostic benefits, compared to conventional devices, due to their capability to sense inside or beside the body, thanks to the use of electroactive polymers as sensors.

7.3 Current Capabilities and Recent Advances

Set out below are some of the main advances achieved in recent decades concerning electroactive polymer sensors and the technologies associated with their use. The study focuses on piezoelectric polymers as a representative example of this kind of material, since these are the most used as sensors, particularly PVDF (and its copolymers). However, some consideration is also given to the use of other materials that possess a wide range of applications for the future with respect to diagnostic devices, as do pseudo-ferroelectric polymers and cellular ferroelectrets.

As a case study to show the full development of a medical device based on the properties of these materials, using state-of-the-art technologies, we have taken the example of a splint for detecting intraoral pressures for the early diagnosis of bruxism and other occlusal pathologies.

As a brief introduction we can say that bruxism is a condition consisting of a usually involuntary clenching or grinding of the teeth that generally leads to wear on the teeth, orofacial pain and additional problems in the temperomandibular joint and even the neck. The condition is prevalent in between 10% and 20% of the adult population and diagnosis is usually based on aspects of dental wear when the teeth are already worn and the prognosis of the condition is more severe. In order to be able to diagnose the condition earlier, faster, more effectively and save dental costs, we propose that instrumented splints should be designed and used for a precise detection and recording of the intensity and duration of interdental pressure episodes, and that are also sensitive to different types of bruxism.

Such a device, which we have included here as a case study, can also be used for carrying out studies to go more deeply into the different factors associated with bruxism and even reach a quantitative definition of the condition.

If careful attention is paid to the issues set out in the case study, similar development processes can be applied to the production of all kinds of instrumented prostheses and implants intended for measuring the forces or contact pressures between different parts of the body, providing the piezoelectrics are carefully chosen and the signal is adjusted properly to the range of forces or pressures involved.

7.3.1 Synthesis and processing of piezoelectric polymers

Synthesis

Poly(vinylidene fluoride) or PVDF $-(CH_2 - CF_2)_n-$ is synthesised from vinylidene fluoride, VDF, by means of a process of free radical polymerisation. The process can be initiated by various initiators or by the action of a source of radiation over the gaseous VDF. However, due to the large amount of energy liberated during polymerisation, more controlled polymerisations in emulsion or suspension are usually used (according to procedures described in detail in references such as Jungnickel (1996)).

The material thus obtained is in an α phase, not a piezoelectric phase and has many applications for the manufacture of pipes and plumbing components due to its high resistance to corrosion by acids, bases and UV radiation. It is also marketed as a powder (KYNAR 500 or HYLAR 5000) for the production of high quality paints for protecting metals, like those used in the construction of the Petronas Towers (Kuala Lumpur, Malaysia) or the Taipei 101 building (Taipei, Taiwan).

However, if it is to be used to design active devices that make use of its piezoelectric (or pyroelectric) sensor capabilities, it needs additional processing to induce its change to phase β that has the required properties, as we shall now see.

Processing

The outstanding piezoelectric (Kawai, 1969) and pyroelectric properties (Bergman *et al.*, 1971) of poly(vinylidene fluoride) or PVDF (and its copolymers) is obtained by inducing a change in its initially randomly oriented crystalline structure (phase α), so as to reach the ferroelectric phase β. By stretching the PVDF film in a 4:1 ratio using a traction machine, we pass from the PVDF phase to the β phase that has very marked piezoelectric properties.

Stretching in both directions helps get a more uniform thickness, increases isotropy and gives greater stability to phase β. Once stretched, the film is polymerised through the action of a very strong electric field (around 2000 V/m), to force the dipoles to face the same direction, which helps enhance the final properties of the sensor.

PVDF in its β phase presents both piezoelectric properties (suitable for pressure sensors) and pyroelectric properties (suitable for temperature sensors, as explained in Chapter 8). In addition, its pyroelectric coefficients let forces be measured in different directions, as will be explained further on.

Depending on whether electro-mechanical or electro-thermal coupling is used to produce sensors, ferroelectric polymers have different fields of application. This has led us to dedicate almost two complete chapters (7 and 8) to these materials, separating the study according to the sizes involved, but achieving a general performance model.

To obtain the sensors used in the following sections on characterisation, conditioning, integration and tests, we took 40 μm thick poly(vinylidene fluoride) PVDF biaxially stretched film (Bi-ax. PVDF) (that was subjected to the above process) from Piezotech S.A., with Au-Pt electrodes deposited by sputtering, as Fig. 7.3 shows. The basic characteristics are set out in the following table that lets the PVDF properties (uniaxially and biaxially stretched) be compared with those of the poly(vinylidene fluoride–trifluoroethylene) copolymer or P(VDF–TrFE).

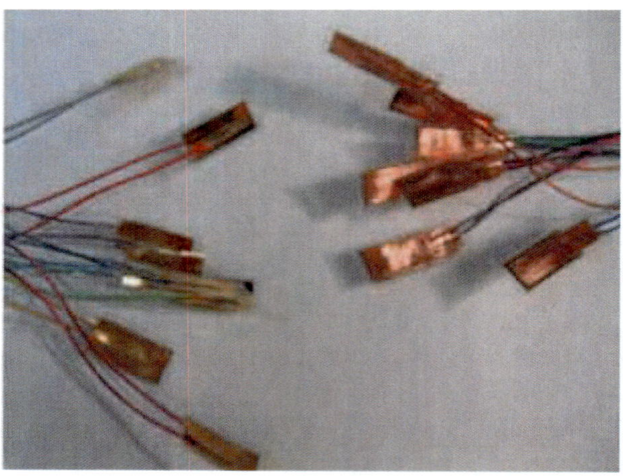

Figure 7.3 Piezoelectric sensors with preliminary connections and encapsulation.

Table 7.1 Typical Values of the Properties of Some Piezoelectric Polymers

	d_{33} (pC/N)	d_{31} (pC/N)	d_{32} (pC/N)	ϵ (F/m)
Uni-ax. "PVDF"	−20	18	3	$1{,}1{\cdot}1^{-10}$
Bi-ax. "PVDF"	−24	7	7	$1{,}1{\cdot}1^{-10}$
P(VDF-TrFE)	−24	7	7	$0{,}9{\cdot}1^{-10}$

This film was cut, joined to the connecting cables and thoroughly encapsulated to protect it, testing different coatings, as Fig. 7.3 shows, to obtain the characterised sensors that will be used further on in the design example.

These materials reach a temperature called the Curie temperature, above which they lose their polarisation, which means their use as sensors is limited at the top end. However, with the PVDF used the loss of piezo- and pyroelectric properties begins from 80°C.

With copolymers such as P(VDF-TrFE), the loss of polarisation begins from 110°C, in which circumstance the size of the additional fluoride atom directly aids crystallisation in phase β. However, the dielectric constant of the material in this last example is somewhat less and leads to a drop in the capability to generate a charge.

In any case, throughout the process to incorporate the sensors into the devices being produced (the intraoral splint in this case) this issue must be kept in mind and care taken not to exceed this temperature.

7.3.2 Characterisation and Modelling of Piezoelectric Polymers

Basic equations of piezoelectricity

One of the bases for using piezoelectric materials is a detailed analysis of the basic equations (the result of many characterisations) to be able to model and predict their behaviour. As will be shown below, apart from helping in future decisions about the design of a specific device, these equations are of enormous help when selecting the materials that are suitable for the application under development.

A brief summary of these equations is included here and are referred to in various sections of the book. However, more specific references can be consulted if more information is required (Nye, ed., 2006; Bar-Cohen, 2006; Hafez, 2006; IEEE Standards on Piezoelectricity).

We can firstly take the one-dimensional electromechanical and isotropic behaviour of this kind of material that is governed by different laws.

Hooke's law. In a solid body subjected to traction, the stress σ [N/m^2] is proportional to the longitudinal deformation ε [m/m] = $\Delta l/l$, where l is the original length and Δl the increase in length according to Hooke's law:

$$\sigma = E \cdot \varepsilon, \text{ sometimes represented as } \varepsilon = s \cdot \sigma$$

E is the elasticity modulus of the material or the Young modulus, and s [m^2/N] = $1/E$ is the elasticity or the "elastic compliance" in the references cited.

It must be pointed out that the materials only behave in this linear manner below the elastic limit and there are numerous exceptions to this kind of behaviour.

Electric displacement. In an isotropic medium, the electric displacement field $\boldsymbol{D}$ [C/m^2] is proportional to the electric field $\boldsymbol{E}$ [V/m] in the following ratio:

$$\boldsymbol{D} = \epsilon \cdot \boldsymbol{E} = \epsilon_0 \cdot \epsilon_r \cdot \boldsymbol{E} = \epsilon_0 \cdot (1 + \chi) \cdot \boldsymbol{E}$$

where

ϵ. is the electric permittivity of the material [F/m];
$\epsilon_{0,}$ the electric permittivity of the vacuum [F/m];
$\epsilon_{r,}$ the relative permittivity [F/m]; and
χ, the dimensional electric susceptibility of the material.

The direct piezoelectric effect. Piezoelectric materials generally show additional electric displacement (called polarisation in some references) $\boldsymbol{P}$ [C/m^2], which is proportional to the force σ [N/m^2] applied, whose constant of proportionality d [C/N] is the so-named electric coefficient, as can be seen from the following equation:

$$\boldsymbol{P} = d \cdot \sigma$$

Therefore, these materials have a total electric displacement that is given by

$$\boldsymbol{D} = d \cdot \sigma + \epsilon \cdot \boldsymbol{E}$$

In materials with spontaneous polarisation, this must be included in the foregoing equation as the addend, and the above-mentioned polarisation can only be interpreted as a change in the polarisation of the material due to mechanical effects.

The inverse piezoelectric effect. Piezoelectric materials also show an additional deformation ε [m/m] that is proportional to the electric field applied $\boldsymbol{E}$ [V/m], whose coefficient of proportionality is once again d [C/N]. Therefore, the total deformation in these materials is given by

$$\varepsilon = s \cdot \sigma + d \cdot \boldsymbol{E}$$

Taking the three directions of space and extending the above to anisotropic materials, the above one-dimensional equations can be generalised in the following written tensorial form (omitting the summations according to the Einstein notation). In these, the subscripts i, j, k, l, can take on the values 1, 2, 3, to refer to the different directions of space. According to convention the third direction is usually chosen parallel to the direction of polarisation of the material.

$$\sigma = E \cdot \varepsilon \rightarrow \varepsilon_{ij} = s_{ijkl}\, \sigma_{kl}$$

$$\boldsymbol{D} = \epsilon \cdot \boldsymbol{E} \rightarrow D_i = \epsilon_{ij}\, E_j$$

$$\boldsymbol{P} = d \cdot \sigma \rightarrow P_i = d_{ijk}\, \sigma_{jk}$$

$$\varepsilon = d \cdot \boldsymbol{E} \rightarrow \varepsilon_{jk} = d_{ijk}\, E_i$$

In these equations the 81 s_{ijkl} elements constitute a fourth order tensor, the 27 piezoelectric coefficients d_{ijk} constitute a third order tensor and the 9 coefficients of σ_{jk}, ϵ_{ij}, ε_{ij}, constitute 3 third order tensors.

Thanks to the existence of symmetries, instead of the tensorial notation it is usual to use a simplified matrix notation or Voigt notation to study these phenomena so as to reduce the number of subscripts used, with more compact equations being obtained.

The procedure is summarised here, although the references mentioned may be consulted for greater detail. Specifically, of the nine components of the force and deformation matrices, only six are independent and the following change of subscripts can be made in these matrices, which leads to these matrices being vectorised:

$11 \rightarrow 1$	$22 \rightarrow 2$	$33 \rightarrow 3$
23 and 32 $\rightarrow 4$	31 and 13 $\rightarrow 5$	12 and 21 $\rightarrow 6$

Likewise, the last two suffixes of the tensors s_{ijkl}, y, d_{ijk} are replaced, which results in the constitutive equations being expressed as

$$\{\mathbf{S}\} = [\mathbf{s}]\,\{\mathbf{T}\} + [\mathbf{d}]^t\,\{\mathbf{E}\}$$
$$\{\mathbf{D}\} = [\mathbf{d}]\,\{\mathbf{T}\} + [\epsilon]\,\{\mathbf{E}\}$$

where

$\{\mathbf{S}\}$ is the strain vector;
$\{\mathbf{T}\}$, the stress vector;
$\{\mathbf{E}\}$, the electric field vector;
$\{\mathbf{D}\}$, the electric displacement vector;
$[\mathbf{s}]$, the elasticity matrix or the "elastic compliance matrix" of the material;
$[\mathbf{d}]$, the piezoelectric coefficients matrix;
$[\mathbf{d}]^t$, the transfer piezoelectric coefficients matrix; and
$[\epsilon]$, the matrix of the electric permittivity of the material.

This can be rewritten as follows, in accordance with the components of each vector or matrix:

$$\begin{Bmatrix} S_1 \\ S_2 \\ S_3 \\ S_4 \\ S_5 \\ S_6 \end{Bmatrix} = \begin{bmatrix} s_{11} & s_{12} & s_{13} & s_{14} & s_{15} & s_{16} \\ s_{21} & s_{22} & s_{23} & s_{24} & s_{25} & s_{26} \\ s_{31} & s_{32} & s_{33} & s_{34} & s_{35} & s_{36} \\ s_{41} & s_{42} & s_{43} & s_{44} & s_{45} & s_{46} \\ s_{51} & s_{52} & s_{53} & s_{54} & s_{55} & s_{56} \\ s_{61} & s_{62} & s_{63} & s_{64} & s_{65} & s_{66} \end{bmatrix} \begin{Bmatrix} T_1 \\ T_2 \\ T_3 \\ T_4 \\ T_5 \\ T_6 \end{Bmatrix} + \begin{bmatrix} d_{11} & d_{12} & d_{13} \\ d_{21} & d_{22} & d_{23} \\ d_{31} & d_{32} & d_{33} \\ d_{41} & d_{42} & d_{43} \\ d_{51} & d_{52} & d_{53} \\ d_{61} & d_{62} & d_{63} \end{bmatrix} \begin{Bmatrix} E_1 \\ E_2 \\ E_3 \end{Bmatrix}$$

$$\begin{Bmatrix} D_1 \\ D_2 \\ D_3 \end{Bmatrix} = \begin{bmatrix} d_{11} & d_{12} & d_{13} & d_{14} & d_{15} & d_{16} \\ d_{21} & d_{22} & d_{23} & d_{24} & d_{25} & d_{26} \\ d_{31} & d_{32} & d_{33} & d_{34} & d_{35} & d_{36} \end{bmatrix} \begin{Bmatrix} T_1 \\ T_2 \\ T_3 \\ T_4 \\ T_5 \\ T_6 \end{Bmatrix} + \begin{bmatrix} \epsilon_{11} & \epsilon_{12} & \epsilon_{13} \\ \epsilon_{21} & \epsilon_{22} & \epsilon_{23} \\ \epsilon_{31} & \epsilon_{32} & \epsilon_{33} \end{bmatrix} \begin{Bmatrix} E_1 \\ E_2 \\ E_3 \end{Bmatrix}$$

The piezoelectric coefficients matrix of a material contains many null terms depending on the material's class of crystallography, as other studies have shown (Nye, ed., 2006). This fact has some fundamental implications when choosing a material to be used as an electromechanical transducer in a specific application.

As an example of this importance, we can briefly analyse the use of a piezoelectric sensor in the form of a film whose surface is perpendicular to direction "3" of polarisation. In these film sensors, the voltage is usually measured between the two sides of the film. Therefore, a traction (or compression) in the "1" direction generates a voltage in the direction of polarisation in line with the d_{31} coefficient, a traction in direction "2" generates a voltage in the direction of polarisation in line with the d_{32} coefficient and a traction in direction "3" generates a voltage in the direction of polarisation in line with the value of coefficient d_{33}.

If the d_{33} coefficient were to be null, this film could not be used to measure the perpendicular pressures on its surface, which is necessary for finding intraoral pressures.

Likewise, there are other piezoelectric materials that do not allow measuring shear stress or that can only be used as actuators in one direction. Shown below are the coefficient matrices for the two materials belonging to different crystal classes, the above one PVDF (orthorhombic class mm^2 crystallography phase β polymer) and below the quartz one (hexagonal phase β, with crystal class 622), in which the right directions for measuring pressures can be verified by a visual inspection (Nye, ed., 2006).

$$\begin{pmatrix} 0 & 0 & 0 & 0 & d_{15} & 0 \\ 0 & 0 & 0 & d_{24} & 0 & 0 \\ d_{31} & d_{32} & d_{33} & 0 & 0 & 0 \end{pmatrix} \quad \text{PVDF piezoelectric matrix}$$

$$\begin{pmatrix} 0 & 0 & 0 & d_{14} & 0 & 0 \\ 0 & 0 & 0 & 0 & -d_{14} & 0 \\ 0 & 0 & 0 & 0 & 0 & 0 \end{pmatrix} \quad \text{Quartz piezoelectric matrix}$$

This often influences choosing poly(vinylidene fluoride) or PVDF as a sensor. In its phase β, this material is ferroelectric and therefore possesses piezoelectric properties and its piezoelectric coefficients allow measuring stress in different directions. The material has remarkable medical applications, as can be seen in the section on *in vivo* tests.

Characterisation: Typical procedures and equipment

The mechanical and piezoelectric properties of piezoelectric material can be found by different methods of characterisation, some of which are set out in the IEEE Standards on Piezoelectricity. There are also some standard shapes for the samples for these procedures.

The choice of techniques to be used is highly dependent on the shapes of the samples and the available instruments, for which reason it is not advisable to recommend just one measuring technique.

To supplement the information given in this book it is important to consult the documents produced by the IEC (International Electrotechnical Commission) and CENELEC (European Committee for Electrotechnical Standardization), with particularly excellent documents for the study of multilayer materials with piezoelectric properties intended for the development of sensors and actuators, also with application for the development of medical devices.

The first experiments with piezoelectric materials determined the elastic and piezoelectric constants by using static tests, charging the samples and reading the displacements and charges or voltages generated.

However, due to the problems of controlling the shaping conditions, as very thin piezoelectric film was used, (tens of microns), static tests are becoming obsolete for characterising new materials.

Notwithstanding, when characterising the behaviour of these materials as parts of more complex devices, the static tests using ad hoc test benches, like those shown in preceding sections, continue to be of interest and are sufficiently accurate for most applications.

When characterising new piezoelectric materials greater accuracy is usually had by using dynamic tests that also enable the behaviour of more complex geometries to be evaluated. The electrical properties of the piezoelectric resonators or vibrators are dependent on the mechanical or piezoelectric properties of the material subjected to vibration and on the geometry of the vibrating sample.

The values of the mechanical and piezoelectric constants can therefore be found by making samples with specific geometries vibrate (by subjecting them to a frequency scan) and comparing the measures taken with known behaviour models. Measuring basically consists in finding the electrical impedance of the resonators according to frequency.

Additional information on characterisation can be found in the following subsections, as well as in the references included at the end of the chapter.

7.3.3 Aspects Related to Signal Conditioning of Piezoelectric Polymers

The two most usual working modes for a piezoelectric or pyroelectric sensor are in an open circuit or a short circuit (as specified in the "Piezo Film Technical Manual" of "Measurement Specialties"). In the first case the metallised faces of the sensor are used as the armatures of a condenser and the voltage resulting from the charge generated ($V = Q/C$) between them is measured (open circuit) using an electrometric amplifier. This electrometric amplifier consists of a voltage amplifier with an input resistance of more than 1 TΩ and an input current of less than 1 pA. In the second case, the sensor always "sees" a voltage of 0 V between its faces and transfers the charge to a condenser of known value where the voltage drop ($V = Q/C$) between armatures is measured. In every case, the use of operational amplifiers supplies a low impedance voltage output that can continue to be processed easily.

Measuring the voltage drop over the sensor itself presents several problems. The capacity of the sensor has a high tolerance due to the fact that it not only depends on the physical characteristics of the PVDF film used, but also on the elements surrounding it and its spatial shape. Also, in order to find the capacity over which the charge is distributed we also need to add the capacity of the connecting wires and the amplifier input. All this causes the dispersion of the device's sensitivity to be high.

However, using a charge amplifier the voltage between the sensor terminals is kept permanently at zero. This eliminates the effect of any parasite capacities and resistance. Moreover, the charge is transferred to a condenser of known capacity and tolerance which means the dispersion sensitivity is less than if working with an open circuit and it is not necessary to impose any especially rigorous conditions on the manufacture of the medical device. A charge amplifier was chosen for the developed prototype in the case study set out here due to its advantages. More details regarding the amplifier components and other conditioning systems can be found in the references (Lafont *et al.*, 2008, 2009; Martínez *et al.*, 2010).

It is especially important to consider the effects of the charge amplifier when predicting and modelling the device's behaviour as the use of appropriate models can be of help for choosing the various conditioning components.

The model specified below taken from a system for measuring intraoral pressures is a direct result of the basic piezoelectricity equations already explained, although certain simplifications have been made regarding the direction of stress. Other simplified models have also been used to model the conditioning electronics, particularly the charge amplifier, following certain suggestions in the "Piezo Film Technical Manual" of "Measurement Specialties".

However, certain considerations concerning the joint modelling of the stiffness and damping of the protective coatings together with some issues concerning the application of stress on the measuring system are a novel contribution and enable a proper fit of the model to be achieved.

Figure 7.4 shows a diagram of a piezoelectric sensor subjected to a normal charge on its surface. The resulting charge displacements on applying a force to the piezoelectric sensor can be represented by the equivalent electric circuit, which is also depicted. In essence, the material behaves as an intensity generator that supplies a condenser in proportion to the force applied. When connected to an external circuit, this condenser discharges in proportion to the equivalent resistance of that circuit.

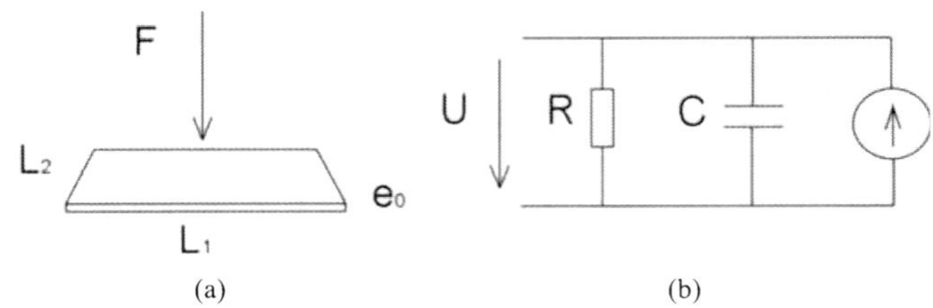

Figure 7.4 (A) Piezoelectric sensor. (B) Circuit diagram of piezoelectric sensor model.

The force F [N] on the sensor acts as an intensity generator to power a condenser of C [F] capacity in accordance with the expression:

$$C = C(F) = \epsilon \cdot (L_1 \cdot L_2)/e$$

where

ϵ is the electric permittivity of the sensor;

$L_1 \cdot L_{2,}$ the effective area of the sensor; and

e the sensor thickness.

In turn, the thickness of the sensor, e [m], is dependent on the initial thickness, e_0 [m], of the pressure applied, σ [Pa] and on the material's elasticity modulus, E [N/m^2], through the following expressions:

$$\sigma = F/(L_1 \cdot L_2); \qquad e = e_0 \cdot (1 - \sigma/E)$$

The current intensity, I [A], generated by applying the force F, is dependent on the transversal piezoelectric coefficient of the sensor d_{33} [C/N] according to:

$$Q = d_{33} \cdot F \rightarrow I = dQ/dt = d_{33} \cdot dF/dt$$

When the sensor is connected to an external circuit, the latter is discharged in proportion to the equivalent resistance R of this external circuit (the input resistance to the oscilloscope in the first tests performed). The intensity thus generated is given by the expression:

$$I = d_{33} \cdot dF/dt = U/R + C \cdot dU/dt$$

where U [V] is the voltage received by the circuit connected to the sensor.

These equations can be simply modelled using programs like Simulink – Matlab, that allow simulating complex systems through the successive connection of sub-systems.

When simulating the pressure inputs on the sensor (successive bites) it is important to keep in mind that "step" type pressure signals do not correspond to real physical events, since although the perpendicular episodes of bruxism are produced suddenly, this muscular contraction is never instantaneous. On the other hand, the sensors receive a slightly dampened signal that is delayed by the effect of the viscoelastic properties of the materials forming the various protective coatings used and the PVDF itself.

In order to take account of these effects, a one-degree-of-freedom mechanical subsystem with mass, stiffness and damping is included in the model. This subsystem allows the "Simulink" square wave generator to be adapted to the signal that is actually received by the sensor (free of perpendicular flanks), as Fig. 7.5 shows.

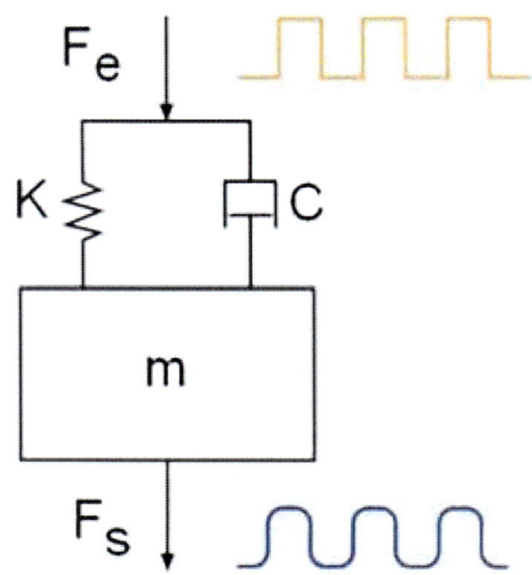

Figure 7.5 Damping subsystem diagram.

The main values associated with the use of conditioning electronics also need to be incorporated, particularly the value of the input resistance marking the velocity of piezoelectric discharge and the value of the capacity of the reference condenser C_f that determines the amplification obtained, in accordance with the following equations:

$U = Q/C_f$ (open circuit voltage)

The sensor thus amplified presents a $1/C_f$ amplification factor and a time constant $R \cdot C_f$ ("Measurement Computing", Elwenspoek and Wiegerink, 2001), which lead to a behaviour in line with the following equation:

$$d_{33} \cdot (dF/dt) \cdot (1\ [F]/C_f) = U/R + C_f \cdot dU/dt$$

(it marks how the voltage evolves in the actual circuit)

Figure 7.6 shows the block diagram for the full model. It includes the modifications due to the use of amplification and conditioning as well as the mentioned subsystem to fit the square wave generated using "Simulink" to the actual pressure acting on the surface of the sensor.

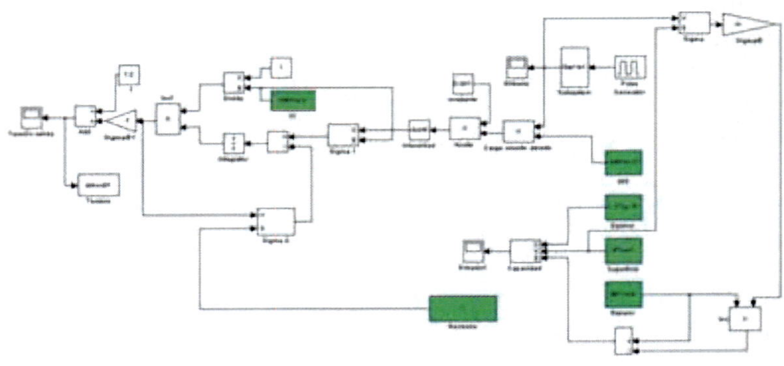

Figure 7.6 Improved electromechanical model.

This model and various simulations have helped estimate the right values for the charge amplifier condenser in the 1 to 100 nF range and the input resistance value at around 10 TΩ. The values finally chosen were as a result of the *in vitro* and *in vivo* tests that are set out in the following sub-sections. They also allowed validating the proposed behaviour model with a view to future redesign work.

Figure 7.7 shows a simulation of a splint calibration procedure. This procedure, as explained in the final *in vitro* tests, consists in placing the splint on a test bench and subjecting it to square pressure signals and supplying the pneumatic muscles of this bench with 1, 2, 3 and 4 bar and carrying out different repetitions for each intensity.

To simulate this calibration procedure, the pressure powering the pneumatic muscles needs to be converted into force applied to the sensor. To do this, the calibration straight line of the pneumatic muscles operating the test bench is used in combination with the test bench geometry data set out in the following sub-section.

Figure 7.7 shows the simulated results of the sensor response for pneumatic muscle power supply pressures of 1, 2, 3 and 4 bar corresponding to the forces on each sensor integrated into the splint of around 290, 550, 820 and 1080 N, respectively.

Each of the three repetitions shows the simulated response compared with the application of these forces. The increasing voltages correspond to higher pressures.

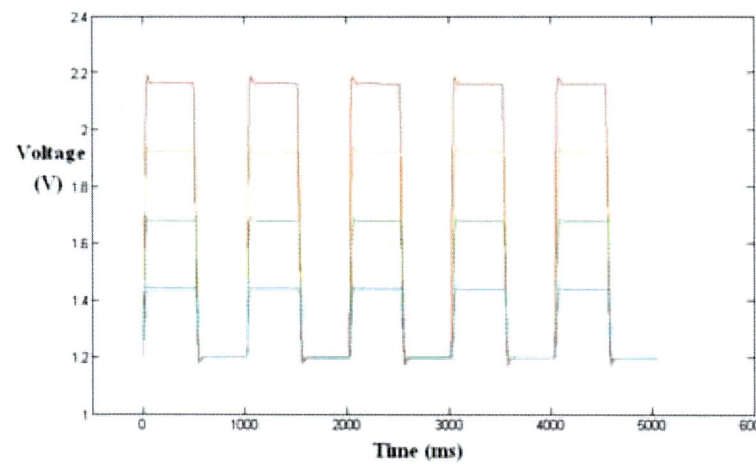

Figure 7.7 Simulation results of the fitted model. Voltage found as a result of muscle power supply pressure (4 bar – in red, 3 bar – in yellow, 2 bar – in green, 1 bar – in blue).

As explained, developing behaviour models allows simulating the response of these polymers integrated as sensors into medical devices. This is enormously useful when designing and selecting the conditioning electronics components. However, these simulations must be validated by integrating the sensors into actual devices and performing the ensuing *in vitro* and *in vivo* tests, as will be explained in the following sub-sections.

7.3.4 Integration of Polymer Piezoelectric Sensors into Biodevices

Some of the main requirements to be met during projects to develop implantable diagnostic devices integrating this kind of polymer sensor are listed below:

- To protect the sensors and the intracorporeal electronics (portable and wireless "Holter" devices) and prevent their coming into direct contact with body mucous and tissues.
- To make sure the intracorporeal electronics and the pressure sensors are tightly sealed to ensure proper system functioning.
- To improve the useful life of the devices, at least sufficiently for carrying out the *in vivo* tests so that a final duration can be attained that is similar to that of other standard implants that it is intended to replace in the market.
- To select and use materials that are compatible with body mucous and tissues.
- To select and use manufacturing processes that do not damage the sensors or the intraoral electronics.
- To optimise the distribution of the electronic components inside the intracorporeal device to ensure the proper functioning of any future portable or wireless systems.

As additional improvements for protecting and encapsulating sensors and to guarantee a longer-lasting seal, we suggested using 150 micron thick polyurethane layers supplied by "3M" corporation, with the results shown in Fig. 7.8.

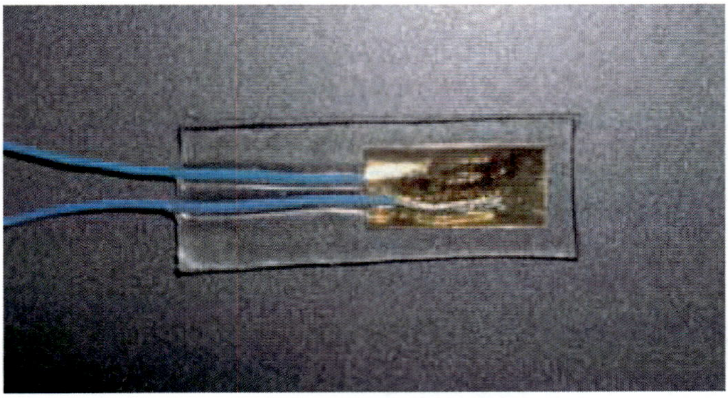

Figure 7.8 Improvement in encapsulating piezoelectric sensors.

The results of our team using this protection were good for calculating intraoral pressures, as we shall explain further on.

The sensors must also be integrated into the end devices by using transformation or manufacturing processes that do not affect their properties. Low temperature processes must be sought that do not lead to the material's Curie temperature being exceeded, above which the material begins to lose its piezoelectric properties.

Of all the procedures we used to integrate these sensors into intraoral devices, such as discharge splints or Michigan devices, it is worth pointing out the following:

- Dual layer thermoshaping for sandwich-type structure with encapsulated electronic components.
- Monolayer thermoshaping with ensuing component encapsulation using additional photopolymerisable material (e.g., Delta Splint® Kit marketed by Kuss Dental).
- Monolayer thermoshaping with ensuing component encapsulation using the addition of polymerisable acrylic material by pressure deposition.
- Dual shaping of the photopolymerisable material in dental moulds including the components at the core of the material.

Some prototypes produced by using these procedures are illustrated in Figs. 7.9 to 7.11. Plaster and resin models of the dentures of the patients taking part in the research were used. Two stages of vacuum thermoshaping were carried out on these models using two acrylic wafers between which the PVDF sensors were positioned.

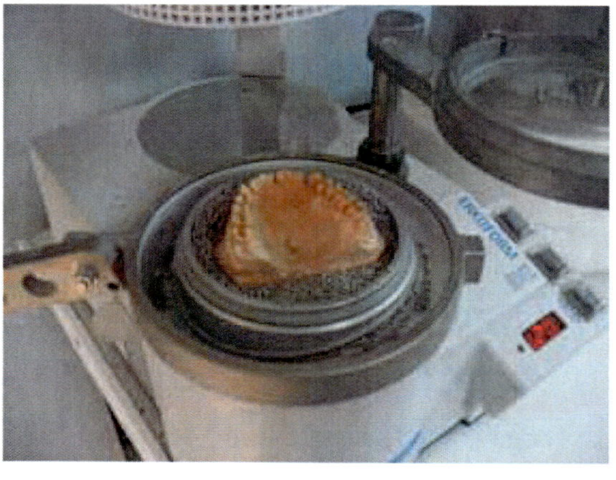

Figure 7.9 Denture model placed in a vacuum thermoshaping machine.

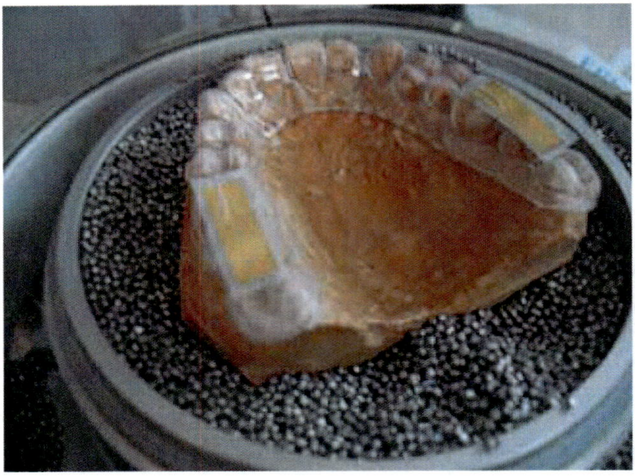

Figure 7.10 Sensors placed on the first layer before carrying out the second thermoshaping.

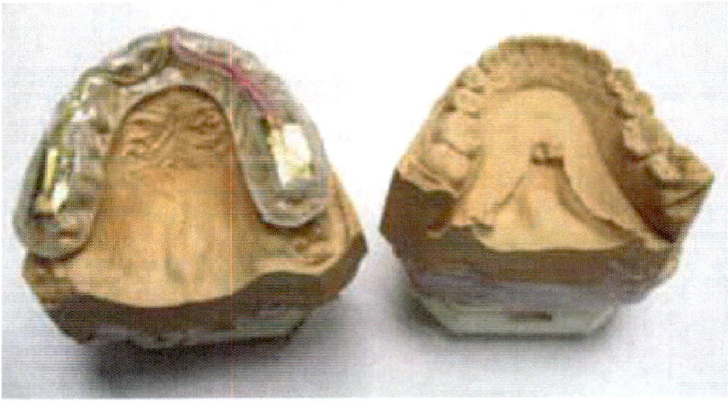

Figure 7.11 Prototypes with encapsulated sensors ready for testing (Lafont *et al.*, Biodevices, 2009).

These encapsulations also help limit the movements of the connecting wires around the sensors as their capacitive effects could negatively affect measurement.

7.3.5 *In vitro* and *in vivo* Trials

***In vitro* trials**

Validating the behaviour of a device intended to diagnose a condition by pressure measurement can be effectively done by designing ad hoc test benches powered by pneumatic actuators. These actuators can be directly controlled from a PC with the help of a signal generator to activate the electrovalves that open and close the pressurised air supply.

Tests can also be conducted simply at different pressures adjusted to the *in vivo* conditions in which the end device will have to operate. Shown in Fig. 7.12 is an example of a bench that was used to evaluate the response of the splints for diagnosing bruxism explained in the case study.

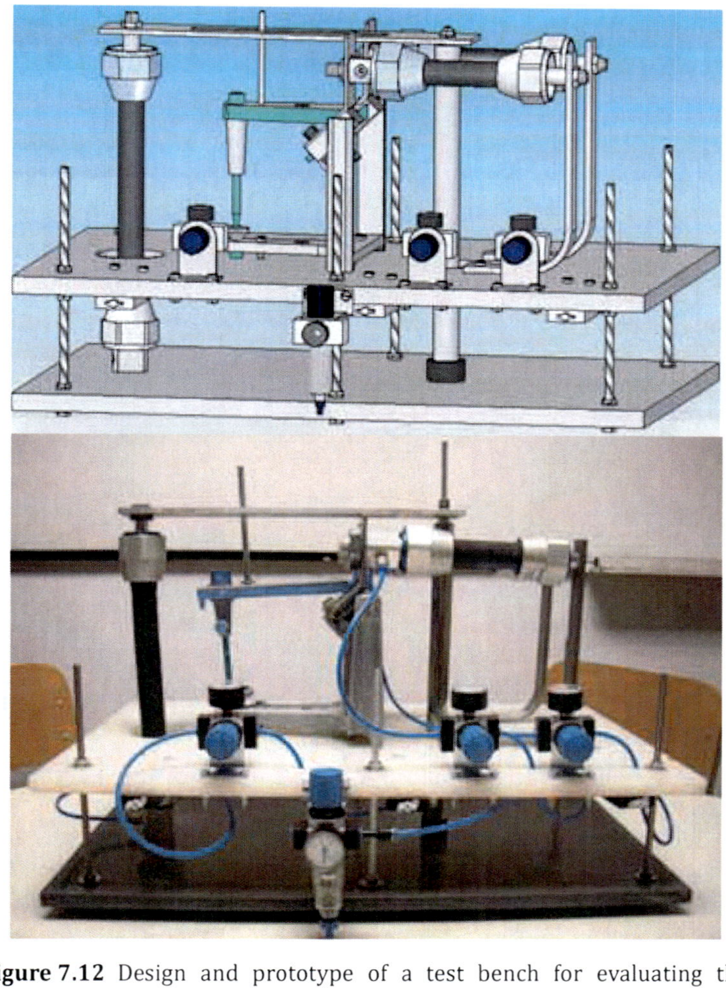

Figure 7.12 Design and prototype of a test bench for evaluating the devices.

Four repeated "bites" were used to calibrate each splint with a force equal to the application of a power pressure of 4, 3, 2 and 1 bar (1 bar = 105 Pa) for the simulator's pneumatic bite muscle with a 5 s duration followed by a 5 s rest. The four repetitions for each pressure value applied are important for checking the repeatability of the measuring system.

The force applied to the splint in proportion to the pressure applied to the pneumatic muscle is obtained from the characteristic curve (power supply pressure – force applied) of the pneumatic muscle while also taking into account the test bench geometry.

Figure 7.13 shows the results of calibrating a splint as an example, depicting the measured voltage according to the pressure steps applied to the pneumatic muscle and their size.

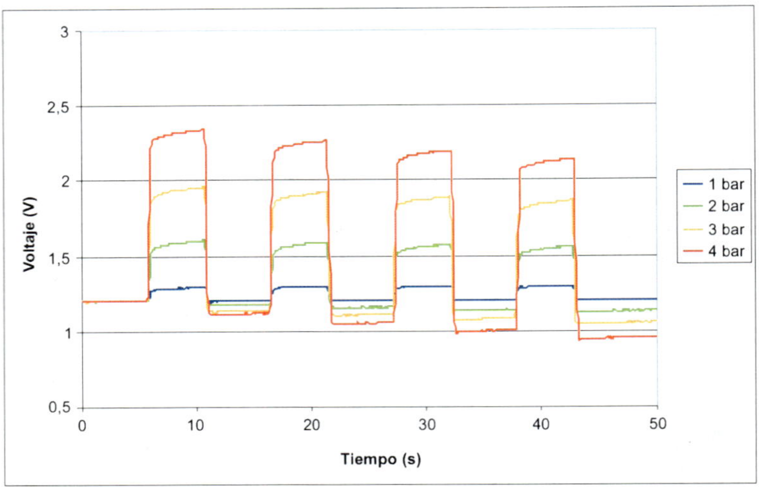

Figure 7.13 Results of calibration process for a personalised splint.

It can be seen how every pressure application is accompanied by an increase in ΔV voltage in respect to the reference value. This can be set out as a splint calibration table that is ordered according to the different pressures applied, as Table 7.2 illustrates. In this example of calibration it is important to highlight that for a specific pressure size applied the increase in voltage recorded has a standard deviation of less than 2% in every case.

By representing the mean ΔV values (together with their standard deviation) for the different pressure levels applied the calibration curve (straight) of the splint is found, as Fig. 7.14 shows.

Table 7.2 Example of a Splint Calibration Table

	Δ*V* for different applied pressures (4 repetitions)			
	1 bar	**2 bar**	**3 bar**	**4 bar**
1st	0.0733	0.3638	0.6909	1.0913
2nd	0.0879	0.3699	0.7312	1.0804
3rd	0.0781	0.376	0.7349	1.0926
4th	0.0879	0.3698	0.7385	1.0986
Mean	0.0818	0.3699	0.7239	1.0907
Standard deviation	0.00633	0.00431	0.01921	0.00656

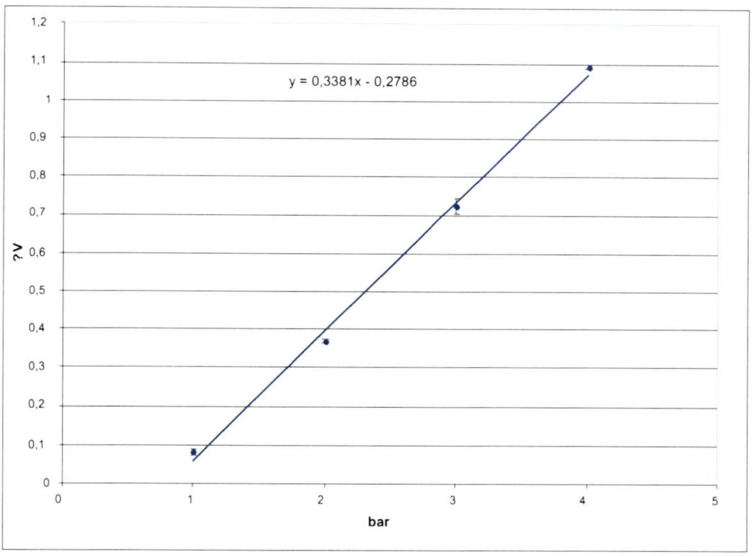

Figure 7.14 Calibration curve of a splint (relationship between increase in voltage and pressure applied during the test).

In every case, the standard deviations given by the tests are comparable to the errors resulting from other links in the measurement chain (pneumatic installation, conditioning electronics, connections, data acquisition card or computer). The calibration curves obtained not only help show the remarkable repeatability of the bite force detection system but also the linearity of the range applicable to human patients. Although a calibration test needs to be performed for each splint produced (since we are dealing with a customised, handmade process), it is important to point out that these characterisation tests can be programmed and carried out practically automatically, thanks to our test bench.

In fact, each calibration gives two characteristic curves of the splint; one for each sensor, although herein we have set out the results given by the right sensor of each splint due to the similarity of the results mentioned earlier on.

It is also important to check that the thermal effects in these tests (and the pyroelectric behaviour of the PVDF) do not have any noticeable effects on the pressure measurements. Using encapsulation helps, to a large extent, to mitigate the phenomena of thermoelectric coupling, but this is something that must be checked. This can be done, for example, by immersing the device in water at different temperatures or test procedures similar to those described in Chapter 8.

The following sub-section explains the *in vivo* tests and the use of pre-calibrated splints to quantify the bite episodes of the different patients taking part in the research.

In vivo trials

Having checked that the system is correctly adjusted and safe, considering the range of forces or pressures to be measured and the possible effects of the system on the body, we can then proceed with the *in vivo* tests with the available prototype or prototypes, in this case using instrumented discharge splints to measure intraoral pressures.

The tests must be conducted in a laboratory under proper conditions of hygiene and safety. In our case, if possible, there should be access to toilets and the following personal items should be on hand:

- Toothbrush and toothpaste
- Dental mouthwash
- Disposable tissues
- Disposable cups
- Running water, or if not, bottled water
- A washbasin or failing that, individual spittoons
- Sterile gloves for assistants
- Antibacterial liquid soap
- Antiseptic mouthwash

The laboratory must also be suited to recording signals and not have any other communication systems in use that could interfere with the conditioning and handling of the signals generated by the sensors during testing.

It is also important to ensure that the participants conduct the tests in the same conditions, following a common protocol that makes it easy to repeat the tests and compare the results.

The best way to ensure this is to use a protocol of computer guided tests that require the patient being assessed to carry out a series of movements and apply some forces in a particular way so that the forces applied can be recorded and the data synchronised with the orders contained in the protocol. In order to manage this protocol and record the data simultaneously a computer "guideline program" was designed with the following functionalities:

- To identify and code both the patient and the test performed
- To set the parameters for each test, such as duration times and the number of repetitions in each case
- To characterise the maximum force of each patient
- A patient guide to show them how to make perpendicular, transversal, rhythmic or high speed bite movements
- To record and synchronise the data related to each of the movements or bite types mentioned

To make the tests easier it is also recommended to establish a schedule to manage the work of producing the splints (or the device under development), calibration and to receive the participants in the test laboratory.

All this is of undoubted help for meeting project schedules and avoiding any unnecessary delays while at the same time making an optimal use of staff and materials.

When the system had been optimised through the *in vitro* tests and the first *in vivo* data, systematic tests were carried out on eight patients showing bruxist behaviour on their instrumented splints. The full test comprises five modules that assess "maximum bite force", "bites of different duration", "rhythmic bites", "chattering" and "grinding of the teeth". They are specially designed to detect different kinds of bruxism and episodes of different length.

A Bruxcare company, Grindalert headband recorder was also used during the medical tests to detect muscular movements by "S-EMG" (surface electromyography). The intention was to compare the detection capability of an instrumented splint to that of an "S-EMG" to highlight the benefits of our system, particularly regarding discriminating between the different kinds of bruxism and detecting transversal bruxism. One of the results obtained with one of the participants is shown below by way of an example. The simulated bruxism episodes were carried out in line with the guideline program's instructions which display the mouth movements to be made on a screen.

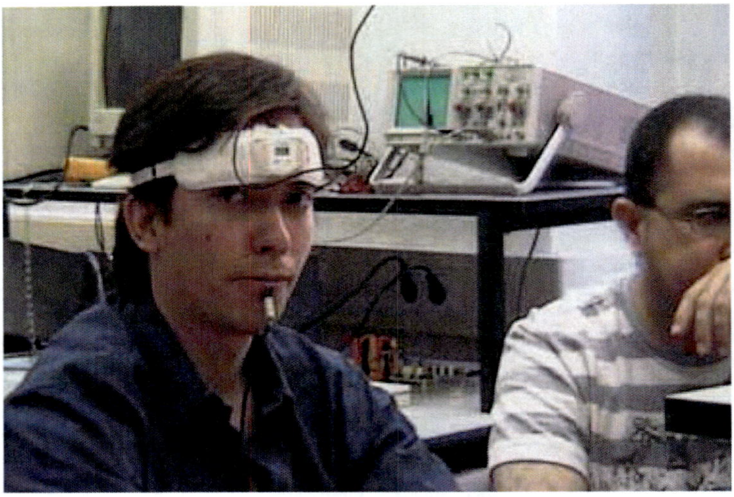

Figure 7.15 *In vivo* tests. Patient with instrumented splint and "S-EMG" recorder.

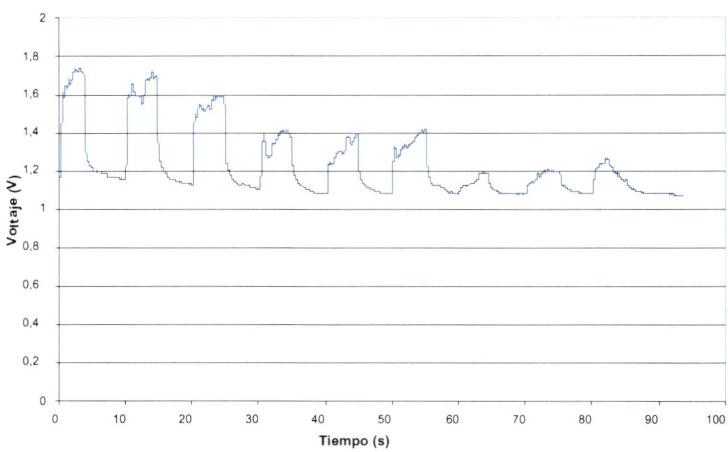

Figure 7.16 Perpendicular bruxism test. For each bite force three repetitions: clenching forces at 50%, 25% and 10% of what the patient considers to be their maximum bite.

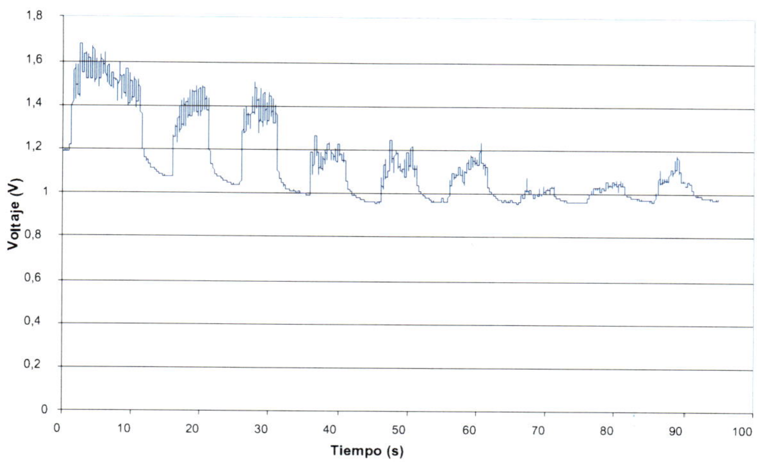

Figure 7.17 Transversal bruxism test. For each bite force three repetitions: clenching forces at 50%, 25% and 10% of what the patient considers to be their maximum bite, together with lateral jaw movement.

In any case, it is important to emphasise the capability of the developed system to detect not only different kinds of bruxism but also its advantages for quantifying their intensity from the calibration of the instrumented splints. These diagnostic capabilities were made possible by the use of piezoelectric polymers as sensors. It is these that have contributed to making the system accurate and repeatable while enabling the durability and size of this kind of system to be optimised.

Sensor failure rate due to problems of manufacture, encapsulating or their integration into the splints was less than 10% for the splints in the final *in vivo* tests.

Additional information, including a summary of the *in vivo* tests performed on simulated patients, showing the recordings of the left sensors (in red) and right sensors (in blue) of each splint used, can be found in the references (Díaz Lantada, 2009).

We hope the methodology adhered to in this case study on the measurement of intraoral pressures and the diagnosis of bruxism may be of use for future developments of diagnostic devices based on the use of electroactive polymers as sensors. Aimed at facilitating these projects, also included below is some brief information on the different commercial polymer sensors available.

7.3.6 Commercial Polymer Pressure/Force Sensors

The reason for choosing Piezotech S.A. as a supplier for the PVDF sensors used in the case studies explained was due to their advantages regarding the processing they perform, which is protected by a patent from the "Institut Saint-Louis", taken out by Bauer, which succeeds in attaining notable piezoelectric properties that are highly stable over time.

Moreover, the Curie temperature of the material is high enough to withstand later processing for it to be encapsulated in the diagnostic devices used. For other designs requiring pressures to be measured at higher temperatures or that are to be subjected to hot processing during their integration into the end device, other "P(VDF–TrFE)" copolymers can be used whose Curie temperature can be adjusted to higher values.

Other suppliers, like "Ktech Corp." supply a range of pressure and impact sensors in polymer and ceramic materials, pre-prepared for taking measurements. In addition, some polymers can also be used as actuators for applications like those dealt with in the preceding chapter.

However, there are still few suppliers of piezoelectric polymers (compared to suppliers of piezolelectric ceramics) and the variety of commercial polymers with these properties is also small, it being almost exclusively limited to PVDF, some or other copolymer like P(VDF–TrFE) and certain PVDF-Nylon mixtures.

Table 7.3 lists a short comparison between polymer materials and ceramic film used as sensors (Bar-Cohen, 2004; Díaz Lantada, 2009; Ealo, 2009; www.memsnet.org), although for further detailed information the different manufacturers should be consulted or the specific characterisation tests should be performed.

Table 7.3 Properties of Different Piezoelectric Materials for Sensing

	Piezoceramics				Piezopolymers	
	SiO_2	$LiNbO_3$	$BaTiO_3$	PZT	PVDF	P(VDF–TrFE)
Density (g/cm^3)	2.7	4.6	5.7	7.4	1.8	1.8
Dielectric constant: ε_r	4.5	28	1300	250–4500	11	9

Main piezoelectric coefficient: $\|d_{max}\|$ (10^{-12} C/N)	2	6	180	50–700	20–35	20–35
Curie temperature (°C)	570	1200	140	300	80–140	100–160
Young Modulus: *E* (MPa)	70000	76000	67000	63000	400–2000	400–2000

7.4 Main Challenges

This section deals with the main fields of study, where more research efforts are being made, in order to promote the expansion throughout the industry of electroactive polymers as pressure/force sensors for biodevices and biomedical purposes.

7.4.1 Combining Sensing and Actuating Capabilities

Manufacturing multilayer materials formed by superposing different films of piezoelectric materials is leading to the production of composites that combine actuating and detecting capabilities, usually joining the direct piezoelectric effect of polymers (as sensors) with the inverse piezoelectric effect of ceramics (as actuators), more detail of which is given in Chapters 13 and 14.

Moreover, some recent studies have been linked to the development of general behaviour models that assist design tasks by using materials that can intrinsically behave as sensors and as actuators or "self-sensing actuators", as do ferroelectric polymers (Janocha and Kuhnen, SMART 09, 2009).

Developing new sensor actuators possessing these characteristics together with the production of behaviour models that let the behaviour of these devices be accurately predicted and help control them (preventing any effects of hysteresis and non-linearity), may turn out to be decisive factors for promoting medical applications for these alternatives.

Of all these applications, worth mentioning is the discovery of active catheters capable of detecting foreign bodies, the manufacture of minimally invasive micro-pincers for assessing the potential damage to tissues during an operation and other surgical devices.

7.4.2 Response Stability: Mechanical, Environmental and Temporal Effects

One drawback of polymers as structural materials or materials subjected to stress is the appearance of stress relaxation and creep phenomena (even under small-size low charges), as well as considerable effects of temperature changes on their properties (rises of around 40°C can lead to reductions in the elasticity modulus of more than two orders of magnitude).

With the passage of time (even a few days or weeks), polymers become subjected to processes of enthalpic relaxation or physical ageing due to the adaptation of the polymer chains, which during shaping had remained in a state of unstable balance, which usually results in the material becoming much more fragile.

Also, various environmental effects such as exposure to UV rays, humidity or the presence of other corrosive agents encourage the appearance of secondary polymerisations and chemical ageing, usually leading to a reduction in the material's mechanical strength.

All these possible influences on the long-term behaviour of polymers, especially in the case of new materials intended for detection, must be very precisely characterised so that the long-term response of the associated devices can be modelled.

As these polymers with detection capabilities are often of recent appearance, their properties are often not characterised with all the accuracy of detail that might be wished and the suppliers' data sheets do not provide all the required information. For this reason, these aspects should be very closely examined.

7.4.3 Wireless Communication of the Signals Obtained

In recent years, wireless sensor networks (WSN) have emerged as a promising form of technology for monitoring installations, machines and structures (Lynch *et al.*, 2006; Kim *et al.*, 2007; Feltrin *et al.*, 2009). The main benefits are they can be rapidly implemented and their little influence on the system being monitored (due to their lack of wires). However, certain problems of consumption due to said wireless transmission limit the autonomy of these systems and are an obstacle to producing complex sizes or obtaining very accurate data.

Notwithstanding the medical applications being put forward for wireless sensor networks like those dealt with in this chapter are growing fast. The feasibility has been demonstrated of intracorporeally monitoring various body pressures (blood pressure, contact pressure between joints, quality of contact between prostheses and bones etc.) as has the wireless transmission of this information to the exterior for subsequent analysis (Biodevices Conferences, 2008, 2009, 2010; Biosignals Conferences, 2008, 2009, 2010).

Different communication protocols, like Bluetooth or Zig-Bee, as well as different types of links, ranging from radio to NFC or RFID, have been successfully tested (González Bris and Díaz Lantada, 2009).

Each has its own advantages over the others concerning aspects such as scope, attenuation by body tissue, and stability of the link or size of the associated electronics. Therefore, it is not clear that any one will take the place of another on the market.

So, the coming years will undoubtedly see major improvements in these links and protocols that will lead to the design of implantable devices (small size, high autonomy and with little impact on the body) with the ability to monitor different physiological signals that use wireless communication.

7.4.4 Alternative "Pseudo-Piezoelectric" Materials

As a general rule, ferroelectric materials (with piezo and pyroleectric properties) have oriented electric dipoles and are therefore polar materials. However, non-polar materials, that is, materials that do not possess permanent molecular dipoles, can also exhibit behaviour that is very similar to ferroelectric behaviour, as has been demonstrated with different foamed plastics.

To achieve this state, the interior cavities of the polymer are subjected to high electric fields that generate tiny microplasma discharges in them, similar to a flash of lightning. The resulting material possesses positive and negative electric charges on the opposite surfaces of its interior cavities and is called ferroelectret (Lindner *et al.*, 2004; Ealo, 2009).

Although the prefix "ferro" is because it behaves like ferroelectric materials, the term "electret" is related to Sessler's definition which states that an electret is a dielectric material that exhibits a quasi-permanent electric charge distribution. That is, the charge decay time constant is much greater than the period of use or research with the material.

Cellular polypropylene (PPc) was the first material to be denominated as a ferroelectret. It was initially developed by the Finnish Research Centre (VTT) and patented in 1987 by Kirjavainen. To date, it is the only ferroelectret that is consistently produced regarding quality and quantity (distributed under the trade name of EmfitTM, the internal structure of which is shown in Fig. 7.18).

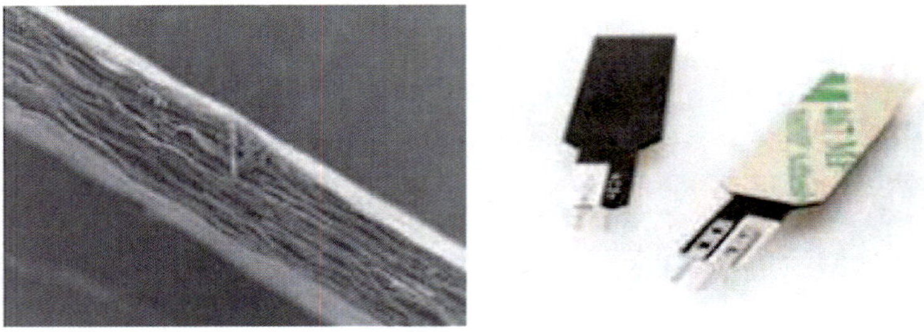

Figure 7.18 SEM picture of Emfit pseudo-piezoelectric film and commercial sensors (www.emfit.com).

When compressed, the various layers of material (70–80 μm thick) come close to one another and behave as a capacitor-sensor in which the armatures of the condenser come together and separate under variable pressures, which gives rise to their pseudo-piezoelectric behaviour ($d_{33} \approx 20\text{–}300 \cdot 10^{-12}$ C/N). Apart from their numerous industrial uses, one of the main medical applications proposed to date is as sensors to detect epilepsy and record bed occupancy in hospitals.

A major drawback of ferroelectrets manufactured with PPc is the low thermal stability of the charge density trapped at temperatures above 50°C. However, at ambient temperature and moderate humidity, its charge density can remain invariable for decades. The higher the storage temperatures and humidity, the greater the speed of decay of the charge density.

Recently, other materials possessing these pseudo-piezoelectric characteristics have been manufactured using PET, COC, CIP and PTFE, although lower charge densities have been obtained than with PPc.

7.4.5 Some Considerations on Piezoresistive Polymers

The piezoelectric sensors dealt with in the chapter up to now exhibit detection mechanisms similar to those of capacitive pressure sensors. These usually behave in a stable manner in the face of thermal effects and their energy consumption is very small. This has boosted their use as sensors compared to other piezoresistive polymer-based alternatives (Elwenspoek (ed.) and Wiegerink, 2001).

However, the measured electric capacity usually shows very low values, which mean that conditioning electronics, like those already referred to, need to be used. The sensitivity thus obtained is more than by using piezoresistive sensors. However, these sensors can sometimes be produced in smaller sizes and more simply integrated, which is essential for certain medical applications.

Piezoresistive polymers are normally produced by incorporating certain amounts of conductive particles into the core of the material during the polymerisation process, which after being carefully distributed (mechanical shakers, ultrasound dispersion and other processes) become embedded in the material itself.

Typical conductor polymers on the market are various epoxy resins, elastomers, such as rubbers and silicones, numerous adhesives and paints and inks, with fillings (particles dispersed in their interior) usually comprising Ag, Ni, Pt or C. Applying pressure to these materials increases the number of contacts between the metal particles present in the polymer and reduces the electrical resistance values from figures of around thousands of Ω/cm to a few dozen Ω/cm. Some of the main companies marketing sensors based on this kind of material are Tekscan, Interlink and Fibron Technologies.

One noteworthy use of these materials in diagnostic devices is the recent use of piezoresistive sensors like those shown in Fig. 7.19, for detecting intraoral pressures by their integration into discharge splints González Bris and Díaz Lantada, 2009).

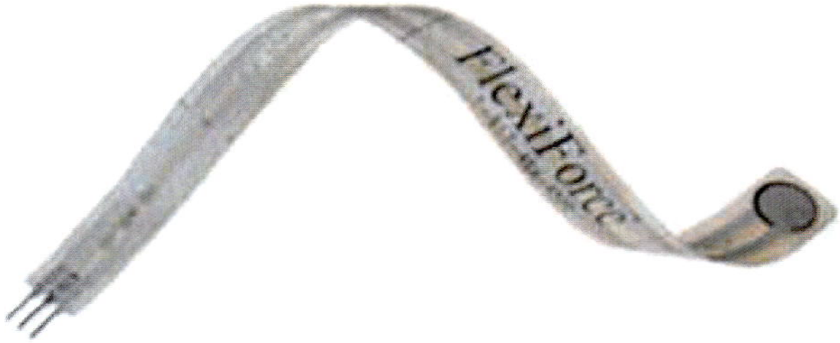

Figure 7.19 Flexiforce sensor Model A201. Tekscan (www.tekscan.com).

A particularly relevant and novel example of piezoresistive polymers is quantum tunnelling composites or QTCs. These are composites with an elastomeric polymer matrix and metal filler particles (usually nickel). In a state of rest, these metal particles are not in contact and the polymer is insulating, but when the material is appropriately deformed, the particles come together (without actually touching) and the electrons can "leap" from the irregularities of some particles to those of other particles without any need for contact due to the quantum tunnel effect.

This causes the electrical resistance of the material to fall drastically (from an initial figure of millions of Ω/cm to a figure of a few Ω/cm).

QTCs were discovered by the scientist David Lussey in 1997, when he was attempting to discover an adhesive to conduct electricity. The surprising properties of this new material led to Peratech Ltd. being set up for research work into these materials and to seek technology transfer applications for them.

Among the benefits of these QTCs, it must be stated that since they are insulating in an unstressed state, the conditioning electronics associated with the devices do not consume energy while no pressure is applied. This helps minimise the size of the power supply system required, which opens up the way to many uses, particularly those connected with implantable medical devices (Mootanah and Bader, 2006) and aeronautical devices where end size is a determining factor (Bloor, 2005, 2006).

For further information on QTCs the references can be consulted, as well as Chapter 14 which contains an introduction to quantum tunnelling composites as active materials and their applications as sensors in medical devices.

7.5 Improving Results and Conclusions

Electroactive polymers (those showing electromechanical coupling, for the purposes of this handbook) exhibit remarkable biomedical applications, not only as actuators but also as sensors for making much diagnostic work easier and for monitoring physiological signals.

Many devices already show the benefits of using this kind of sensor compared to other more conventional ones (ceramics, optics etc.). In future years, significant advances are expected in the different issues mentioned that will help promote the industrial and social impact of these active polymers.

Recent advances in issues of international co-operation concerning active materials, with the setting up of specific forums like the World Wide EAP Webhub, Scientific.net, Biomat.net and others, are helping to disseminate results and exchange opinions.

Additional information can be found in the following list of references as well as in the websites of the different suppliers included in the annexes of the handbook.

References

Aguado, X.; González, J.L. "La capacidad de salto: problemas de medición y soluciones". Revista de Entrenamiento Deportivo, 9(4), 17–23, 1995.

Bailey-Van Kuren, M. "A demanufacturing projector-vision system for combined manual and automated processing of used electronics". Computers in Industry, 56(8–9), 894-904, 2005.

Bar-Cohen, Y. "Electroactive polymer actuators as artificial muscles: Reality, potential and challenges". SPIE Press. Washington, 2002.

Bar-Cohen, Y. "Electroactive polymer (EAP) actuators as artificial muscles: Reality, potential and challenges". SPIE Press, 2nd Edition. Washington, 2004.

Bauer, S.; Bauer-Gogonea, S.; *et al.* "Piezoelectric polymers". Materials Research Society. MRS The Materials Gateway (www.mrs.org).

Bergman, J.G.; McFee, J.H.; Crane, G.F. "Pyroelectricity and optical second harmonic generation in polyvinylidene fluoride films". Applied Physics Letters, 18(5), 203, 1971.

Bloor, D.; Donnelly, K.; Hands, P.; *et al.* "A metal-polymer composite with unusual properties". Journal of Physics D: Applied Physics, 38, 2851–2860, 2005.

Bloor, D.; Graham, A.; Williams, E.J. "Metal–polymer composite with nanostructured filler particles and amplified physical properties". Applied Physics Letters, 88, 102103, 2006.

Brady, S.P.; Coyle, S.; Diamond, D. "Wireless-based monitoring of body movements using wearable sensors". Symposium S: Smart Nanotextiles, 2006.

Díaz Lantada, A. "Metodología para el desarrollo de dispositivos médicos basados en el empleo de polímeros activos como sensores y actuadores". PhD Thesis. Universidad Politécnica de Madrid, 2009.

Ealo, J. "Transductores basados en ferroelectrets para aplicaciones ultrasónicas en aire". PhD Thesis. Universidad Politécnica de Madrid, 2009.

Elwenspoek, M.; Wiegerink, R. "Mechanical microsensors". Microtechnology and MEMS Series. Springer Verlag. Berlin, Heidelberg, New York, 2001.

Feltrin, G.; Meyer, J.; Bischoff, R. Saukh, O. "Information extraction in structural health monitoring with wireless sensor networks". IV ECCOMAS Thematic Conference on Smart Materials and Structures, SMART 09, 2009.

González Bris, C.; Díaz Lantada, A. "A wearable passive force sensor/active interrogator intended for intra-splint use for the detection and recording of bruxism". 3rd International Conference on Pervasive Computing Technologies for Healthcare 2009. 1–3 April 2009 in London. I.S.B.N.: 978-963-9799-42-4.

Hafez, M. "Polymer based actuators as artificial muscles". FSRM Training in Microsystems Course. Teaching Resources. Zurich 2006.

IEEE Standard on Piezoelectricity, 1988.

Janocha, H.; Kuhnen, K. "Solid-state actuators with inherent sensory capabilities". IV ECCOMAS Thematic Conference on Smart Materials and Structures, SMART' 09.

Jungnickel, B. J. In "Polymeric materials encyclopedia", Ed. Salamone, J.C., CRC Press, 8, 7115, 1996.

Kawai, H. "The piezoelectricity of poly(vinylidene fluoride)". Japanese Journal of Applied Physics, 8, 975–976, 1969.

Kim, S.; Pakzad, S.; Culler, D.; *et al.* "Health monitoring of civil infrastructures using wireless sensor networks". Proceedings of the 6th International Conference on Information Processing in Sensor Networks, IPSN 2007.

Lafont Morgado, P.; Díaz Lantada, A.; *et al.*- "Dispositivos médicos basados en el empleo de polímeros electroactivos". Actas del 8° Congreso Iberoamericano de Ingeniería Mecánica. Pontificia Universidad Católica del Perú. Cuzco, 2007.

Lafont Morgado, P.; Díaz Lantada, A.; Martínez Álvarez, A.; *et al.* "Instrumented splint for the diagnosis of bruxism". International Conference on Biomedical Electronics and Devices Biostec 2008 – Biodevices, 2, 216–222. IEEE Engineering in Medicine and Biology Society. 28–31 January, 2008, Madeira, Portugal.

Lindner, M.; Hoislbauer, H.; Schwodiauer, R.; *et al.* "Charged cellular polymers with ferroelectretic behaviour". IEEE Transactions on dielectrics and Electrical Insulation, 11(2), 255–263, 2004.

Lynch, J.P.; Yang, W.; Loh, K.J.; *et al.* "Performance monitoring of the Geumdang bridge using a dense network of high-resolution wireless sensors". Smart Materials and Structures, 15, 1561–1575, 2006.

Martínez, A.; Barrientos, A.; Díaz Lantada, A.; *et al.*- "Diagnosis of bruxism based on piezoelectric sensors and remote communication IEEE-ICIT 2010 - IEEE International Conference on Industrial Technology, 14–17 March 2010, Valparaíso, Chile.

Mootanah, R.; Bader, D.L.- "Pressure sensors". Wiley Encyclopedia of Biomedical Engineering. John Wiley & Sons, 2006.

Mukherjee, N.- "Development of high sensitivity bending mode polymer piezoelectric devices for inner ear". PhD Thesis, 2003.

Nye, J.F. (ed.)- "Physical properties of crystals: Their representation by tensors and matrices". Oxford University Press. Oxford, 1957, 1985, 2006.

Schena, M. "Haptic stylus utilizing an electroactive polymer". Patent application number 20090184923, 2008.

Wagner, N.; Quartano, L.A.; Nicholson, C.E. "Translating civilian and defense technologies for pediatric critical care and rehabilitation research". Technology and Health Care, 14(1), 49–58, 2006.

Chapter 8

Pyroelectric Materials for Biodevices

Andrés Díaz Lantada
Mechanical Engineering Department, E.T.S.I. Industriales,
Universidad Politécnica de Madrid, c/ José Gutiérrez Abascal 2,
28006 Madrid, Spain
adiaz@etsii.upm.es

8.1 Brief Introduction to Pyroelectric Materials

Pyroelectricity is the ability of certain materials to generate an electrical potential when they are heated or cooled. As a result of this change in temperature, positive and negative charges move to opposite ends through migration (the material becomes polarised) and, therefore, an electrical potential is established.

This kind of phenomenon appears in dielectric materials with spontaneous polarisations due to dipole orientation within their structure. These effects have been known to mankind even since Antiquity, especially regarding ceramic materials and metallic oxides.

The name of pyroelectricity was given by Brewster in 1824 when studying the remarkable properties of some ceramic materials. But research into polymer pyroelectricity is more recent, starting around 1955 with some initial results which were not commercially promising.

New attention was given to this property with the discovery of pyroelectric effects in poly(vinylidene fluoride) (PVDF) and its copolymers by Bergman in 1971, after the discovery of piezoelectricity in these materials by Kawai in 1969.

Handbook of Active Materials for Medical Devices: Advances and Applications
Edited by Andrés Díaz Lantada

www.panstanford.com

During the last decades important progress has been made in creating artificial pyroelectric materials, usually in the form of a thin film, out of gallium nitride (GaN), caesium nitrate ($CsNO_3$), polyvinylidene fluorides (PVDF and copolymers), derivatives of phenylpyrazine cobalt phthalocyanine and other materials.

The main industrial uses are linked to the development of temperature sensors, presence detectors, humidity, leaks or other phenomena that go hand-in-hand with temperature changes (Fig. 8.1). Their use in medical devices is also notable as the following examples will show.

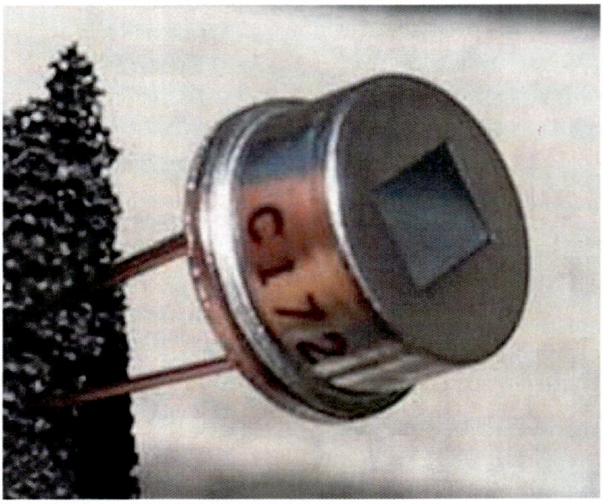

Figure 8.1 Example of pyroelectric sensor (for flame detector and gas analysis). KUBE Electronics AG Model AR172 (www.kube.ch).

Despite their very recent appearance, pyroelectric polymers are replacing pyroelectric ceramics in many applications, such as sensors, particularly in the area of biomedics (De Rossi and Dario, 1983; Brown, 1989). The main reasons behind the interest in promoting the use of polymers as sensors are

- Their greater flexibility makes it easy to integrate them into the end device as well as their ease of adaptation to the surface over which the measurements will be taken.
- They possess a low dielectric constant, low density and a high resistance to impact, all of which make them ideal as sensors.
- They are easier to process than ceramics as large areas can be obtained that can then be cut and shaped to obtain complex forms.

- An absence of toxic components, such as lead and rare earths in their composition, is a plus for their use in the development of medical devices of a diagnostic nature.
- The recent appearance of suppliers that mass produce sensors with remarkable characteristics and repeatability, based on this type of pyroelectric polymer.

The chapter contains a comparison of piezoelectric material properties, both of ceramics and polymers, as an aid to selecting materials to design the devices.

8.2 Potential for Biodevices

Biomedical applications of this kind of material are also related to their being used as temperature sensors, as explained further on.

Thermal cameras

Infrared thermography is a technique for carrying out inspections and non-destructive tests which has multiple applications in the development of machines and products, equipment and facilities maintenance, and troubleshooting. Since all bodies emit (according to their temperature) infrared radiation (IR), which increases in intensity as the temperature rises, variations in this intensity can be detected by using IR sensors.

Thermal cameras can detect radiation in the infrared range of the electromagnetic spectrum (usually between a 900 and 14000 nm wavelength, instead of operating in the visible range of 450–750 nm) and can produce images of this radiation. These cameras are fitted with a sensor matrix (called a microbolometer) that can be developed using pyroelectric materials. Depending on the intensity of the radiation, more or less current is sent to the camera's control electronics, which with the aid of specific software enables temperature maps to be obtained.

Some of the fundamental advantages of the technique are its speed and ease of use, easy to interpret temperature map-based results and the fact that it is a non-destructive technique that does not damage the systems under study (Schindel, 2007; Maldague, 1993).

The medical applications of these apparatuses are many, the most important being to detect tumours or subcutaneous defects and evaluate the progress of muscle or bone injuries (Schindel, 2007). They can be also used as a support tool for other medical devices based on active materials with thermomechanical coupling (Paumier *et al.*, 2008).

Biometric systems

These materials can be used as the component parts of real-time footstep pattern biometric systems used to examine persons recognised by security systems or in more medical spheres, to study the evolution of injuries affecting patient mobility (Fang, 2007).

Assisted surgery

These materials have been used to measure blood temperature during operations to implant coronary stents, in order to correlate temperature profile with blood flow and as a tool for controlling the surgical process (Mochi *et al.*, 2004).

Flow volume sensors

Dymedix Co. has developed nasal flow detectors using PVDF, which, besides their pyroelectric properties enable temperature changes to be detected. This means problems like sleep apnoea or cot death in the newborn can be actively controlled. These devices are placed in the nasal orifices and the patient's respiration induces charges in the polymer according to a particular pattern. If the patient stops breathing the sensor detects the pattern change and through a microcontroller activates an alarm that wakes the patient or alerts their family.

X-ray intensity detectors

Due to the fact that human body tissue heats up through the absorption of X-rays (during X-ray examinations), pyroelectric sensors can be used to estimate the dose of radiation absorbed and assess risk situations. The phenomenon has been tested *in vivo* during mammogram tests with results showing high precision and high sensitivity (De Paula, 2005).

8.3 Current Capabilities and Recent Advances

Set out below are some of the main advances achieved in the last decades concerning pyroelectric materials, mainly ceramics and polymers, and the technologies associated with their use.

8.3.1 Synthesis and Processing of Pyroelectric Materials

Ceramics

Some of the pyroelectric effects in natural minerals have been known since Antiquity. The oldest reference comes from the writings of

Theophrastus where he explains how tourmaline crystals when heated were capable of attracting smoke and bits of straw, although more systematic studies did not begin until the 18th and 19th centuries (Fig. 8.2).

However, the pyroelectric properties of these minerals are not as remarkable for the development of sensors as the properties possessed by synthetic ceramics or the properties being achieved with ferroelectric polymers through appropriate processing.

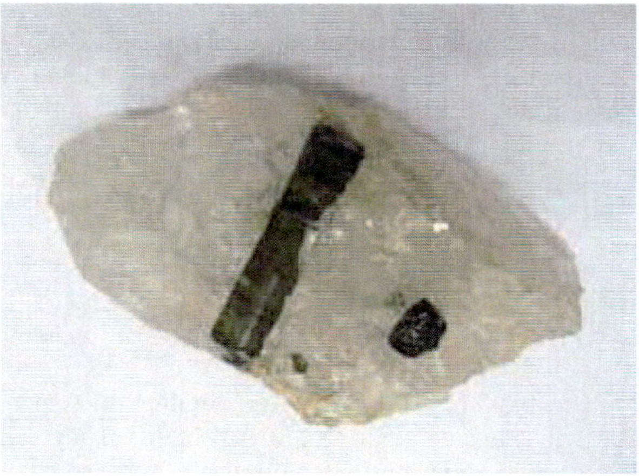

Figure 8.2 Example of a natural pyroelectric material: Tourmaline crystal.

The process for obtaining synthetic pyroelectric ceramics usually begins by using standard procedures for synthesising ceramic materials from different metal and semi-metal oxides.

These are subjected to fusion in a melting pot and exposed to gases at a high temperature and then through controlled cooling, nucleation and the growth of crystals are brought about. Micro-aggregates are thus obtained which are then put under pressure to obtain pellets.

These pellets are then used in sintering processes, normally at temperatures between 1100 and 1400°C, to obtain a film. This is then cut and conditioned to produce the required sensors (Park and Shrout, 1997; Barrel *et al.*, 2009).

Processes have also been described for the deposition of chemical solutions on silicon substrates to obtain ceramic film with pyroelectric properties and very thin thicknesses (nanometres, Suyal, 2002).

Pulsed laser deposition on MgO substrate has also been described to produce $PbTiO_3$ film (Roemer *et al.*, 2008, as well as some of the microstructuring processes discussed in Chapter 13.

One important advantage of thin thickness sensors is linked to their greater flexibility, as they can be adapted to curved surfaces, which is an aid to integrating these materials into more complex detection devices.

Polymers

The polymers that exhibit the most outstanding pyroelectric properties are ferroelectrics (PVDF and copolymers), whose process of synthesis and transformation for obtaining more remarkable features has already been dealt with in the previous chapter (Chapter 7).

Further considerations on processing are included in the sub-section on the main challenges, towards the end of the chapter.

8.3.2 Characterisation and Modelling of Pyroelectric Materials

Basic equations of pyroelectricity

We shall now explain the equations for modelling the thermoelectric behaviour of pyroelectric materials (Nye, 2006). They can also be combined with the equations already set out on piezoelectricity so as to be able to model the materials possessing both properties, as is the case with ferroelectric materials like PVDF polymer) used in much research into sensors.

Pyroelectricity. A pyroelectric material subjected to a uniform, small change of temperature ΔT, usually leads to a change in its polarisation vector $\Delta\mathbf{P}$, in each direction, in accordance with the corresponding pyroelectric coefficient p_i $[C/(m^2{\cdot}K)]$:

$$\Delta P_i = p_i \, \Delta T$$

Thermal expansion. If the temperature of a material changes, associated deformations are also produced that can once again be represented by the tensor or deformation matrix ε_{ij}. When a uniform, small change of temperature ΔT occurs in the material, the deformation is usually homogeneous and all the deformation tensor components are proportional to that ΔT:

$$\varepsilon_{ij} = \alpha_{ij} \, \Delta T$$

where α_{ij} are the thermal expansion coefficients of the material $[1/K]$, which constitute the thermal expansion tensor. Regarding the main axes, the foregoing equations are simplified and become

$\varepsilon_1 = \alpha_1\, \Delta T \qquad \varepsilon_2 = \alpha_2\, \Delta T \qquad \varepsilon_3 = \alpha_3\, \Delta T$

By incorporating these effects into the previously analysed matrix equations, once again using Voigt notation, the thermo-electromechanical couplings of these materials can be modelled:

$$\{\mathbf{S}\} = [\mathbf{s}]\,\{\mathbf{T}\} + [\mathbf{d}]^t\,\{\mathbf{E}\} + \{\alpha\}\,\Delta \mathrm{T}$$
$$\{\mathbf{D}\} = [\mathbf{d}]\,\{\mathbf{T}\} + [\epsilon]\,\{\mathbf{E}\} + \{\mathbf{p}\}\Delta T$$

where

$\{\alpha\}$ is the vector formed by the components α_i with i = 1...6; and

$\{\mathbf{p}\}$ is the vector made up of the components p_i with i = 1...3.

Characterisation of pyroelectric materials

In order to find the pyroelectric coefficient of these materials many techniques have been described based on measuring the voltages, charges or dc current intensities that appear when varying the temperature of the sample being tested.

The main pyroelectric coefficient, which we have defined according to the polarisation (either spontaneously, in most ceramics or induced during processing in ferroelectric polymers) of the material, can be obtained from the current generated by the pyroelectricity with the aid of a simple circuit, the diagram of which is shown in the Fig. 8.3, according to the equation:

$$p_3 = dP_3/dT$$

$$p_3 = \frac{V_{\text{out}}}{R} \cdot \frac{1}{A(dT/dt)}$$

where A is the area of the sensor [m^2] and dT/dt (°C/s) is the heating rate.

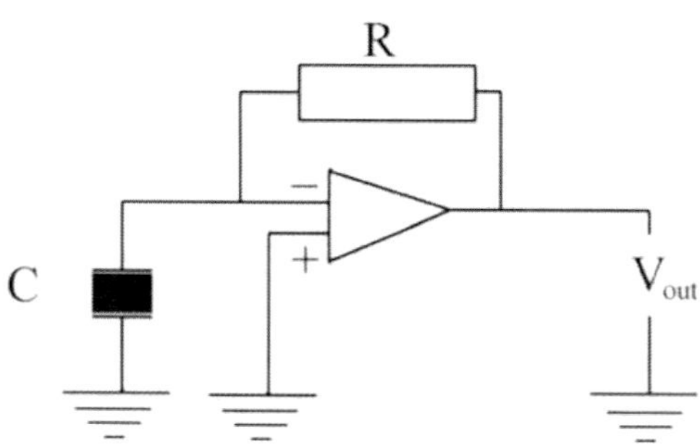

Figure 8.3 Typical circuit for measuring the pyroelectric coefficient. *C:* sample capacitance (F); *R:* resistance (Ω); and V_{out}: output voltage (V).

To measure the material's initial polarisation (either spontaneous or obtained during processing), the charge integration method is appropriate with the aid of a circuit like that in the Fig. 8.4, bearing in mind that the output voltage is given by

$$V_{\text{out}} = \frac{1}{C_{\text{ref}}}\int_0^t i \cdot dt$$

where $i(t) = p_3 \cdot A \cdot (dT/dt)$; the pyroelectric current.

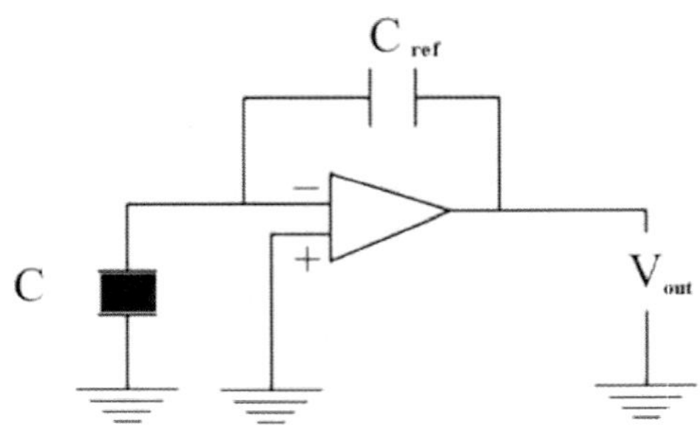

Figure 8.4 Typical circuit for measuring the spontaneous polarisation by charge integration. *C*: sample capacitance (F); C_{ref}: capacitor for integration (F); and V_{out}: output voltage (V).

And the polarisation can be found from the expression:

$$V_{\text{out}} = \frac{A}{C_{\text{ref}}}[P_3(T_C) - P_3(T)]$$

In which the spontaneous polarisation at the Curie temperature $P_3(T_C)$ is usually chosen as null as reference. The changes in polarisation according to the temperature are simply found by using the measuring circuits and equations explained.

Appreciable variations in the pyroelectric coefficient are usually recorded throughout the heating or cooling tests that are associated with phase changes as well as the effects of hysteresis when the Curie temperature is exceeded in an increasing or decreasing direction and according to the specific volume of the material.

Once the properties of the material have been found, it is important to learn to model its behaviour as a part of more complex devices. This is shown in the following pages, once again taking the use of PVDF sensors as an example of its application, due to the importance that polymers are acquiring as sensors and actuators in the development of medical devices and thermo-electromechanical microsystems (MEMS).

Pyroelectric testing material

In order to obtain sensors for a detailed assessment and examination of pyroelectric behaviour, by way of example, we have taken 40 μm thick poly(fluorovinylidene) - PVDF - biaxially stretched film (Bi-ax. PVDF) (similar to that used for instrumented splints) from Piezotech S.A., with Au-Pt electrodes deposited by sputtering. Its basic properties are shown in Table 8.1.

Table 8.1 Typical Values of the Properties of the Polymers Used

	d_{33} (pC/N)	d_{31} (pC/N)	d_{32} (pC/N)	ε (F/m)	p_3 μC/(m²·K)
Uni-ax. "PVDF"	-20	18	3	$1{,}1\cdot 1^{-10}$	-25
Bi-ax. "PVDF"	-24	7	7	$1.1\cdot 1^{-10}$	-25
P(VDF-TrFE)	-24	7	7	$0.9\cdot 1^{-10}$	-25

On the other hand, Table 8.2 shows other physical properties of the sensor as well as of the protective coatings that were used in the behaviour simulations and tests intended to fit the behaviour model described further on.

Table 8.2 Thermal Properties of the Materials Used

	Density (kg/m³)	**Conductivity [W/(m·K)]**	**Specific heat [J/(kg·K)]**
PVDF sensor	1760	0.18	961
PU coating	1270	0.21	1755

The study of this phenomenon is also aimed at analysing the possible influence of temperature on the diagnostic capabilities of certain ferroelectric-based material devices for use as pressure sensors (whose applications were described in Chapter 7). The same conditioning electronics and the same data collection system are used as set out in that chapter.

The developed model of thermoelectric behaviour

The behaviour model for measuring the thermal effects in the device under development includes the following parameters (Díaz Lantada, 2009):

- Sensor thickness

- Effective area of the sensors
- Elasticity modulus of sensor material
- Dielectric constant of the sensors
- Piezoelectric coefficients of the sensor material
- Pyroelectric coefficients of the sensor material
- Equivalent electrical resistance of the sensors
- Equivalent capacity of the sensors
- Thermal conductivity of sensor material
- Specific heat of sensor material
- Density of sensor material
- Thickness of sensor coating material
- Elasticity modulus of sensor coating material
- Thermal conductivity of sensor coating material
- Specific heat of sensor coating material
- Density of sensor coating material
- Equivalent resistance of conditioning circuit
- Equivalent capacity of conditioning circuit
- Electronic amplification factor
- Convection heat transfer coefficients
- Conduction heat transfer coefficients
- Other thermal contact resistances
- Other adjusting factors for the specific application

For some of the sensor or coating materials the model includes the properties mentioned above for each of the materials. The relationships between the different parameters have already been explained since they are a question of basic piezoelectricity and pyroelectricity equations. Listed below are their applications for the study of pyroelectric effects in combination with heat transfer models.

In the same way as the effect of pressure changes, changes in temperature of the PVDF sensor (chosen as an example) act as an intensity generator that is supplying a condenser of C capacity in line with the equation:

$$C = \varepsilon \ (L_1 \cdot L_2)/e$$

Current intensity I, caused by the change of temperature ΔT, is proportional to the pyroelectric coefficient p_3 of the sensor material, as the following equation shows. This equation ignores the previously mentioned thermal dilation effect due to the small increases in temperature to be measured and for which purpose the designed system is intended.

$$Q = p_3\,(L_1 \cdot L_2)\,\Delta T \rightarrow I = dQ/dt = p_3\,(L_1 \cdot L_2)\,dT/dt$$

To measure the temperature changes in the piezoelectric-pyroelectric material of the sensors, the thermal insulation produced by the protective coatings needs to be taken into account. We will now set out a finite difference calculation model for measuring the evolution of the temperature at the core of the sensor, finding an approximate solution to the conduction equation under a non-steady state in the absence of internal heat generation (Chapman, 1990; Perera, 2004) for the sensor scheme of Fig. 8.5:

$$\left(\frac{\partial^2 T}{\partial x^2} + \frac{\partial^2 T}{\partial y^2} + \frac{\partial^2 T}{\partial z^2}\right) k \cdot = \rho \cdot c_\mathrm{p} \cdot \frac{\partial T}{\partial t}$$

Written in this form, each side of the equation represents the amount of heat storage time per unit of volume at a specific point.
where

- k is the conductivity of the material around the point [W/(m·K)];
- T, the temperature of the point [K];
- ρ, the material's density around the considered point [kg/m^3];
- c_{p}, the specific heat of the material around the point [J/(kg·K)];
- x, y, z, the directions of heat propagation; and
- $\frac{\partial}{\partial}$, the partial derivative of one magnitude in respect to another.

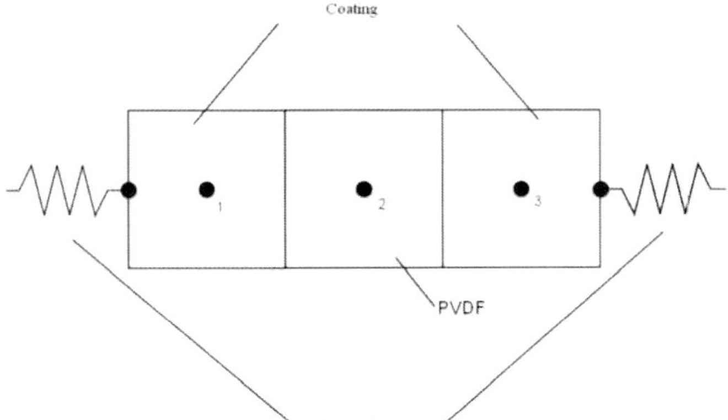

Figure 8.5 Circuit diagram of a PVDF pyroelectric sensor with polyurethane coating.

Shown below is the approximation by finite differences. For the pyroelectric sensor we can take the one-dimensional case without loss of generality:

$$\mathrm{k}\cdot\left(\frac{\partial^2 T}{\partial x^2}\right)=\rho\cdot c_\mathrm{p}\cdot\frac{\partial T}{\partial t}$$

To solve the equation, the sensor is divided into different equally or unequally spaced sections, to each of which a node is assigned whose temperature is representative of the whole associated section. The number of nodes is chosen according to the precision required in the solution. For each point *i* of the node network when applying the formulation explicit to the one-dimensional conduction equation, the following must be true:

$$T_{i'}=T_i+dt\left(\sum_j\frac{T_j-T_i}{R_{ij}C_i}+\frac{q_i}{C_i}\right)$$

where

- T_i is the temperature [K] of node *i* at instant *t*;
- *dt*, the reduced time interval [s] for applying the finite differences calculation to the resolution of the differential equation;.
- $T_{i,}$ the temperature [K] of node *i* at instant $t + dt$;
- $C_{i,}$ the thermal capacity of the cell volume or the section associated with the node *i* and defined by $C_i = V_i\ \rho\cdot c_\mathrm{p}$ where V_i [m^3] is the cell volume, c_p [J/(kg·K)] is the specific heat of the cell material and ρ [$\mathrm{kg/m}^3$] is the cell material density;
- $q_{i,,}$ the amount of heat (external or internal added to the *i* node) [W];
- $\sum_j$, the summation at *j* which extends to all the *j* nodes adjacent to the *i* node; and
- R_{ij}.- the thermal resistance between the *i* node and the *j* [K/W] node. This resistance to heat transfer, depending on the situation of the nodes and the environment of the cells or associated sections, will be defined according to the method of heat transfer.

For convection transfer: $R_{ij}=\dfrac{1}{h_{ij}\cdot A_{cij}}$

where h_{ij} [W/(m^2 K)] is the convection coefficient between the nodes and A_{cij} is the area of heat exchange by convection between the cells associated with the nodes. In the case of heat transfer by conduction or contact, it is sufficient to substitute the values of R_{ij} in the model by applying the following considerations:

For conduction transfer.- $R_{ij} = \dfrac{x_{ij}}{k \cdot A_{kij}}$

where x_{ij} is the distance between the i node and the j node, k is the thermal conductivity between the nodes and A_{kij} is the area of heat exchange by conduction between the cells associated with the nodes.

Taking into account additional thermal resistances through contact – $R_{ij} = \dfrac{R_{tc}}{A_{kij}}$

where R_{tc} is the thermal resistance of contact between the i node and the j node and A_{kij} is the area of heat exchange by conduction between the cells associated with the nodes.

The above equations give a behaviour model for a rapid study of the influence of parameter changes and optimising the device's design process.

These equations were programmed with the aid of "Matlab" to find the evolution of the temperature in the different nodes according to the charge and boundary conditions (Figs. 8.6–8.9). The evolution of the temperature in the middle node, which is that of the sensor, is stored in a vector called "Tempsim" which stores the evolution of the PVDF temperature over time.

This vector is then used as an input to a thermoelectric behaviour model produced by the aid of the "Matlab-Simulink" simulation module which gives the voltage changes at the conditioning electronics output according to the changes of temperature in the sensor material.

This "Simulink" model (Fig. 8.10) includes the charge amplifier amplification factor which gives the ratio between the charge generated by the piezoelectric-pyroelectric sensor or sensors and the voltage generated at the amplifier output (in a similar way to what is included in the piezoelectric behaviour model dealt with in Chapter 7). This voltage is taken as an input to a data acquisition card that enables the evolution of temperature to be represented with the help of computers, oscilloscopes or other signal analysis devices.

The different simulations of response to temperature changes taken from the behaviour models explained, which also allow analysing the influence of different factors on the evolution of the temperature of the sensor, are listed further on. In each case, the sensor was assumed to have an initial temperature of 25°C.

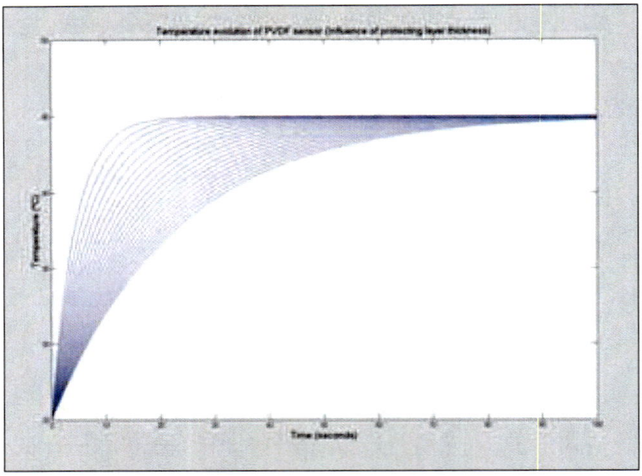

Figure 8.6 Simulation: influence of thickness (100–600 μm) of coating in heat transfer. Convection heating in water at 45°C. Evolution of PVDF temperature.

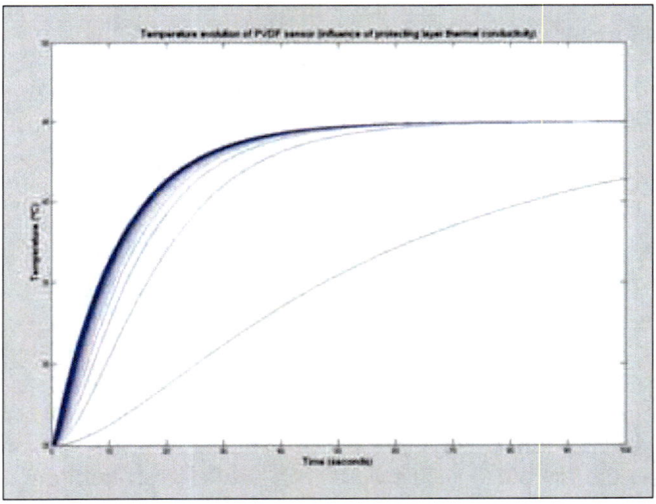

Figure 8.7 Simulation: influence of the conductivity of the coating on heat transfer. Convection heating in water at 45°C. Evolution of PVDF temperature.

Shown below is the Simulink program used to find the voltage response according to the voltage over time that the sensor would give, taking the temperature values over time. The block diagram reveals certain similarities with the piezoelectric simulator shown in the preceding chapter, but with the important difference that the input is a variable obtained by running the Matlab program described instead of a predetermined signal.

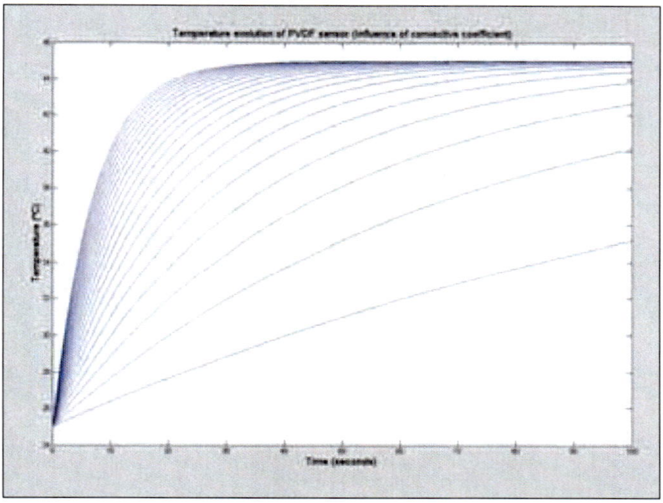

Figure 8.8 Simulation: influence of convection coefficient [5–100 W/(m^2 K)] of the environment. Convection heating in water at 45°C. Evolution of PVDF temperature.

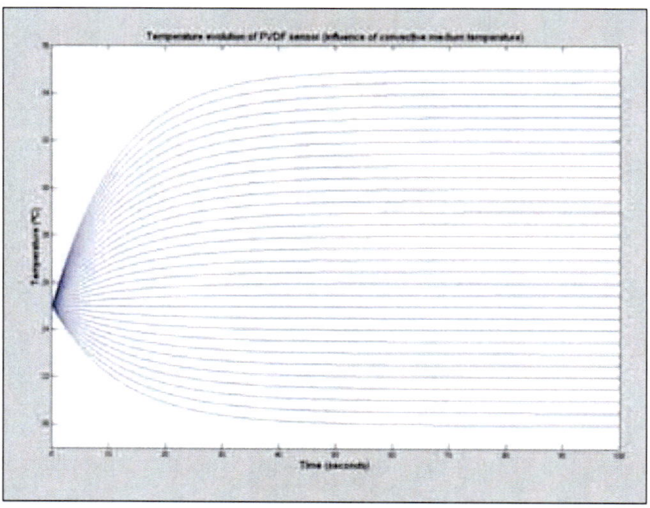

Figure 8.9 Simulation: influence of temperature (20–35°C) of the convective environment. Evolution of temperature of PVDF sensor.

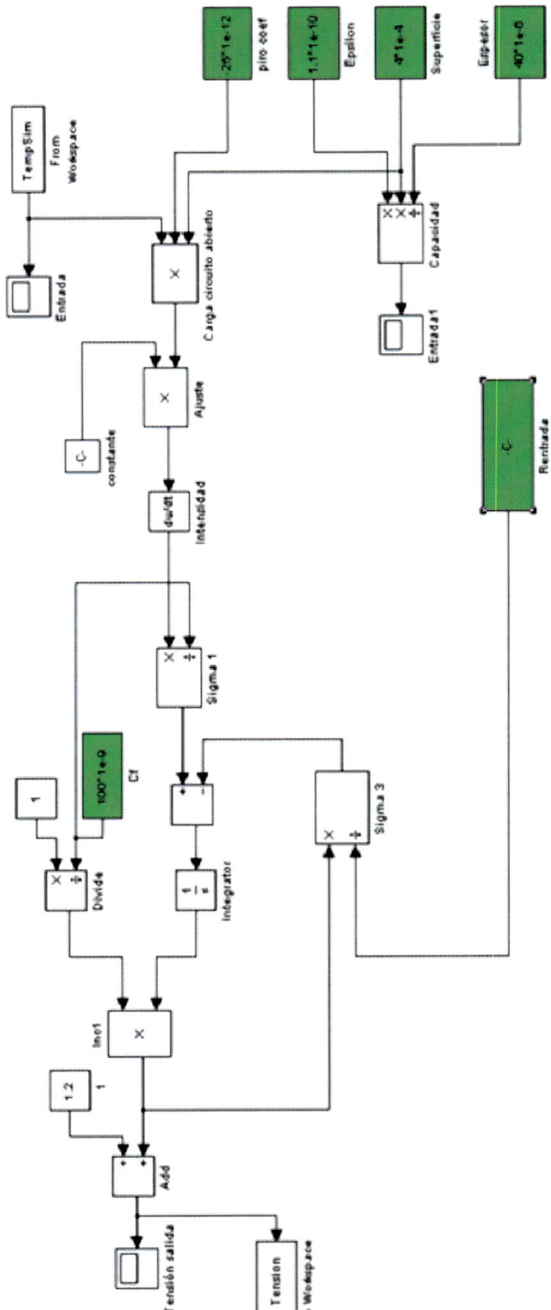

Figure 8.10 Simulink model for simulating pyroelectric sensor behaviour.

Both the pyroelectric coefficient p_3 and the piezoelectric coefficient d_{33} in the PVDF and its copolymers are negative and therefore temperature drops lead to positive voltage rises. Certain references that only study pyroelectric behaviour often take this value through positive convention (Newsome and Andrei, 1996).

However, if we assess the joint behaviour of these ferroelectric polymers compared to pressure and temperature changes, it is important to point out that the compressions as well as the drops in temperature lead to positive voltages, since d_{33} and p_3 are negative.

As an example of the simulations performed, we will now show the different responses given by the "Simulink" simulator in accordance with the model explained for sensors subjected to temperature changes. Later sections will compare the simulations with the tests carried out to validate the model.

As connective environments, we have taken water (as an approximation to *in vivo* behaviour) and air (as an approximation to *ex vivo* applications) and we have also compared the effects of different coating material thicknesses. It can be seen how the sensor, with only a single layer of coating and subjected to water convection (Fig. 8.11) exhibits a much more rapid response than the sensor with three layers of coating and exposed to air convection (Fig. 8.12).

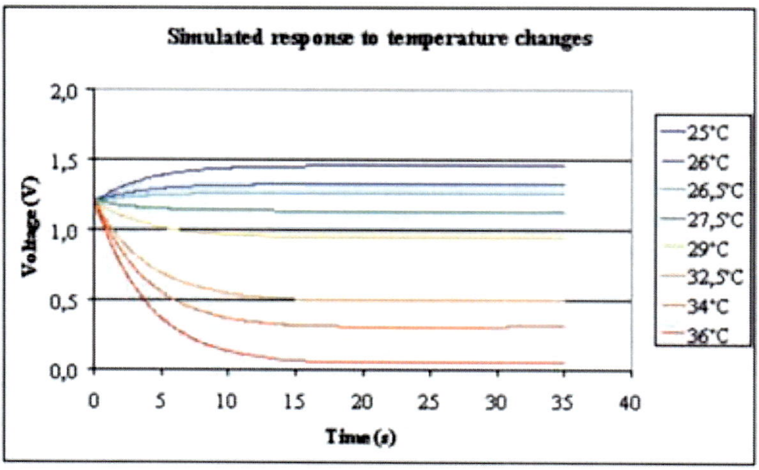

Figure 8.11 Simulation of output voltage due to temperature change in the pyroelectric sensor. Room temperature 27°C. Water temperature in the simulated tests is shown in the key. Sensor with protective monolayer coating (response simulation through introduction into water).

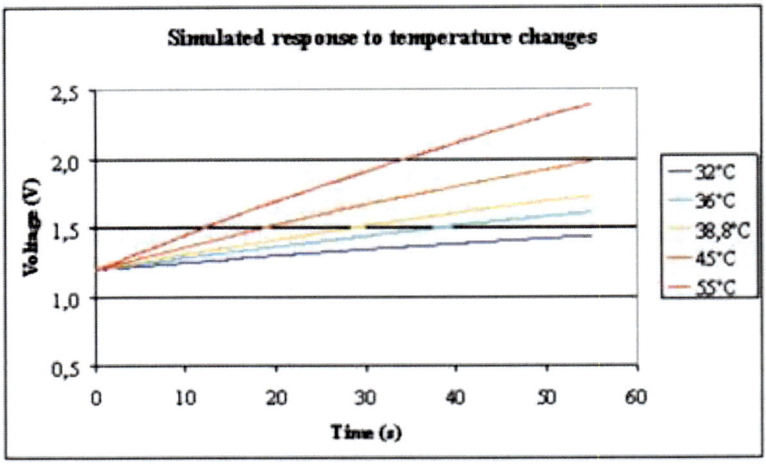

Figure 8.12 Simulation of output voltage due to temperature change in the pyroelectric sensor. Room temperature 26°C. Water temperature in the simulated tests is shown in the key. Sensor with triple-layer coating (response simulation through extraction from water).

8.3.3 Aspects Related to Signal Conditioning of Pyroelectric Materials

As is the case with piezoelectric polymer sensors, the two most usual working modes for a pyroelectric sensor are in open circuit and in short circuit. In the first case, the metallised faces of the sensor are used as the armatures of a condenser and the voltage resulting from the charge generated ($V = Q/C$) between them is measured (open circuit) using an electrometric amplifier. This electrometric amplifier consists of a voltage amplifier with an input resistance of more than 1 TΩ and an input current of less than 1 pA. In the second case, the sensor always "sees" a voltage of 0 V between its faces and transfers the charge to a condenser of known value where the voltage drop ($V = Q/C$) between armatures is measured. In every case, the use of operational amplifiers supplies a low impedance voltage output that can continue to be processed easily.

Measuring the voltage drop over the sensor itself presents several problems. Firstly, the capacity of the sensor has a high tolerance due to the fact that it not only depends on the physical characteristics of the PVDF film used, but also on the elements surrounding it and its spatial shape. Also, in order to find the capacity over which the charge is distributed we also need to add the capacity of the connecting wires and the amplifier input.

All this causes the dispersion of the device's sensitivity to be high, especially if we bear in mind the usual low values of pyroelectric coefficients [around tens or hundreds of $\mu C/(m^2 \cdot K)$] that lead to very small current intensities.

However, using a charge amplifier, the voltage between the sensor terminals is kept permanently at zero. This eliminates the effect of any parasite capacities and resistance. Moreover, the charge is transferred to a condenser of known capacity and tolerance, which means the dispersion sensitivity is less than if working with an open circuit and the manufacture of the devices is simplified.

8.3.4 Integration of Pyroelectric Materials into Biodevices

As with other medical device developments integrating sensors, as well as electronic components for the right conditioning and power supply batteries, the use of manufacturing and fast prototyping technologies is particularly suited to validating geometries and functionalities (Kucklick, 2006; Díaz Lantada, 2009).

One thing that helps integrate these materials as sensors into medical devices, whose geometry is often complex, is the flexibility of the material. For this reason, pyroelectric polymers turn out to be good candidates. Additionally, their formulations are frequently neither toxic nor dangerous, while ceramics sometimes contain toxic components, such as Pb, Mn, Bi and others.

Another area where more progress needs to be made, particularly for applications in which sensors have to be in direct contact with body tissue, is to produce body-compatible electrodes (Kim, 2008), as will be described in the section on future challenges towards the end of the chapter.

8.3.5 Trials and Main Results

In vitro tests

The test bench layout prepared for the pyroelectric tests for the PVDF sensors is shown in Fig. 8.13. It comprises an electric heater, a container with water, an arm to clamp the sensor, and conditioning and data acquisition electronics, all connected to a personal computer.

For measuring temperature a "CME 305" digital thermometer was used with a precision of 0.1°C.

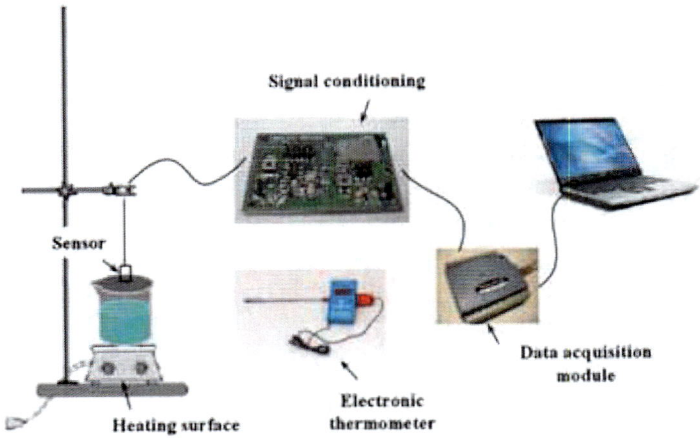

Figure 8.13 Layout of the test bench used.

This test bench stands out for its speed off implementation, ease of handling and low cost, apart from the fact that pyroelectric sensor behaviour can be reliably characterised.

The choice of water as a convective medium was because it was wished to study the response of the sensor when in contact with body fluids. It was also intended to maximise the thermal effects on the sensor by carrying out the tests in contact with water due to its higher convection coefficient, as an alternative to the studies carried out under non-forced air convection.

Included below are different images showing the voltages recorded by monolayer and triple-layer coated sensors through their immersion in water at different temperatures and their subsequent evolution by non-forced air convection(Figs. 8.14 and 8.15). It can be seen how the monolayer coated sensors are faster than the triple-layer coated sensors and how their evolution by water convection is also faster than by air as the simulations had already indicated (Figs. 8.16 and 8.17).

The tests have allowed validating and adjusting the behaviour model as well as the associated "Simulink" simulator (Figs. 8.11 and 8.12). These may be able to be used in future design work for analysing the possible use of alternative materials and selecting the most suitable complementary materials and components (material and coating thickness, conditioning electronics, geometries and distribution).

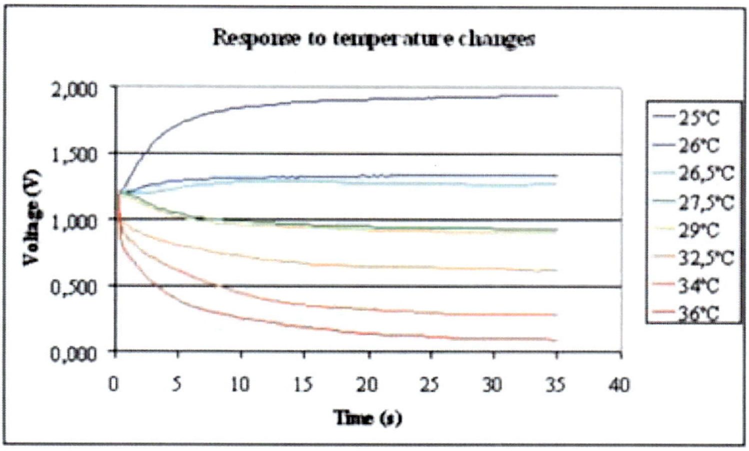

Figure 8.14 Temperature change response tests in the pyroelectric sensor. Room temperature 27°C. Water temperature in the simulated tests is shown in the key. Sensor with monolayer coating (real response through immersion in water).

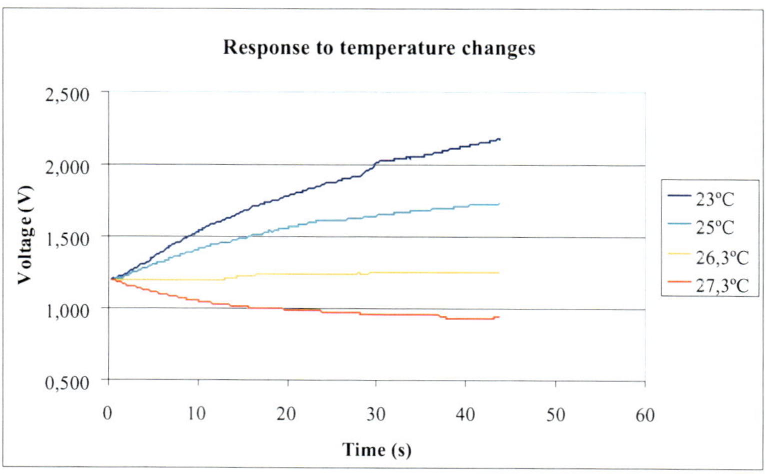

Figure 8.15 Temperature change response tests in the pyroelectric sensor. Room temperature 27°C. Water temperature in the simulated tests is shown in the key. Sensor with triple-layer coating (real response through immersion in water).

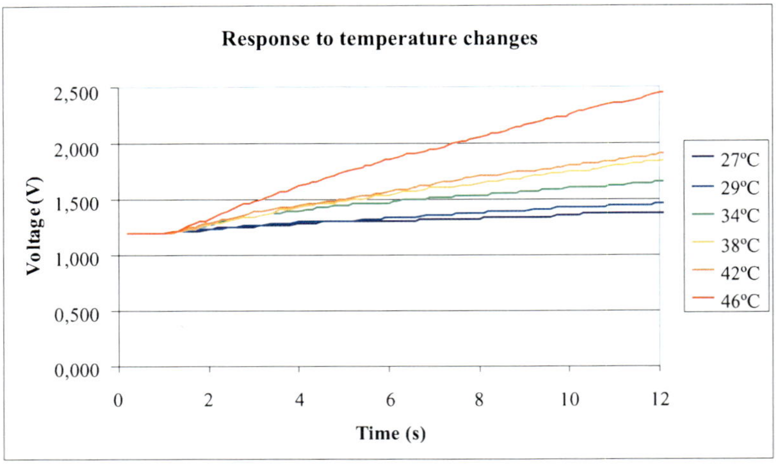

Figure 8.16 Temperature change response tests in the pyroelectric sensor. Room temperature 26°C. Water temperature in the simulated tests is shown in the key. Sensor with monolayer coating (real response through extraction from water).

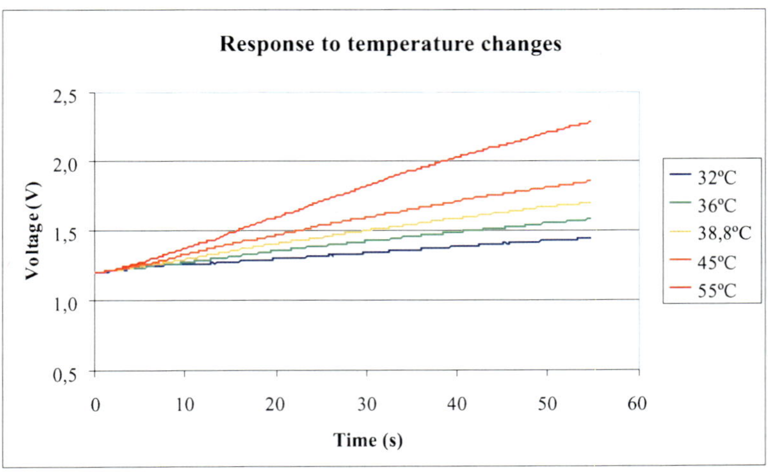

Figure 8.17 Temperature change response tests in the pyroelectric sensor. Room temperature 26°C. Water temperature in the simulated tests is shown in the key. Sensor with triple-layer coating (real response through extraction from water).

To summarise these last two sub-sections, it should be pointed out that a behaviour model has been described for simulating the response of PVDF as a sensor for temperature changes which gives the evolution of the voltage arising from the charge displaced in the conditioned pyroelectric material.

For this purpose, a finite differences calculation model was designed to calculate sensor heating caused by various factors, particularly surrounding environment temperature, the convection coefficient of this medium, the thickness of the protective coating, sensor geometry and other thermal properties of the materials. This model was implemented in "Matlab" for a rapid calculation of the evolution of the temperature of the pyroelectric sensor.

This evolution of sensor temperature is taken as an input to a model produced with "Simulink" which finds the constitutive equations of the pyroelectricity. From these equations, the charge generated, as a function of the evolution of temperature in the material, can be found. The simulator also includes the effects of the charge amplifier and the rest of the signal conditioning, to finally find the evolution of the recorded voltage.

The setting up of a simple, low-cost test bench has also been described, but one which lets pyroelectric sensor characterisation tests be performed rapidly and reliably as well as assessing the influence of different design changes on the response of the these sensors. When the tests have been completed, we proceed to fit the implemented model with Matlab – Simulink, until deviations of less than 5% are reached for 90% of the tests carried out, also including studies of sensibility to changes in coating thickness and to different convection media.

Models like the one used will be of enormous use for future medical and industrial developments since the influence of a wide range of parameters on the behaviour of pyroelectric sensors can be assessed. The number of design iterations can also be simplified and the incorporation of these materials as parts of more complex systems is made easier. Tests benches like the one proposed let prototype and end device performance be directly evaluated, helping to ensure accuracy, repeatability and final quality.

In vivo tests

Regarding the development of *in vivo* tests, it is important to mention the use of sensors and technologies similar to those described for measuring intraoral temperatures (Díaz Lantada, 2009) and for detecting sleep apnoea episodes (Dymedix –Commercial devices).

Orthetic devices (temporary and non-implantable) such as those described in this research can be classified as Class I due to a short-lasting surface contact, which facilitates *in vivo* testing and their subsequent commercialisation.

Other implantable devices with a greater potential for harm require additional controls. This means that commercial developments are still very limited in spite of the recent advances described.

However, implantable medical devices incorporating pyroelectric materials as sensors that require an electrical power supply must meet the requirements laid down in Directive 90/385/EEC pursuant to "Active Implantable Medical Devices", which describes the tests to be passed depending on the class of the device for it to be able to be marketed in the European Union. In other regions, the local regulations must be complied with, although the cited directive forms a good basis in general terms.

8.3.6 Commercial Pyroelectric Sensors

Most ceramic material manufacturers focus on their use as structural or coated materials, but many suppliers of active materials for detection or actuation applications are emerging, many of which supply ceramics.

Smart Material (www.smart-material.com) is a company that develops advanced ceramics with piezo- and pyroelectric properties as well as composites which combine the benefits of polymers and ceramics (mention must be made of their MFC or Macro Fiber Composite film).

This company also supplies support hardware and software characterisation and testing, two fundamental issues throughout the product development process. Other manufacturers of pyroelectric transducers are Silverlight Ltd., Murata Manufacturing Co. Ltd. and Coherent Inc.

Ferroelectrics with piezoelectric and pyroelectric properties are usually used for polymers as they have many applications as sensors in diagnostic devices.

Among the manufacturers most referred to, due to the remarkable properties of their products obtained from the use of specially controlled processing that is protected by patent, we must mention Piezotech S.A. and K-Tech Corporation.

One novel alternative is cellular ferroelectrets, which apart from possessing pseudopiezoelectric properties (as described in the preceding chapter), also exhibit pseudoelectric behaviour, although at present they are being used more as electromechanical transducers than thermoelectric transducers.

To date, the only ferroelectret with more stable and homogeneous properties is EmfitTM film initially developed by the Finnish research Centre (VTT) and patented in 1987 by Kirjavainen, although recent advances augur the appearance of new types of commercial cellular ferroelectrets in the very near future (Lindner *et al.*, 2004; Ealo, 2009.

We include a comparison of the properties of the main materials used as pyroelectric transducers as an aid to the future selection of materials and pre-design work (Table 8.3). However, if more precise data is required the suppliers' characteristics sheets or the characterisation tests themselves must be consulted.

8.4 Main Challenges

8.4.1 Flexibility of Materials

The high flexibility of the transducers facilitates their integration into implantable medical devices, whose surfaces are usually irregular and curved, and also makes the sensors long-lasting.

Ceramics are rigid, fragile materials, particularly if used in the form of thin film. For this reason, pyrocomposites are being produced that combine their excellent pyroelectric properties with the advantages of polymers, as will be explained further on. On the other hand, although polymers have a better flexibility they are more difficult to process to obtain submicrometric film, which limits their potential in industry.

In principle, the thinner the thickness of the pyroelectric transducer, the greater its sensitivity, since the thinner it is the greater the surface/volume ratio and heat transfer is accelerated to a large extent, which leads to a faster response. Therefore, producing very thin pyroelectric polymers may help extend their use in industry as transducers.

To promote these features, the manufacturing processes for obtaining film need to continue improving, such as "dip-coating", "spin-coating", "Langmuir-Blodgett" techniques and other methods of preparing "self-assembled monolayers" and especially "dry and vacuum" vapour deposition techniques.

Table 8.3 Properties of Different Pyroelectric Materials (under Standard Conditions)
Note (For additional data consult the references or the suppliers).

	Pyroceramics					Pyropolymers	
	GaN	$CsNO_3$	$PbTiO_3$	$NaKC_4H_4O_6 \cdot 4H_2O$	TGS	PVDF	P(VDF-TrFE)
Density (g/cm^3)	6.1	3.6	7.5	1.8	1.7	1.8	1.8
Dielectric constant: ε_r	6–11	14–26	40–80	12–40	15–35	11	9
Pyroelectric coefficient: $\lvert \boldsymbol{p}_{max} \rvert$ [$\mu C/(m^2 \cdot K)$]	7.5	4.5	250	Around 20–30	330–650	20–35	20–35
Curie temperature (°C)	270–400 (Mn doped)	420	400–450	Ferroelectric only from 255 to 297 K	45–60	80 –140	100–160
Young Modulus: *E* (MPa)	94000–324000	n.a.	115000–135000	10000–30000	30000	400–2000	400–2000

Recent advances (Takashima *et al.*, 2008) have shown it is possible to use VDF oligometers (manufactured by Daikin Technologies Ltd.) to produce approximately 500 μm thick polymer pyroelectric sensors of outstanding flexibility and sensitivity.

8.4.2 Absence of Toxic Components and Composites

Many pyroelectric ceramics have toxic components such as Pb, Se, Sb, Mn and others, which means their use as active implantable devices is not always recommendable. Certain improvements have been achieved by dispersing ceramic nanoparticles in polymer matrices, which protect the body tissues (Sakamoto *et al.*, 1998, 2001; Xie, 2008), but their biocompatibility still needs to be carefully examined.

For this reason, pyroelectric polymers that are naturally free of Pb and other dangerous elements are being closely examined, as in many cases they are compatible with body tissue (Shimizu, 2009).

To complement the body compatibility of pyroelectric polymers intense work is being done to improve the materials and technologies used for electrode deposition in order to achieve coatings that are apt for direct transducer-tissue contact. This is enormously important for optimising the size and sensitivity of the diagnostic devices in question.

These deposition technologies are not only oriented towards preventing the body from coming into contact with possible harmful elements, but also for properly adapting the mechanical impedances, with stiffer electrodes in the zone in contact with the transducer and more flexible ones in the zone in contact with body tissue, which benefits this transducer-tissue relationship (Kim, 2008).

These advances will lead to new ideas being developed for the use of pyroelectric sensors as parts of active implantable devices in order to aid assessing any potential harm to tissues adjacent to the implant through heating. Some of these proposals have already been protected under patent, like US7289856, which describes the use of a pyroelectric sensor to contribute to the safe functioning of a pacemaker (Annapurna, 2004).

8.4.3 Pyroelectrics for High Temperatures

For high temperature applications polymer materials have serious drawbacks with respect to ceramic materials as pyroelectric sensors. However, ceramics with Curie temperatures of over 400°C are not frequent, a temperature that set the limit of applications for pyroelectric sensors until a few years ago. AlN is a special case whose pyroelectric coefficient increases proportionally at T^3 up to 150°C and maintains this figure with slight changes from 150 to 670°C (Yan, 2007).

The production of ceramic pyroelectrics by sintering has been recently described, such as $0.15BiScO_3–0.85(Pb_{1-3x/2}Bi_x)(Ti_{0,98}Mn_{0,02})O_3$, which because of the incorporation of Mn and the modification of Bi enables Curie temperatures of up to 520°C to be reached, some 120 to 150°C higher than the typical temperatures for materials like PZT or $PbTiO_3$ (Chen, 2008).

Doping Bi_3NbTiO_9-based ceramics with W to obtain $Bi_3NbTi_{0,95}W_{0,05}O_9$ has also turned out to be very effective recently (Barrel *et al.*, 2009).

Variations on the proportion and type of dope are enabling the Curie temperatures of these materials to be adjusted in a range of between 300°C and 600°C, and future advances in material science and manufacturing technologies are inspiring confidence that this kind of sensor will be produced with a wider range of use.

8.4.4 Combining Polymer and Ceramic Properties

Piezocomposites and pyrocomposites are seeking to combine the excellent high piezo- and pyroelectric coefficient properties of ceramics with the remarkable flexibility of polymers and their advantages for possible mass production (injection moulding, extrusion and other thermoshaping). Therefore, by using piezo- or pyroelectric ceramics as a disperse component in a polymer matrix, novel solutions can be found for specific applications.

The advances in the use of PZT powder dispersed in a polyurethane matrix to produce a transducer with a pyroelectric coefficient of around 70 $\mu C/(m^2 \cdot K)$, has already been described. This is significantly more than for PVDF, with suitable flexibility and mechanical strength (Sakamoto *et al.*, 1998, 2001).

Transducer film has also recently been obtained through the incorporation of PbSe nanoparticles into the core of an organic polymer (chitosan obtained from the shells of crustaceans). This has helped make good use of the sensor properties of the ceramic particles and also enhance their biocompatibility (Xie *et al.*, 2008).

Certain novel studies have also shown the effects of modifying the concentration of $CsNO_3$ as a filler material in a poly(vinyl alcohol) (PVA) matrix for obtaining ferroelectric film (Nautiyal *et al.*, 2009), having discovered optimal properties from a ferroelectric point of view for a 50% weight of filler.

If development work on the new materials is to be promoted it is essential to continue researching into modelling and simulating behaviour to predict the effects of the main factors of influence on transducer response (matrix properties, filler properties, distribution, geometry and size) (Díaz Lantada, 2009).

8.4.5 Competition from New Principles: Quantum Sensors

Quantum sensors are devices, which due to the nanometric level structure of the material used as a transducer, give rise to certain quantum phenomena that help increase the sensitivity and resolution of these devices.

Unlike thermal sensors, quantum detectors do not rely on the conversion of incoming radiation to heat. They are capable of converting incoming photons directly into an electrical signal. When photons in a particular range of wavelengths are absorbed by the detector, they create free electron-hole pairs, which can be detected as electrical current.

The signal output of a quantum detector is very small and is normally masked by the noise generated internally to the device at room temperatures. Since this noise within a semiconductor is partly proportional to temperature, quantum detectors are operated at cryogenic temperatures down to 77 K (liquid nitrogen) or 4 K (liquid helium) to minimise noise.

This cooling requirement is a significant disadvantage in the use of quantum detectors, especially for biomedical applications, as it increases the size of the device. However, their superior electronic performance still makes them the detector of choice for many thermal imaging applications. Some systems can detect temperature differences as small as 0.05°C.

Of all the materials typically used in the manufacture of thermal quantum sensors, we should mention InSb, PbS, PbSe and PtSi, whose effects on the body require more study to improve the their options for use in active implantable medical devices.

Other kinds of quantum sensors will be analysed in detail in Chapter 14, with a particular emphasis on other electromechanical and thermomechanical couplings.

8.5 Improving Results and Conclusions

This chapter has presented an introduction to pyroelectricity and its main applications in the development of biodevices, focusing also on modelling the properties of pyroelectric materials, specially polyvinylidene fluoride or PVDF as representative of pyroelectric polymers, due to their increasing expansion in industry as sensors.

Consequently some results related with sensor behaviour modelling, signal conditioning and characterisation trials are presented, as a way of providing researchers in this area with some basic help for studying these materials and developing new biodevices.

The main biomedical applications (both commercially available and in progress) are discussed, together with the most important current limitations and present areas of research. Future advances related to materials processing and sensor manufacture, together with improvements in the miniaturisation of conditioning electronics, will promote the capabilities of biodevices based on the use of pyroelectric materials as sensors.

It is important to note that this type of material can also be applied to medical devices in combination with other families of active materials, especially those based on thermal activation (shape-memory alloys, shape-memory polymers bimetallic actuators). Thus, pyroelectric sensors could be used as a way of monitoring temperature and optimising activation of the active part of the device.

Additional information can be found in the following list of references as well as in the websites of the different suppliers included in the annexes of the handbook.

References

Annapurna, K. "Medical electrical lead containing a pyroelectric material". US Patent 7289856, 2004.

Barrel, J.; Mac Kenzie, K.J.D.; Stytsenko, E.; Viviani, M. Development of pyroelectric ceramics for high-temperature applications. Materials Science and Engineering B, 161(1–3), 125–129, 2009.

Bergman, J.G.; McFee, J.H.; Crane, G.F. "Pyroelectricity and optical second harmonic generation in polyvinylidene fluoride films". Applied Physics Letters, 18(5), 203, 1971.

Brown, L.F..- "The theory and design of piezoelectric/pyroelectric polymer film sensors for biomedical engineering applications". Biomedical Sciences Instrumentation, 25, 119–126, 1989.

Chapman, A. J. "Transmisión del calor". Librería Editorial Bellisco. Madrid, 1990.

Chen, Y.; Zhu J.; Xiao, D.; Qin, B.; Jiang, Y. Bismuth-modified BiScO3–PbTiO3 piezoelectric ceramics with high Curie temperature. Materials Letters, 62(20), 3567–3569, 2008.

De Paula, M.; Carvalho, A.; Brassalotti, A.L.; Alter, A. J.; Sakamoto, W. K.; Malmonge, J. A.; Almeida, A..- "Microcontrolled pyro-electric instrument for measuring X-ray intensity in mammography". Medical & Biological Engineering & Computing, 43(6), 751–755, 2005.

De Rossi, D.; Dario, D. "Biomedical applications of piezoelectric and pyroelectric polymers". Ferroelectrics 49(1), 49–58, 1983.

Díaz Lantada, A. "Metodología para el desarrollo de dispositivos médicos basados en el empleo de polímeros activos como sensores y actuadores". PhD Thesis. Universidad Politécnica de Madrid, 2009.

Díaz Lantada, A.; Lafont Morgado, P.; Lorenzo Yustos, H.; *et al.* "Modelling and trials of pyroelectric sensors for improving its application for biodevices". Special Session on Active Materials for Medical Devices. Biodevices 2009 – International Conference on Biomedical Electronics and Devices. IEEE Engineering in Medicine and Biology Society. INSTICC Press, 2009.

Ealo, J. "Transductores basados en ferroelectretos para aplicaciones ultrasónicas en aire". PhD Thesis. Universidad Politécnica de Madrid, 2009.

Fang, J. S.; Hao, Q.; Brady, D.; Guenther, B.; Hsu, H. "A pyroelectric infrared biometric system for real-time walker recognition by use of a maximum likelihood principal components estimation (MLPCE) method". Optics Express, 15(6), 3271–3284, 2007.

Kawai, H. "The piezoelectricity of poly(vinylidene fluoride)". Japanese Journal of Applied Physics, 8, 975-976, 1969.

Kim, D.H.; Richardson-Burns, S.; Povlich, L.; et al. "Soft, fuzzy, and bioactive conducting polymer for improving the chronic performance of neural prosthetic devices". Indwelling Neural Implants, 2008.

Kucklick, T.R. "The medical device R&D handbook". CRC Press, Taylor and Francis Group. Florida, 2006.

Lindner, M.; Hoislbauer, H.; Schwodiauer, R.; et al."Charged cellular polymers with ferroelectretic behaviour". IEEE Transactions on dielectrics and Electrical Insulation, 11(2), 255–263, 2004.

Maldague, X. "Nondestructive evaluation of materials by infrared thermography". Springer Verlag. London, 1993.

Measurement Specialties.- "Piezo film sensors: Technical manual". Sensor Products Division, 1999 (www.msiusa.com).

Mochi, M.; Giovanetti, G.; Francesconi, R.; Hartwig, V. "A study for a portable IR sensor to detect the blood temperature during coronary bypass implantation". CNR – University Pisa. Technical Report, 2004.

Nautiyal, A.; Sekhar, K.C.; Pathak, N.P.; Nath, R. "Ferroelectric and phase transition studies in cesium nitrate: poly(vinyl alcohol) composite films". Applied Physics A, (published online) 14 March 2009.

Newsome, R.W.; Andrei, E.Y. "Measurement of the pyroelectric coefficient of poly(vinilidene fluoride) down to 3 K". Physical Review B, 55(11), 7264–7271, 1996.

Nye, J.F. "Physical properties of crystals: Their representation by tensors and matrices". Oxford University Press. Oxford, 1957, 1985, 2006.

Park, S.E.; Shrout, T.R. "Ultrahigh strain and piezoelectric behavior in relaxor based ferroelectric single crystals". Journal of Applied Physics, 82(4), 1804, 1997.

Paumier, G.; Siv, S.; Bancaud, A.; *et al.* "Thermoresponsive polymer-based microdevice for nano-liquid chromatography". International Conference on Biomedical Electronics and Devices Biostec 2008 – Biodevices, 1, 178–181. IEEE Engineering in Medicine and Biology Society. INSTICC Press, 2008.

Perera, R. "Introducción al método de los elementos finitos". Sección de Publicaciones de la E.T.S.I. Industriales – Universidad Politécnica de Madrid. Madrid, 2004.

Roemer, A.; Millon, E.; Seiler, W.; *et al.*. "Correlation between structural and mechanical properties of $PbTiO_3$ thin films grown by pulsed-laser deposition". Applied Surface Science, 252(13), 4558–4563, 2008.

Sakamoto, W.; Shibatta-Katesawa, S.; Kanda, D.; *et al.*. "Piezoelectric effect in composite polyurethane-ferroelectric ceramics". Physica Status Solidi, 172(1), 265–271, 1998.

Sakamoto, W.K.; Kanda, D.; Das-Gupta, D. "Dielectric and pyroelectric properties of a composite of ferroelectric ceramic and polyurethane". Materials Research Innovations, 5(6), 257–260, 2001.

Schindel, B. "Thermographie in der Theorie und Praxis". Online book 2007, (www.irPOD.net).

Shimizu, N. "High-sensitivity infrared sensor goes lead-free, bendable". Nikkei Electronics Asia Newsletter, 2009.

Singh, S.; Thakur, O.P.; Prakash, C.; Raina, K.K. "Improved piezoelectric properties via mechano-chemical activation in modified PCT ceramics". Materials Chemistry and Physics, 94(1), 7–12, 2005.

Suyal, G.; Bharadwaja, S. S. N.; Cantoni, M.; *et al.* "Properties of chemical solution deposited polycrystalline neodymium-modified $Bi_4Ti_3O_{12}$". Journal of Electroceramics, 9, 187–192, 2002.

Takashima, K.; Horie, S.; Mukai, T.; *et al.* "Piezoelectric properties of vinylidene fluoride oligomer for use in medical tactile sensor applications". Sensors and Actuators A: Physical, 144(1), 90–96, 2008.

Xie, J.K.; Jiao, K.; Liu, H.; *et al.* "DNA Electrochemical Sensor Based on PbSe Nanoparticle for the Sensitive Detection of CaMV35S Gene Sequence". Chinese Journal of Analytical Chemistry, 36(7), 874–878, 2008.

Yan, W.S.; Zhang, R.; Xiu, X.Q.; *et al* Temperature dependence of the pyroelectric coefficient and the spontaneous polarization of AlN. Applied Physics Letters, 90, 212102, 2007.

Chapter 9

Active Ceramics in Biodevices

Andrés Díaz Lantada
Mechanical Engineering Department, E.T.S.I. Industriales, Universidad Politécnica de Madrid, c/ José Gutiérrez Abascal 2, 28006 Madrid, Spain
adiaz@etsii.upm.es

9.1 Introduction

The word "ceramic" comes from the Greek word "keramos", whose Sanskrit root means "to burn". In its strictest sense it refers to clay in all its forms. However, the modern use of this term includes all non-metallic inorganic materials that can be shaped by the action of heat. Until the 1950s the most important ceramic materials were the traditional clays used in pottery, bricks, tiles and the like, together with cement and glass, but in the second half of the 20th century an enormous amount of work went into developing technical ceramics to improve the properties of conventional ceramics. Typical ceramics that can be mentioned are various metal carbides and oxides like silicon carbide, tungsten carbide, silicon dioxide, ferrite, zinc oxide, yttrium oxide, barium and copper, among many others.

Generally speaking, ceramic materials are hard and highly resistant to compression, although their porosity and fragility limit some applications. Some of them, refractory ceramics, are able to withstand very high temperatures and are also good thermal insulators. This means they can be used in a wide range of applications, such as shields for aircraft engines, furnaces and installations that operate at high temperatures. Their electrical properties usually place them

Handbook of Active Materials for Medical Devices: Advances and Applications
Edited by Andrés Díaz Lantada

www.panstanford.com

in the category of insulating materials, although the progress made in the last 50 years has led to the development of ceramic semi-conductors, conductors and super-conductors, opening up new horizons for applications in the electronics industry.

On the other hand, the advances in micromanufacturing technologies since the 1970s have been very closely linked to active or "intelligent" ceramics that can be used as transducers to develop sensors and actuators. These properties combined with the progress in micromanufacturing technologies and the possibility to produce microstructured materials have helped strengthen the impact of ceramic materials on the development of devices for different tasks in health sciences (see Chapter 13). So, in the last decades numerous microstructured "passive" ceramic coatings have been put to good use and have helped to enhance the tribological and biological properties of many implants and prostheses and to optimise such challenges as the final osteointegration and biocompatibility of these devices. "Active" ceramics have also gradually been taking centre stage and helping as transducers to contribute or enhance different diagnostic or therapeutic solutions.

As an approach to the extensive family of active ceramic materials, in the previous chapter we have already dealt with pyroelectric ceramics. These present thermo-electrical coupling of properties, which makes them candidates as temperature sensors. Other ceramics present electro-optical, magneto-mechanical or magneto-thermal behaviour, among others, which will be examined in the following chapters.

However, the term "active ceramics" is mainly used for ceramic materials with coupling of mechanical and electrical properties. The most widespread active ceramics are piezoelectric, which can change their geometry and transmit mechanical forces when they receive electrical stimuli and can displace charges (and generate potential differences) when subjected to deformations or mechanical force. This makes them ideal for activation and detection tasks and even "self-sensing actuators", as will be seen throughout the chapter.

Some excellent examples of these kinds of ceramics, as already mentioned in previous chapters, are quartz (with some types included in Fig. 9.1), topaz, tourmaline, Rochelle salt, barium titanate ($BaTiO_3$) and lead zirconate titanate or "PZT" system ($Pb[Zr_xTi_{1-x}]O_3$; where $0 < x < 1$). These properties can also be found in some natural materials like bone, tendons, gossamer or, to a lesser degree, wood, as well as some electroactive synthetic polymers already dealt with in the handbook.

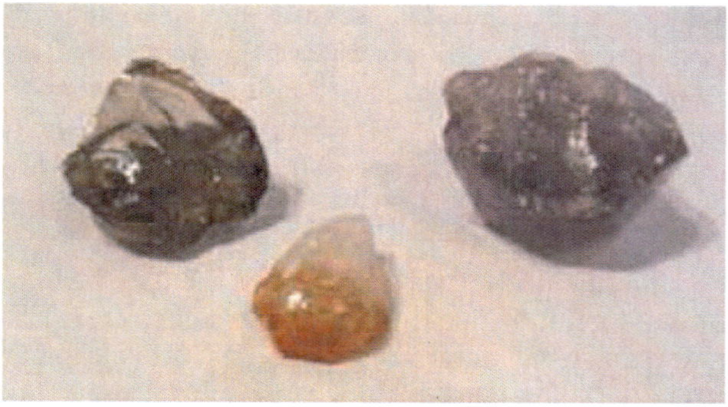

Figure 9.1 Different varieties of quartz (smoked, citrine and amethyst) as a piezoelectric material.

Therefore, this chapter is somewhat similar to Chapter 7, which took a detailed look at piezoelectric polymers like "PVDF" and its copolymers and at its most innovative applications in the medical industry. Notwithstanding, this chapter will focus more closely on piezoelectric activation rather than on the subject of electroactive polymers as sensors, since piezoelectric ceramics have some advantages as actuators over their polymer counterparts (which, in turn, make better sensors, as we have already explained).

Electroactive ceramics were discovered before other families of active materials and have been showing promising results since the 1880s (with the first research done by the brothers Pierre and Jacques Curie) and particularly outstanding results since the 1960s. This has allowed decades of in-depth examination of the problems concerning the synthesis, processing, characterisation, modelling and simulation of these "intelligent" ceramics. This means that the appearance of commercial devices has been a gradual ongoing process, mainly actuators or sensors, in the form of film (and more recently in the form of multilayer film) supplied by over twenty multinational companies.

The following section starts with an analysis of the most recent major proposals for medical applications concerning active device development using ceramic materials as electromechanical transducers.

9.2 Applications in Medical Devices

Besides the benefits linked to the ceramic coatings of numerous prostheses, either to increase resistance to wear or to enhance body compatibility, also worthy of mention is the use of active ceramics with piezoelectric properties, mainly as component parts of medical devices capable of detection or activation (Cheremisinoff, 1990; Haertling, 1999; Davis, 2003; Schwartz, 2006). Some of the most implemented active ceramics used in such devices are calcium titanates, barium or lead, lead zirconate-titanate ("PZT") or tungsten and bronze alloys.

On the other hand, being able to deposit them in the form of thin layers in combination with polymer or metal substrates also endows these materials with numerous capabilities (Albella, 2006; Janas and Safari, 2005). Some major applications are listed below, firstly looking at their applications as sensors and then as actuators.

Pressure sensors

In order to evaluate the pressure or contact forces between different parts of the body, suitably prepared piezoelectric ceramics can be used to measure footstep pressure for use in rehabilitation or high performance physiotherapy (Pons *et al.*, 2007). They are particularly suited to monitoring the evolution of lesions and for analysing progressive improvements until the optimal state is reached in top athletes.

Active orthopaedic devices

Their use as transducers in inertial sensors has been tested for various orthopaedic devices, such as motorised leg orthosis that require a real-time electronic control by means of information from inertial sensors (Moreno *et al.*, 2006).

Monitoring patients

Piezoelectrics processed in thin film form are light and convenient for being used to monitor patients. Some of the physiological magnitudes that can be monitored are any body movements that are capable of deforming the material (and so generate a voltage), as is the case with cardiac and respiratory movements and other involuntary movements. These kinds of sensors can be used directly on patients or embedded in mattresses, carpets or other structures. The signals generated can be managed remotely, which means that a larger number of patients can be supervised in special circumstances (Dent and Smith, 2009).

Electronic stethoscopes

Stethoscopes are acoustic instruments used in medicine, kinesiology, phonoaudiology, veterinary science and nursing for listening to the sounds inside a human or animal body. It is generally used to listen to heart sounds or respiratory sounds, although it is sometimes used to listen to intestinal noise or unusual murmurs in arteries and veins.

The use of piezoelectric film has also led to the development of electronic stethoscopes. These consist of a piezoelectric microphone, a signal amplifier and a connection to other devices such as a PC so that the signals recorded can then be analysed (Dent and Smith, 2009). These devices enable more objective approaches to be taken that can supplement the traditional procedure which simply amplifies the acoustic signal so that the doctor can make an assessment based on their experience (listening). Moreover, these electronic devices are especially suitable for making assessments in noisy surroundings (ambulances, emergency services and others).

Active cochlear implants

These are high-precision, high-tech active implantable health products that help bring back hearing to persons whose cilia cells of the cochlea are damaged, by stimulating the ganglionar cells (of the auditory nerve) whose mission is to send coded information to the brain.

The use of electromechanical transducers that can generate electric stimuli in response to mechanical impulses (sound pressure waves, in this case) have played a major role in the development of these implants. Piezoelectric ceramics and piezoelectric polymers have both been used to find different solutions (Mukherjee *et al.*, 2000). They have evolved remarkably since the first implant in 1957, culminating in the present-day devices from firms like Advanced Bionics, Cochlear and Med-el o MXM.

Sensors in heart pacemakers

Piezoelectric sensors can also be used to monitor patient activity from the inside of heart pacemakers. A cantilever microstructure is usually integrated into the interior of the pacemaker on which a piezoelectric material is deposited or adhered. This microstructure vibrates according to the activity of the patient, which causes the piezoelectric material to deform and generate a signal that helps manage the device and adjust the stimulation frequency (Dent and Smith, 2009).

As the signal is generated by the piezoelectric material itself, it is often unnecessary to use a battery to provide more power, so this makes the material ideal as it helps minimise the end size of the implantable devices.

Compact rehabilitation systems

Piezoelectric ceramics posses the capability to be used in small size rehabilitation systems that send the patient mechanical requests by means of various piezoelectric actuators. Their use has also been put forward for exoskeletons intended to control degenerative illnesses like Parkinson disease (Pons *et al.*, 2007).

Medical imaging systems

Piezoelectric ceramics have been used for some time as precision actuators to move medical imaging systems and in electronic and atom force microscopes (Mc Keighen, 1989). In order to expand the movement achieved/applied voltage ratio, multilayer ceramic stacks can be used to pass from around 1 to 5 nm/V to values of 1 μm/V.

Their use in combination with other transducers (like the piezoelectric transducers described in Chapter 10) can lead to optimal quality outcomes.

Drug delivery systems

There are different types of micropump designs, with and without valves, for the controlled delivery of drugs based on the use of a piezoelectric ceramic actuator (usually PZT) which operates a membrane whose job is to absorb and then drive the fluid in question (Feng and Kim, 2004). The flow volume can vary depending on the operating frequency and the flows can reach levels as small as 1 to 10 μL/min.

Development of other micro-electro-mechanical systems (MEMS)

In the last decade, in-depth research has been conducted into developing a kind of actuator commonly called a "microcantilever", which is basically a resonant cantilever structure with self-diagnostic or "self-sensing" capabilities. The first to emerge were monolayer ones but cantilevers with a larger number of layers of different materials are gradually being used, into which additional functionalities can be integrated (different kinds of combined activation and detection).

Ceramic piezoelectric materials, particularly PZT, are proving to be highly suitable as active layers of these cantilevers for producing controllable vibrations and exciting different vibration modes in these structures according to the movements required (Yao *et al.*, 2004). They can be used for microactuator development in numerous spheres of health sciences (minimal invasive surgery, biology and biochemistry, for manipulating cells etc.).

Figures 9.2 and 9.3, respectively illustrate bimorphous ceramic sensors for measuring deformations (and to a certain extent, vibrations) and a piezoelectric ceramic accelerometer specially designed for vibration and noise tests. By simply adapting conventional applications to these materials, solutions can be found to numerous medical needs related to monitoring forces and accelerations in different organs or as an aid to evaluating the way different implants respond.

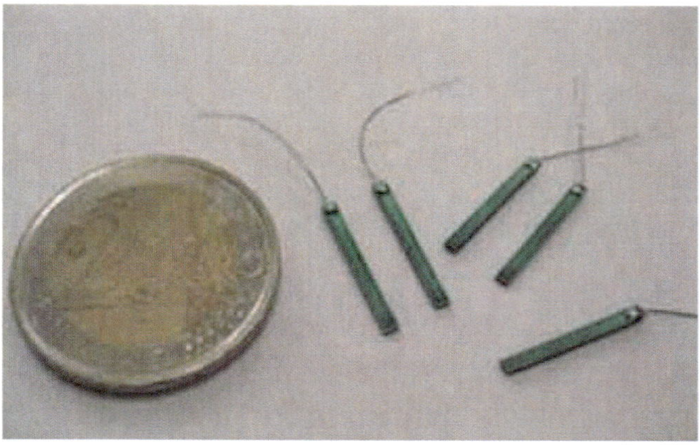

Figure 9.2 Bimorphous ceramic sensors for measuring vibrations.

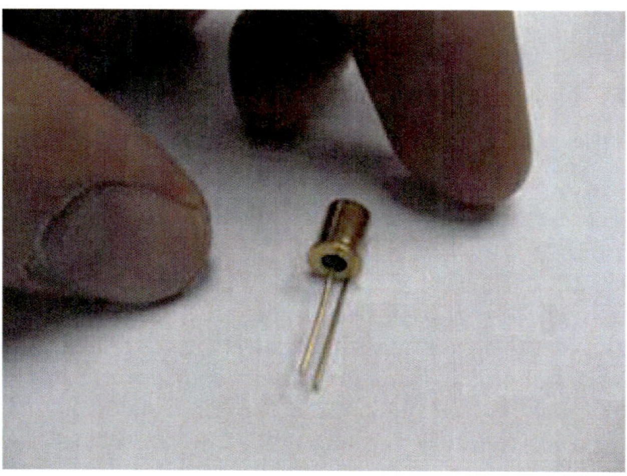

Figure 9.3 Piezoelectric ceramic accelerometer with protective encapsulation.

In fact, one of the great benefits of electromechanically active ceramics as with shape-memory alloys is that their working principles have been used in industry for decades. Therefore, it is easier to adapt them to solving medical needs than it is for other families of more innovative intelligent materials.

However, it is important to point out that within the family of active ceramics new developments and advances are ongoing, leading to materials with surprising and little known capabilities. Therefore, characterisation and modelling work combined with rapid prototype production are still relevant issues.

The following sections offer a more detailed explanation of certain points, like the synthesis, processing, modelling, simulation and integration of these materials into more complex devices before going on to analyse the main current research trends and major current needs, with a view to encouraging these materials to be used in the Medical Industry.

9.3 Current Capabilities and Recent Advances

9.3.1 Synthesis and Processing

A range of ceramic minerals naturally possess piezoelectric properties. These are quartz, minerals from the tourmaline, topaz, Rochelle salt group and some phosphates like $AlPO_4$, in addition to many biological materials like wood, bones, tendons or gossamer.

But those giving most rise to a large number of applications are some artificially fabricated piezoelectric crystals or ceramics, among which we can mention $GaPO_4$, $La_3Ga_5SiO_{14}$, $BaTiO_3$, $PbTiO_3$, PZT or $Pb[Zr_xTi_{1-x}]O_3$ (with $0< x <1$), $LiNbO_3$, $KNbO_3$, $LiTaO_3$, Na_2WO_3, $Ba_2NaNb_5O_5$ or $Pb_2KNb_5O_{15}$.

The process for obtaining synthetic piezoelectric ceramics usually begins with a conventional process to synthesise ceramic materials from different metal and semi-metal oxides subjected to fusion in a crucible and exposed to high temperature gases, which through controlled cooling gives rise to nucleation and crystal growth. Thus, microagregate is obtained which is then subjected to pressure to obtain ceramic pellets. These pellets are then used in sintering processes at temperatures that are usually between 1100 and 1400°C. Film is thus obtained, which after a suitable cutting and curing process results in the required sensors or actuators (Park and Shrout, 1997).

Deposition processes have also been described for precursor chemical solutions as silicon substrates for the production of ceramic film with piezoelectric properties and with very thin thicknesses (nanometres, Suyal, 2002). Laser pulsed deposition has also been used on MgO substrate to produce micrometric $PbTiO_3$ film (Roemer *et al.*, 2006).

One major advantage of obtaining thin sensors or actuators is their greater flexibility, which enables them to adapt to curved surfaces and helps integrate these materials into complex geometry devices (which is often the case with medical devices that have to adapt to body structures and tissues) for use in activation or detection.

It should be mentioned that toxicity of devices containing lead is driving research into alternative piezoelectric designs like NaKNb, with similar properties to PZT and a high Curie temperature (above which piezoelectric properties disappear), like $BiFeO_3$ or $NaNbO_3$, although their properties still need to be investigated as well as the consequences arising from their use. These aspects are also slowly promoting the use of some piezoelectric polymers such as PVDF and its copolymers.

9.3.2 Characterisation and Modelling

A piezoelectric material's mechanical and piezoelectric properties can be found through different methods of characterisation, some of which are described in the IEEE Standards on Piezoelectricity. There are also standard geometries of samples for these procedures. The choice of the techniques to be used depends very much on the geometries of the samples and the tools available. It is therefore inappropriate to recommend a single measuring technique.

To supplement the information in the IEEE document, the documents produced by the IEC (International Electrotechnical Commission) and CENELEC (European Committee for Electrotechnical Standardization) should be referred to. These documents are excellent for the study of multilayer materials with piezoelectric properties for sensor and actuator development.

The first experiments with piezoelectric materials found their piezoelectric and elastic constants by using static tests to charge the samples and measure the displacements and charges or the voltages generated. However, due to the difficulties of controlling the boundary conditions particularly when using piezoelectric thin film (tens of microns), static tests are becoming obsolete for characterising new materials.

However, for characterising the behaviour of these materials as the component parts of more complex devices, static tests using ad hoc test benches, like those shown in the preceding sections, are still of interest and their accuracy is sufficient for most applications.

For characterising new piezoelectric materials better accuracy is usually had by performing dynamic tests, as these also enable the behaviour of more complex geometries to be evaluated. The electrical properties of piezoelectric resonators or vibrators are dependent on the piezoelectric and mechanical properties of the material under vibration and the geometry of the vibrating sample.

Therefore, the values of the mechanical and piezoelectric constants can be found by vibrating specific geometry samples (by subjecting them to a frequency scan) and comparing the measurements taken with known behaviour models. Measurement basically consists in finding the electrical impedance of the resonators according to the frequency.

The behaviour of piezoelectric ceramics can be modelled using the following set of equations that we saw when dealing with piezoelectric polymers in Chapter 7. In this chapter, we sought to generate a voltage in response to mechanical stimuli, whereas with piezoelectric ceramics, what is often sought is to generate deformations (and the associated mechanical forces in constrained systems) by means of an electrical stimulus as input.

The equations describing these systems are similar, although during the actuator design procedure we need to proceed in the opposite direction from what is prescribed for piezoelectric sensors (Nye, 2006). We again include these equations as a brief reminder, but without the thermal effects described in the preceding chapter.

$$\{\mathbf{S}\} = [\mathbf{s}]\ \{\mathbf{T}\} + [\mathbf{d}]^t\ \{\mathbf{E}\}$$
$$\{\mathbf{D}\} = [\mathbf{d}]\ \{\mathbf{T}\} + [\epsilon]\ \{\mathbf{E}\}$$

where

$\{\mathbf{S}\}$ is the deformation vector;

$\{\mathbf{T}\}$, the stress vector;

$\{\mathbf{E}\}$, the electric field vector;

$\{\mathbf{D}\}$, the electric displacement vector;

$[\mathbf{s}]$, the elasticity matrix or the "elastic compliance" of the material;

$[\mathbf{d}]$, the piezoelectric coefficients matrix;

$[\mathbf{d}]^t$, the transfer piezoelectric coefficients matrix; and

$[\epsilon]$, the matrix of the electric permittivity of the material.

The piezoelectric coefficient matrix of a material normally contains many null terms depending on the material's class of crystallography, as other studies have shown (Nye, 1957, 1985, 2006). This fact has some fundamental implications when choosing a material to be used as an electromechanical transducer in a specific application. It is important to note that there are many piezoelectric materials that do not allow generating deformations and pressures perpendicular to their surface, while many others are not capable of generating shear strains and stresses. Many of them can only be used as an actuator in one direction.

As a case study, we will now show the modelling of an accelerometer for measuring vibrations. It is normally based on using a piezoelectric ceramic crystal or film (with a stiffness k and damping c), on which an inertial mass (m) is placed, the whole set being encapsulated for protection. The accelerometer, outlined in Fig. 9.4, is attached to a surface of the system under study. The position of the body of the accelerometer in respect of the reference inertial system is marked by an x. The position of the mass is called x_m and the subtraction $x_m - x = x_r$ gives us the relative position of the mass in respect to the body of the sensor. This also serves to analyse the deformation undergone by the piezoelectric material, whose deformation is responsible for generating the electric signal, as demonstrated by the following equations.

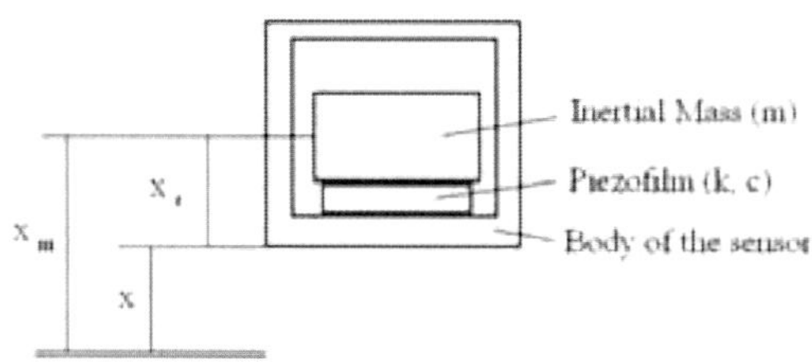

Figure 9.4 Outline of a piezoelectric accelerometer.

The piezoelectric is connected to the conditioning electronics and measured. It can then be modelled as a current generator to power a condenser that discharges to the measuring system via the input resistance.

The inertial force of the mass is transmitted onto the piezoelectric sensor so that such force will produce a charge displacement Q, in accordance with the value of the piezoelectric coefficient d_{33}, a charge that flows through the circuit in Fig. 9.5 and enables the voltage U to be read. The differential equations governing the relationships between the different electromechanical effects are listed below, but without the effects arising from the use of a charge amplifier, so that we can focus our attention on the piezoelectric behaviour.

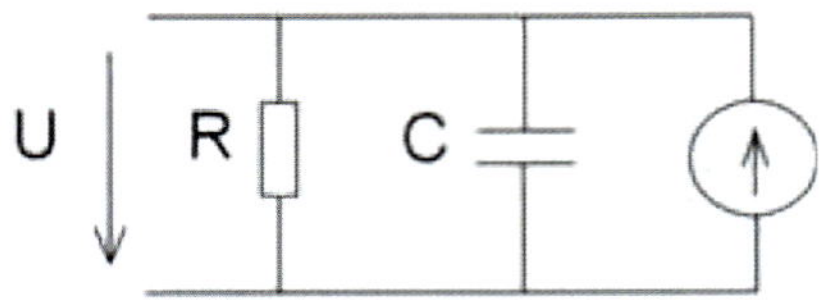

Figure 9.5 Electrical diagram of piezoelectric sensor behaviour.

$$m\, d^2x/dt^2 = -\,(m\, d^2x_r/dt^2 + c\, dx_r/dt + k\cdot x_r)$$

$$k\ x_r(t) = F(t)$$

$$Q = d_{33} \cdot F \rightarrow dQ/dt = d_{33} \cdot dF/dt = I$$

$$U/R + C \cdot dU/dt = I = d_{33} \cdot dF/dt$$

$$dU/dt + [1/(R{\cdot}C)]\ U = (d_{33}/C)\ dF/dt$$

By taking these equations a "Simulink" model was constructed, as shown in Fig. 9.6. This may be of help for a quick examination of the different influencing factors and the effects associated with their variations. The top part of the diagram mainly shows the mechanical behaviour of a vibratory system that is the equivalent of an accelerometer powered by an acceleration at its base.

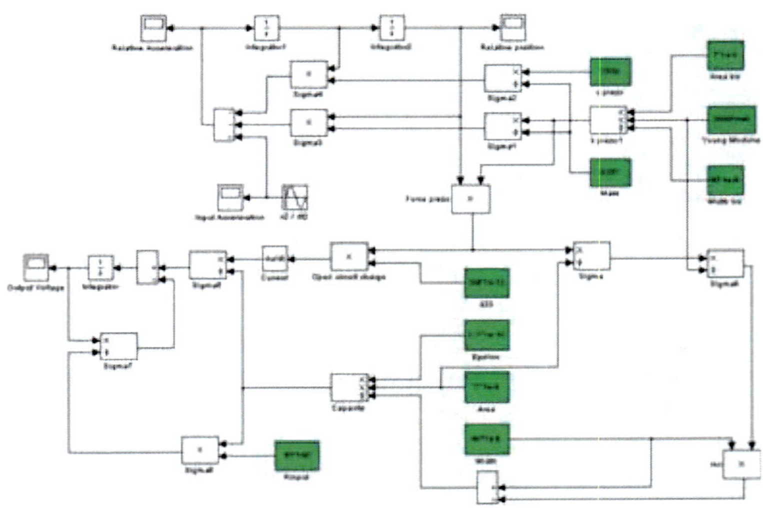

Figure 9.6 Electromechanical model in Simulink for modelling piezoelectric accelerometer behaviour (for ceramics as well as polymers).

The bottom part of the diagram represents the excitation of the piezoelectric and the generation of the corresponding output voltage. We decided to include the diagram here in case it might be of use to other researchers wishing to model these effects.

Figure 9.7 shows an example of the response of the sensor or voltage read (lower image) in response to sinusoidal acceleration as system input. The values of the different constants used for the example, associated with a standard piezoelectric part, are detailed below.

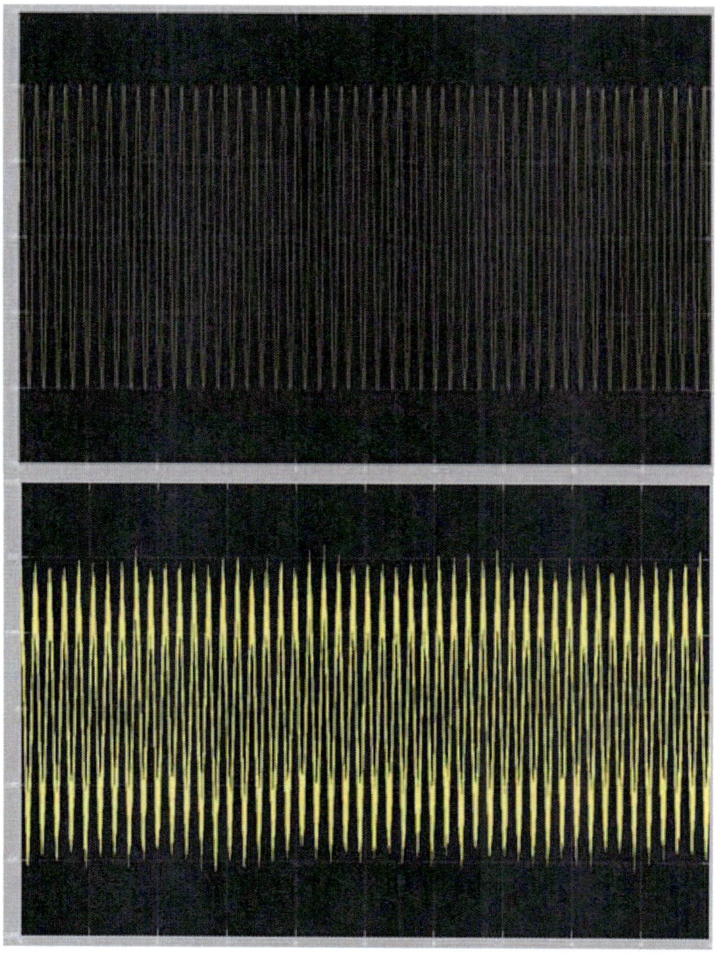

Figure 9.7 Input acceleration (upper image) and output voltage of the accelerometer (lower image) before filtering and conditioning.

$d_{33} = 24$ pC/N $\varepsilon = 1.1\ 10{-}^{10}$ F/m $E = 2000$ MPa

$k = E\ \ w/A$ (where w is the sensor thickness and A its area)

$c = 2\ (k\ \ M)^{1/2} \cdot \xi = 1700$ N$\cdot$ s/m $\rightarrow\ \xi = 0.085$

Using conditioning electronics, usually with a charge amplifier, anti-aliasing filter and other adjustment filters, in combination with an analogue-digital converter and a PC data collection card, enables a more convenient man-machine interface to be had for analysing the use of these materials and achieving more suitable designs.

The polymer materials used in accelerometers generally have a higher and less stiff damping value than ceramic materials. The piezoelectric coefficient in ceramics like PZT is usually higher than for polymers like PVDF. However, the slightest stiffness in the polymer causes higher deformations to appear and a stronger output signal. This, together with the lower fragility of polymer materials, is resulting in the gradual proliferation of piezoelectric polymer accelerometers in Industry. Once the single dimension system has been analysed, it is a simple matter to connect Simulink blocks, like those in Fig. 9.6, to achieve a fuller model that can be used to simulate triaxial accelerometers for measuring accelerations in the three directions of space.

9.3.3 Simulation Tools as an Aid to Device Development

With the information from characterisation tests it is simple to simulate the behaviour of an active ceramic actuator integrated into a complex device and analyse the influence of the actuator and device geometries on the final response of the complete system. To perform these simulations, finite elements calculation programs can be invaluable, as was also shown in previous chapters. These tools are extremely valuable in these systems for predicting the influence on global system response of the mass and geometry of the piezoelectrics used. This can sometimes be extremely complicated if only analytical vibration theory models are used.

We will now show a case study of a piezoelectric actuator for activating passive membrane movement, one circular and the other rectangular, for fluidic devices (diaphragm pumps and others). This case study is closely related to that dealt with in Chapter 7, where activation is produced by an electroactive polymer membrane.

At the end of the section is a comparison between the two alternatives, which helps to show how in most active medical device development problems different principles can be used to solve them (based on different "intelligent" materials) to reach satisfactory solutions.

Since the topic of electroactive polymers has already examined and the theoretical models sufficiently compared with the theoretical models (Blevins, 1979) and simulations, here we will focus on comparing the results of the simulations between electroactive polymer-based devices and those based on membranes activated by active ceramics.

To implement the FEM models in Figs. 9.8 and 9.9, NX-7 was used ("Siemens – PLM Solutions"). The standard properties of elastomers were applied in the passive membrane zone and the standard characteristics of piezoelectric ceramics in the actuator zone. The data on designed geometries, meshings and properties of the materials is shown below.

To simulate polymer membrane, in the first case a 20 mm diameter, 0.2 mm thick membrane was designed similar to the one used in Chapter 6 to perform the comparative study included further on. The ceramic actuator for that first case was a 4 mm diameter, 0.4 mm thick ceramic plate. In the second case, a 20 mm × 10 mm, 0.2 mm thick rectangular membrane was designed with a 4 mm × 2 mm, 0.4 mm thick ceramic actuator.

The mechanical properties used for the polymer membrane material are

Young modulus: 0.5 MPa
Poisson ratio: 0.4
Density: 900 kg/m^3

The mechanical properties used for the ceramic actuator material are

Young modulus: 20000 MPa
Poisson ratio: 0.35
Density: 3400 kg/m^3

Standard 2D meshed plate elements were used for the membranes with 0.5 mm side squares, and for the ceramic actuators, 3D tetrahedral meshes were used with a standard size of 0.3 mm. In the contact interfaces between the actuators and the membranes a "surface to surface contact" boundary condition was used to simulate the adhesive used in the actual devices.

The models prepared for the simulation are shown in Figs. 9.8 and 9.9. Supported edges were used as boundary conditions that allow using very thin plate elements to perform an approximate simulation of thin membrane behaviour. In these simulations and taking account of sufficiently small deformations, we discarded making calculations under the hypothesis of "large deformations" and neither did we include stress stiffening effects.

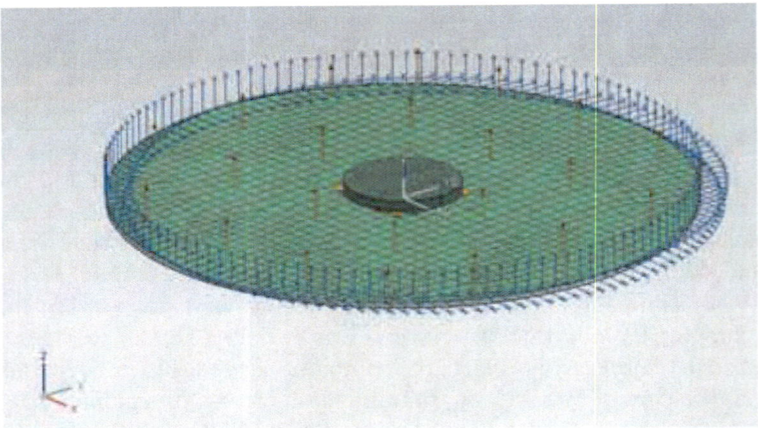

Figure 9.8 Finite elements model to simulate the response of a passive elastomer circular membrane with an integrated piezoelectric to activate it. Thin plate supported on its boundary as an approximation. Piezoelectric adhesive-membrane contact simulation.

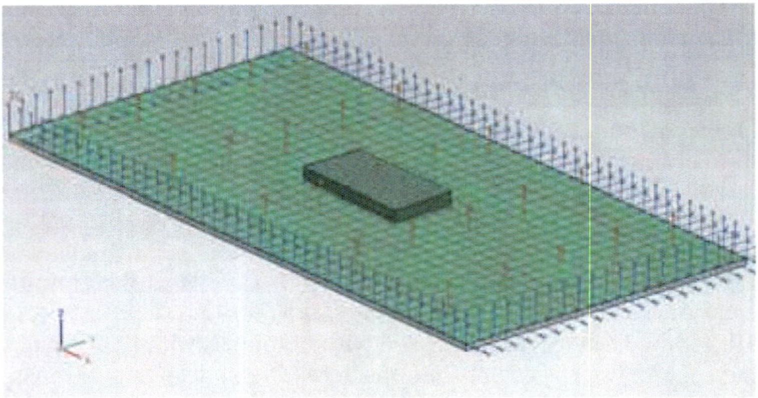

Figure 9.9 Finite elements model to simulate the response of a passive elastomer rectangular membrane with an integrated piezoelectric to activate it. Thin plate supported on its boundary as an approximation. Piezoelectric adhesive-membrane contact simulation.

It is important to point out that to simulate these effects and other non-linearities there are calculation programs, like ANSYS and Abaqus, which at present are the most efficient for adding increasing complexities to the models. However, as an initial approximation, the results shown here can be used for design work due to the similarities between the membrane models attached at their boundary with stiffening effects through stress and the thin plate models supported on their boundary (Blevins, 1979).

Figures 9.10 and 9.11 show the results of the dynamic simulation performed showing the first vibration modes for the different membrane and actuator settings. The frequencies at which these different modes appear can be seen in Fig. 9.12 and help predict the power frequencies to be applied to the piezoelectric actuators in order to obtain the different activation modes.

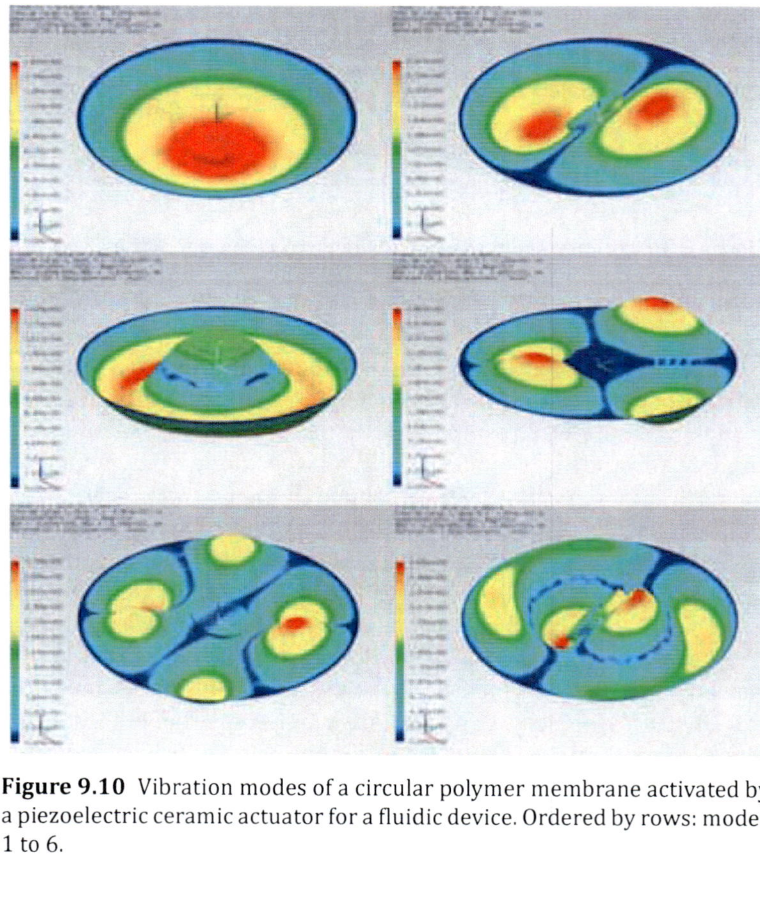

Figure 9.10 Vibration modes of a circular polymer membrane activated by a piezoelectric ceramic actuator for a fluidic device. Ordered by rows: modes 1 to 6.

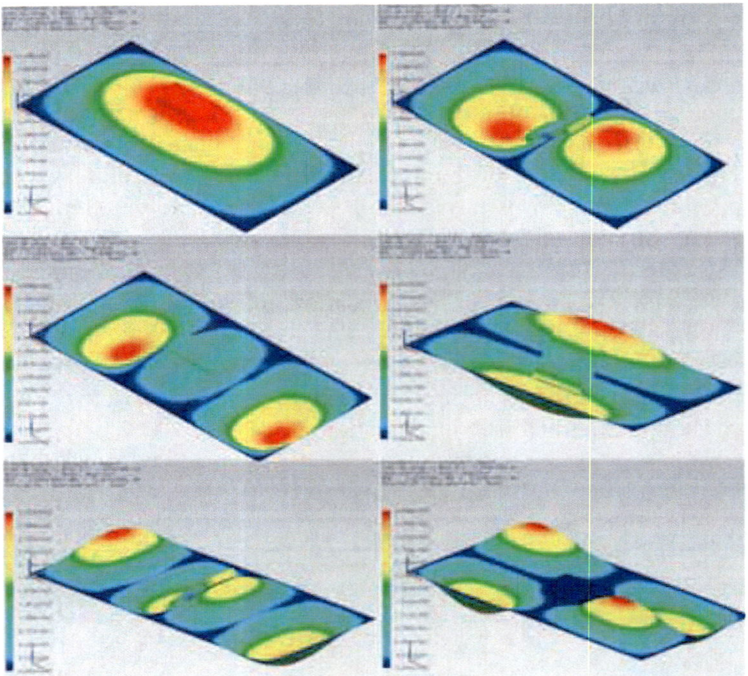

Figure 9.11 Vibration modes of a rectangular polymer membrane activated by a piezoelectric ceramic actuator for a fluidic device. Ordered by rows: modes 1 to 6.

It must be stated that that the fit between the calculations or simulations for vibration frequencies (relative to the different modes) and the test results with actual devices are usually more suitable for the first modes, since for the modes that appear at higher frequencies the slightest change in the boundary conditions can have a decisive influence on the associated frequency.

In the case studies presented, the inclusion of the piezoelectric on the polymer film (passive) causes the total system mass to be somewhat larger than that of the analogue example shown in Chapter 6 in which the polymer film was the active component. It can be seen how the inclusion of this additional mass makes the system dealt with here respond more slowly, resulting in the natural vibration frequencies (listed in the summary in Fig. 9.12), associated with each mode being less than those calculated for the example in Chapter 6 ("Circular EAP" and "Rectangular EAP").

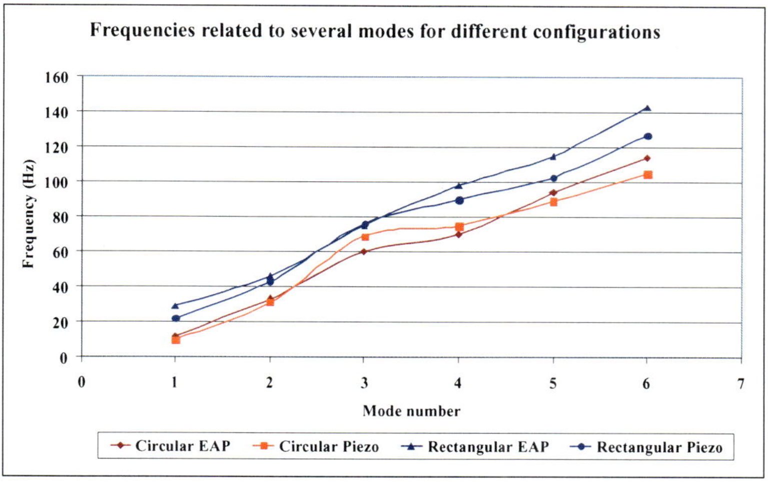

Figure 9.12 Simulation results: Frequencies related to several modes for different settings. Comparative study between EAP membranes and passive membranes excited by piezoelectric ceramics.

On the other hand, what is evident is the higher stiffness of the ceramic material which is practically unaltered in comparison with the deformations attained by the polymer membrane. This probably helps to stiffen some vibration modes, fostering their appearance at higher frequencies. This may help to understand some of the obvious differences in Fig. 9.12, between the lines associated with the electroactive polymer-based devices and those based on passive membranes activated by the active ceramics described here ("Circular Piezo" and "Rectangular Piezo").

We must again underline that the different mode geometries are an aid for designing the casing geometry, which together with the polymer film and the piezoelectric actuator make up the active device under development. For example, in the case of a diaphragm pump for controlled drug delivery or to assist pumping body fluids, the position of the nodes (zero vibration zones) and antinodes (marked amplitude zones) help position the piezoelectric actuator(s), as well as the aspiration channels (for fluid input) and propulsion (for fluid output) of the pump. So, the most suitable thing is to place the actuator (or actuators) in the marked amplitude zone, since if it is placed on the nodes (or nodal zones) in the mode to be excited, the deformations induced in the polymer film will be much smaller. Using adequate diffusers in the input and output channels will lead to a positive pumping in the right direction, as stated in various handbooks on microsystems (Koch, 2000; Maluf, 2000; Gad-el-Hak, 2002).

Since the boundary conditions of the polymer film have a decisive influence on the values of the natural vibration frequencies and are difficult to simulate, we must insist on the importance of using prototypes to help validate or correct the initial design predictions based on the theoretical models or simulations. Some of these boundary conditions for a fluidic device are the bonding of the piezoelectric part and the surrounding fluids. Therefore, rapid prototyping and manufacturing tools will prove to be invaluable, as we have already seen from other chapters. FEM tool simulations are also very useful for viewing the geometry associated with each mode and the design considerations for the device depending on the mode to be excited for activation. On the other hand, theoretical models, together with FEM simulations are enormously useful for predicting the main dimensions of the various device components when dealing with complex geometries.

These examples have served to demonstrate the effectiveness of a structured design methodology that uses equations from theoretical models to pre-select concepts, materials and working principles, perform simulations for evaluation, and compare and enhance geometries. It is also important to carry out tests to verify, adjust and optimise the designs in a controlled manner.

Programs like Matlab–Simulink are ideal additional simulation tools for evaluating the response of an electromechanical system, even under non-linear conditions, as we have shown in various examples throughout the handbook.

9.3.4 Device Integration: *In vitro* and *in vivo* Tests

In the conditioning of piezoelectric ceramic sensors similar principles are followed similar to those described in Chapter 7, when it deals with piezoelectric polymer sensors like PVDF and its copolymers. However, the values of the different components should be designed in accordance with the piezoelectric coefficients of these active ceramics and the output voltage required.

Using charge amplifiers usually helps to obtain more stable output signals in the presence of external noise which reduces the capacitor effects of other measuring system components, such as wires and other protective coatings.

Piezoelectric ceramic actuator management requires power electronics or a signal generator to be used to power the actuator and a voltage, and a current and frequency regulator controlled from a PC with the aid of man-machine interface software.

The advantage is that more and more commercial systems are appearing to activate piezoelectrics, many of which are plug and play so that control can be had from a personal computer with the aid of easily manageable software or using one's own programs for more specific applications.

On occasions, if the system is operating at high frequency, the heat generated by the actuator can limit its range of application. This again underlines the importance of performing thorough characterisations for the materials right from the beginning and when they are integrated into the device, before embarking on any *in vivo* testing. Thermographic cameras are ideal for evaluating these thermal effects, as previous chapters have shown.

When including active ceramics as actuators or sensors on structures or metallic, ceramic, polymer or composite structures or parts, it is advisable to use adhesives that have been carefully chosen for the materials to be bonded, seeking to use biocompatible adhesives, especially for devices that will be implantable. To ensure a good choice, the online catalogues and selectors of the major manufacturers can be referred to (Loctite, Henkel, among others).

Should the actuators be associated with fluidic devices, suitable insulation must be used to avoid leakage. The connection zone between the sides of the piezoelectric must be carefully protected to avoid short-circuits when they come into contact with fluids as this would result in a malfunction.

In this respect, elastomer coatings with pressure additives have proved to be effective, as was shown in Chapter 7.

Progress in rapid manufacturing and prototyping technologies (sometimes called "layer manufacturing technologies" or "free-form fabrication technologies") is enabling complex geometry ceramic parts to be produced directly (Brady, 1997) and even micrometric dimensions (Zhang *et al.*, 1999), as will be examined in Section 9.4 on the main research trends.

9.3.5 Materials and Commercial Devices

In spite of the ongoing progress in this field and the fact that most proposals for application are still under development, more and more piezoelectric ceramic-based medical devices are appearing on the market for the diagnosis or treatment of different conditions.

However, they can also be used to assist in study tasks, research work and teaching, in practical workshops or test benches.

One of the outstanding products are piezoelectrically activated diaphragm micro-pumps, available from some companies (thinXXS Microtechnology) which are often supplied as a test kit for regulating pressure and flow according to the voltage, current intensity and frequency applied to the piezoelectric part. These commercial micro-pumps can be used as an aid when testing individually developed microfluidic systems, usually lab-on-a-chip devices and electrophoresis systems, among others.

A good alternative for teaching workshops or beginning research into these materials is to acquire development or evaluation kits for the different technologies so that the effectiveness of the different materials, dimensions and settings of ceramic actuators can be compared, like those marketed by CEDRAT Group and other manufacturers.

These development kits are also valuable for evaluating the use of ceramics as an alternative to other metallic, ceramic, polymer or composite actuators based on electric, magnetic, thermal and other principles (for which some development kits have been referenced in the specific chapters).

9.3.6 "Pseudo-active" Ceramic Materials in Biodevices

Up to now in this chapter, we have concentrated on active ceramics with electroactive coupling properties, mainly piezoelectric ceramics, since ceramics with thermomechanical coupling were analysed in depth in the previous Chapter 8. Nonetheless, it is a good idea to take a careful look at some of the chemical activity exhibited by some microstructured and nanostructured ceramics, as they posses promising capabilities for developing a wide range of sensors suitable for use in the different spheres of health sciences.

Quite often, chemical sensors for gas detection reveal deficiencies when they are required to detect different gaseous species, but to which, their response is the same (Hunter, 2000). To improve on this highly specific ceramic membrane-based gas sensors have been developed (zeolites and other porous crystalline materials).

These are selective membranes, which let certain molecules pass through to reach the sensing element depending on the pore size attained (while avoiding the passage of gas molecules that are not required to be detected). This pore size can usually be regulated from 2 to 15 Å depending on the amounts of SiO_4 and AlO_4 used in their manufacture (through the superimposition of SiO_4 and AlO_4 three-dimensional tetrahedral networks) (Hunter et al., 2000; Gad-el-Hak, 2002).

9.4 Main Challenges and Study Trends

9.4.1 Enhancing Mechanical Response

An issue to be attended in coming years is to enhance the mechanical response of piezoelectric ceramic actuators. This improved response entails achieving larger displacements and developable forces from lower voltages during activation. In this respect, the synthesis and processing processes are being improved to obtain multilayer piezoelectric structures that will strengthen the mechanical response of insulated films.

To give just one example, the new actuators from Noliac Group are achieving optimised responses with multilayer piezoelectrics that attain a displacement of around 0.01 mm with a 5 × 5 × 10 mm actuator, by applying only 60 V, which means the sphere of application of these materials is making considerable headway.

These advances are providing solutions for various sectors of industry. The following are just some of their possibilities as actuators:

- Micro- and nano-positioning
- Vibration and noise control
- Valves and pumps — drug delivery
- Optics and photonics
- Ultrasonic motors
- Instrumentation
- Ultrasonic welding
- Ultrasonic cleaning

And as sensors, some of their possibilities are

- Vibration and shock measurement
- Pressure and force measurement
- Flow and distance measurement
- Sound and noise measurement
- Communication devices
- Sonars

- Energy source/generators
- Gas igniters

Ongoing research must also be done into how they can be gradually made less fragile and how the behaviour of these materials can be improved under fatigue. As commented in Chapter 7, one of the advantages of polymers as sensors on ceramic materials is that they are more flexible and less fragile, but this limits the sphere of application of ceramics as pressure sensors.

The emergence of new composites, possibly with a polymer matrix and piezoelectric ceramic filling could be very valuable for producing actuators/sensors with electromechanical coupling that can be tailored to specific applications according to the properties of the matrix and the percentage of filling.

9.4.2 Optimising the Power and Control Systems for Activation

Although ceramic sensors or actuators, particularly piezoelectrics can be quite accurately modelled by using the basic piezoelectricity equations previously described, while their being integrated into more complex systems as actuators can result in some non-linearities in the behaviour of the whole set due to a range of effects such as boundary conditions, the number and positioning of the actuators, the materials used in different parts of the device or the presence of fluids, to name but a few.

If these complex systems are to be modelled in real time and their control systems managed, we must once again point out the benefits of using artificial neural networks that have been properly trained using the results of tests with actual devices as well as effective modelling tools, as some research has described in detail (Guo *et al.*, 2003; Park and Washington, 2004).

As an example of these tools' potential for modelling intelligent materials with high non-linear behaviour, further on, the handbook includes a detailed example on the modelling of quantum tunnelling composites, in Chapter 15.

The use of these materials as energy collectors for their associated medical devices is also the object of increasing study, as will be detailed further on when we discuss combining active ceramics with other materials (Guyomar and Lallart, 2009).

9.4.3 Combining Activation and Detection Capabilities: Developing Active Self-Sensing Systems

Different actuators based on multifunctional materials can simultaneously furnish information on the force and displacement generated by the actuator itself, as well as on the input electrical magnitudes (voltage and current intensity applied), for which reason they are called self-sensing actuators. The materials that fall into this category are piezoelectric ceramics, piezoelectric polymers and magnetostrictive alloys, although, up to date, most of these applications are related to piezoelectric ceramics (Janocha and Kuhnen, 2009).

By continuously monitoring the input and output magnitudes in these kinds of actuators and comparing them with behaviour models adjusted in the initial reference stages, real-time systems can be implemented to evaluate the "health" or the stability of buildings, bridges and other structures. These are usually called "health monitoring systems" and are the principle application of the phenomenon. The implementation of health monitoring systems for implantable medical devices subjected to considerable mechanical demand and gradual deterioration (as with hip and knee prostheses and many others) is practically direct due to the designs that exist for other industrial applications. However, the integrity of the activation–detection must be ensured as well as making a proper assessment of its biocompatibility.

To promote these combined activation and detection capabilities, research must continue into the issues linked to these device manufacturing processes which attempts to take advantage of additive fabrication (layer manufacturing technologies and other rapid manufacturing technologies like selective laser sintering) that enable especially complex active ceramic geometries to be quickly obtained using CAD-CAM approaches (computer-aided design and manufacture). Positive results are beginning to emerge. In fact "free-form fabrication" approaches have been successfully used to produce piezoelectric parts in PZT (Gureev *et al.*, 2000; Guo, 2002).

The production of piezoelectric ceramics through sintering has also been recently described, such as $0.15BiScO_3$–$0.85(Pb1-3_x/2Bi_x)(Ti0,98Mn0,02)O_3$ which by including Mn and modifying the Bi, Curie temperatures of up to 520°C can be reached, around 120 to 150°C higher than the typical temperatures for materials like PZT or $PbTiO_3$ (Chen *et al.*, 2008).

9.4.4 Combined Use with Other Intelligent Materials

Apart from being able to use active ceramics as self-sensing actuators, in the preceding point we remarked on the fact that their combined use with other "intelligent" materials will gradually increase the complexity of the associated medical devices as well as the detection or activation capabilities in response to an increasing number of stimuli for a comprehensive management of the target pathologies.

In order to improve the energy management of the many devices described in other chapters, ceramic resonators can be used as energy collectors. This will enable the size of the associated devices to be reduced due to a lesser dependence on batteries ("energy harvesting kits" are becoming more frequently sold, like those offered by some manufacturers included in the annexes, to provide a back-up for a wide range of equipment) (Guyomar and Lallart, 2009).

The advantages of self-sensing ceramic actuators can be strengthened by developing multilayer structures to combine piezoelectric ceramics and polymers, PZT and PVDF, for example. In this way, the ceramic layer(s) can be entrusted with activation and the polymer layer(s) can be devoted to detection. This will put the optimal qualities of each type of piezoelectric to the best use and lead to devices that are more suited to structural monitoring.

In-depth research into the medical applications of these "intelligent" structures will give an enormous boost to their applications in industry, other than in the more usual spheres of use such as aeronautics, architecture or civil engineering.

We will again reiterate the importance of a detailed observation of Nature as a practically infinite source of solutions to technological problems. It is not unusual to find natural piezoelectric materials whose capabilities can be used to replace or supplement the piezoelectric ceramics described in this chapter.

Specific materials like wood, gossamer, collagen, tendons, bones, dentine and tooth enamel, to name but a few are piezoelectric materials. It is by no means unreasonable to imagine that future active implantable devices intended for monitoring different behaviours or conditions will discard piezoelectric sensors and replace them by direct connections to body structures and tissues that can collect sufficient information through their electromechanical properties. In fact, using such information from body structures and tissues that are used as transducers instead of conventional transducers might well be one of the most marked lines of research for the future of active implantable devices. If this is to be achieved, electrodes directly integrated into body tissues and structures and also connected to certain components for a wireless exchange of information to the exterior will come into more frequent use, as has recently been demonstrated *in vivo* (Warwick, 2008).

But what continues to be evident is the need to miniaturise electronic amplifying and signal control devices, as well as investigating ways to improve intracorporeal power systems (to palliate the risks involved with implantable power systems) and remote power systems (based on magnetic fields, as already used in some prostheses and implants) (González Bris and Díaz Lantada, 2009).

If these advances are to continue, we must again insist on the need to form teams to develop devices. These teams must have expert engineers in a whole range of branches of technology and professionals from various areas of health sciences, as well as the fortunately ever increasing number of biomedical engineers. They must all work in close collaboration to foster communication between team experts and spearhead these kinds of research projects.

9.4.5 Use of Bioactive Ceramics

The term "active ceramic" often refers to specific ceramic materials whose structure and properties are similar to those to be found in hard body tissues with which they can form stable chemical-physical bonds. We think it would be more correct to call these materials "bioactive ceramics", since the concept of active ceramics used in this handbook makes frequent reference to ceramic materials that present a coupling of mechanical and electrical (or thermal and electrical) properties. However, these bioactive ceramics must be briefly mentioned.

They are basically microstructured ceramic coatings (broadly speaking, passive microstructures), which in the last few decades have contributed to improving the tribological and biological characteristics of numerous implants and prostheses and helped optimise certain aspects, such as the osteointegration and final compatibility of these devices (Ducheyne, 1994; Kasuga, 2005; Lee *et al.*, 2006).

Bioactive porous ceramic coatings are obviously not an example of mechanical activity but chemical activity. This is ideal for optimising the integration process of a range of implants into the body, facilitating cell growth around the implant and enabling drugs to be included to stop rejection. Some of the major research has focused on evaluating the effects of the roughness and porosity of these bioactive ceramic coatings on the final biocompatibility of the devices by analysing the facility with which the cells adjacent to the implant can form bonds and grow around it to provide long-term stability (Neo *et al.*, 1992; Yokozeki *et al.*, 1998; Kasuga, 2005).

Some microstructured ceramics have also proved their usefulness for manufacturing self-cleaning anti-bacterial flooring which is becoming extensive in clinics and hospitals due to the positive results shown (www.active-ceramic.com). Some designs are even based on the superhydrophobic surfaces of some organisms and plants, like lotus petals whose surface texture helps them keep clean and prevent colonies of fungi, parasites and other microorganisms that could cause infections from proliferating on their surface.

To encourage these developments, above all, in the field of microimplants and micro-electromechanical systems (MEMS), recent advances in adapting rapid prototyping and manufacturing technologies to the "micro" field for the direct production of complex geometries by taking the information from CAD programs are looking very promising. The usual method for the direct production of ceramic parts is to take photosensitive polymers as starting material, whereas with laser microstereolithography, ceramic parts can be obtained directly. This is a major step forward in favour of ceramic applications (passive and active) in the development of complex parts and devices (based on "free-form fabrication") (Zhang *et al.*, 1999).

Chapter 7 includes a short introduction to fractal surfaces and their possible use for implant production with surface structures whose roughness and porosity are controlled right from the design stage, which can potentially be supplemented by these "free-form fabrication" technologies to produce enhanced bioactive implants.

9.5 Improving Results and Main Conclusions

This chapter has focused on the study and applications of active ceramics, particularly those that possess coupling of electrical and mechanical properties, such as electromechanical actuators and sensors mainly intended for applications in the biomedical sector.

In fact, one of the great benefits of electromechanically active ceramics, as with shape-memory alloys, is that their working principles have been used in Industry for decades. Therefore, it is easier to adapt them to solving medical needs than for other families of more innovative intelligent materials. However, it is important to point out that within the family of active ceramics new developments and advances are ongoing, leading to materials with surprising and little known capabilities. Therefore, characterisation and modelling work combined with rapid prototype production are still relevant issues.

Issues regarding the synthesis, processing, characterisation, simulation and integration of these kinds of materials into more complex medical devices have been carefully described, ending the chapter by highlighting the main action lines and possibilities for improvement in order to promote the use of these ceramics in Industry.

Top priorities for study are various pieces of research linked to the development of ceramic actuators with enhanced electromechanical response, to the combined use of activation and detection capabilities and to their being combined with other intelligent materials to produce multifunctional systems, apart from the ongoing search for new applications for these materials and the ensuing research.

Other activities present in certain ceramic materials that also have major uses in the biomedical industry have also been briefly examined, such as ceramics with chemical activity used to develop highly specific sensors, or bioactive sensors that are usually used to coat implants to make insertion easier when they come into contact with biological tissues.

We will now once again insist on the need to form teams to develop active implantable medical devices. These teams must have expert engineers in a whole range of branches of technology and professionals from various areas of health sciences, as well as the fortunately ever increasing number of biomedical engineers. They must all work in close collaboration to foster communication between team experts and spearhead these kinds of research projects.

To help bring this about, it is important to gradually include piezoelectric ceramic-related subjects (and "intelligent" materials in general) in the various Master's and PhD programs, in faculties of technology and biotechnology as well as in faculties of medicine and biology.

Additional information can be found in the following list of references as well as in the websites of the different suppliers included in the annexes of the handbook. We hope this will be of use to researchers interested in these materials and their applications, as well as for establishing future contacts among research centres.

References

Albella, J.M. "Preparación y caracterización de recubrimientos y láminas delgadas". PhD Program "Ciencias Físicas de la Universidad Autónoma de Madrid – Instituto de Ciencia de los Materiales de Madrid (CSIC)", Teaching Resources. Madrid, 2006.

Blevins, R.D. "Formulas for natural frequency and mode shape". Litton Educational Publishing, 1979.

Brady, G.A.; Halloran, J.W. "Stereolithography of ceramic suspensions". Rapid Prototyping Journal, 3(2), 61–65, 1997.

Chen, Y.; Zhu J.; Xiao, D.; Qin, B.; Jiang, Y. Bismuth-modified BiScO3–PbTiO3 piezoelectric ceramics with high Curie temperature. Materials Letters, 62(20), 3567–3569, 2008.

Cheremisinoff, N. "Handbook of Ceramics and Composites". Marcel Dekker. New York, 1990.

Davis, J.R. "Handbook of materials for medical devices". ASM International. United States, 2003.

Dent, J.; Smith, P. "Thin film piezoelectric film technology in medical device applications". Application Solutions. ECN e-Newsletter (www.ecnmag.com), 2009.

Ducheyne, P. "Bioactive ceramics". Journal of Bone and Joint Surgery, 76-B, 861–862, 1994.

Feng, G.H.; Kim, E.S. "Micropump based on PZT unimorph and one-way parylene valves". Journal of Micromechanics and Microengineering, 14, 429–435, 2004.

Gad-el-Hak, M. "The MEMS Handbook". CRC Press. Florida, 2002.

González Bris, C.; Díaz Lantada, A. "A wearable passive force sensor/active interrogator intended for intra-splint use for the detection and recording of bruxism". 3rd International Conference on Pervasive Computing Technologies for Healthcare 2009. London, April 2009.

Guo, D. "Gelcasting based solid freeform fabrication of piezoelectric ceramic objects". Scripta Materialia, 47(6), 383, 2002.

Guo, D.; Li, L.; Nan, C.; Xia, J.; Gui, Z. "Modeling and analysis of the electrical properties of PZT through neural networks". Journal of the European Ceramic Society, 23(12), 2177–2181, 2003.

Gureev, D.M.; Ruzhechko, R.V.; Shishkovskii, I.V. "Selective laser sintering of PZT ceramic powders". Technical Physics Letters, 26(3), 262–264, 2000.

Guyomar, D.; Lallart, M. "Mechanical to electrical energy conversion enhancement and self-powered wireless applications". IV ECCOMAS Thematic Conference on Smart Materials and Structures, Porto, 2009.

Haertling, G.H. "Ferroelectric ceramics: History and technology". Journal of the American Ceramic Society, 82(4), 797–818, 1999.

Hunter, G.W.; Neudeck, P.G.; Xu, J.; Greenberg, P. "Chemical sensors for aerospace applications". Microfabricates Systems and MEMS, V International Symposium, in Phoenix. October, 2000.

Janas, V.; Safari, A. "Overview of Fine-Scale Piezoelectric Ceramic/Polymer Composite Processing". Journal of the American Ceramic Society, 78(11), 639–640, 2005.

Janocha, H.; Kuhnen, K. "Solid-state actuators with inherent sensory capabilities". IV ECCOMAS Thematic Conference on Smart Materials and Structures, Porto, 2009.

Kasuga, T. "Bioactive calcium pyrophosphate glasses and glass-ceramics". Acta Biomaterialia, 1(1), 55–64, 2005.

Koch, M.; Evans, A.; Brunnschweiler, A. "Microfluidic technology and applications". Research Studies Press Ltd., Philadelphia, 2000.

Lee, K.Y.; Park, M.; Kim, H.M.; *et al.* "Ceramic bioactivity: progresses, challenges and perspectives". Biomedical Materials, 1, R31–R37, 2006.

Maluf, N. "An introduction to microelectromechanical systems engineering". Artech House Inc., 2000.

Mc Keighen, R. "Optimizing transducer design for medical imaging". Proceedings of the IEEE Engineering in Medicine and Biology Society 11th Annual International Conference, 2, 404–404, 1989.

Measurement Specialties. "Piezo film sensors: Technical manual". Sensor Products Division, 1999 (www.msiusa.com).

Moreno, J.C.; De Lima, E.R.; Ruíz, A.F.; *et al.* "Design and implementation of an inertial measurement unit for control of artificial limbs: Application on leg orthoses". Sensors and Actuators B: Chemical, 118(1), 333–337, 2006.

Mukherjee, N.; Roseman, R.D.; Willging, J.P. "The piezoelectric cochlear implant: Concept, feasibility, challenges and issues". Journal of Biomedical Materials Research Part B: Applied Biomaterials, 57(2), 181–187, 2000.

Neo, M.; Kotani, S.; Fujita, Y.; *et al.* "Differences in ceramic-bone interface between surface-active ceramics and resorbable ceramics: a study by scanning and transmission electron microscopy". Journal of Biomedical Materials Research, 26(2), 255–267, 1992.

Nye, J.F. "Physical properties of crystals: Their representation by tensors and matrices". Oxford University Press. Oxford, 1957, 1985, 2006.

Park, J.K.; Washington, G. "Prediction of hysteretic effects in PZT stack actuators using a hybrid modeling strategy". SPIE Proceeding Series, Conference on Modelling, Signal Processing and Control, San Diego, 2004.

Park, S.E.; Shrout, T.R. "Ultrahigh strain and piezoelectric behavior in relaxor based ferroelectric single crystals". Journal of Applied Physics, 82(4), 1804, 1997.

Pons, J.L.; Rocon, E.; Forner-Cordero, A.; Moreno J. "Biomedical instrumentation based on piezoelectric ceramics". Journal of European Ceramic Society, 27, 4191–4194, 2007.

Roemer, A.; Millon, E.; Seiler, W.; Ruch, D.; Riche, A. "Correlation between structural and mechanical properties of PbTiO3 thin films grown by pulsed-laser deposition". Applied Surface Science, 252(13), 4558–4563, 2006.

Schwartz, M. "New materials, processes and methods technology". CRC Press, Taylor and Francis Group. Florida, 2006.

Suyal, G.; Seifert, A.; Setter, N. "Pyroelectric nanoporous films: Synthesis and properties". American Institute of Physics, 2002.

Warwick, K. "Outthinking and enhancing biological brains". International Conference on Biomedical Electronics and Devices Biostec 2008 – Biodevices, Keynote Lecture. IEEE Engineering in Medicine and Biology Society. INSTICC Press, 2008.

Yao, L.Q.; Zhang, J.G.; Lu, L.; Lai, M.O. "Nonlinear static characteristics of piezoelectric bending actuators under strong applied electric field". Sensors and Actuators A, 115, 168-175, 2004.

Yokozeki, H.; Hayashi, T.; Nakagawa, T.; *et al.* "Influence of surface microstructure on the reaction of the active ceramics *in vivo*". Journal of Materials Science: Materials in Medicine, 9(7), 381-384, 1998.

Zhang, X.; Jiang, X.; Sun, C. "Micro-stereolithography of polymeric and ceramic microstructures". Sensors and Actuators A, 77(2), 149–156, 1999.

Chapter 10

Magnetoactive Materials for Biodevices

Andrés Díaz Lantada and Javier Echávarri Otero
Mechanical Engineering Department, E.T.S.I. Industriales,
Universidad Politécnica de Madrid, c/ José Gutiérrez Abascal 2,
28006 Madrid, Spain
adiaz@etsii.upm.es, jechavarri@etsii.upm.es

10.1 Brief Introduction to Magnetoactive Materials

This chapter is focused on the study of different kinds of magnetoactive materials that are either able to change their mechanical properties or their geometry in response to changes in the magnetic field around them (which usually enables them to be used as actuators) or that are able to change their magnetic properties as a consequence of changes in the variables of their surroundings (which usually enables them to be used as sensors).

Each magnetic material of this kind has innovative applications for medical device development. These are also examined in detail and references to the main researchers and centres involved in these projects are also included as well as links to some of the major suppliers listed in the annexes.

Regarding the development of actuators, three basic kinds of magnetoactive materials are dealt with:

- Electro/magnetorheological fluids, which are able to change their viscosity in response to variations in the magnetic field around them

Handbook of Active Materials for Medical Devices: Advances and Applications
Edited by Andrés Díaz Lantada

- Magnetorheological elastomers and hydrogels, which can change their stiffness (Young modulus) and their damping according to the magnetic field around them
- Magnetostrictive materials, which have the ability to stretch or compress in a controlled manner in response to the action of the external magnetic field

Regarding the development of sensors, three particularly important kinds of magnetoactive materials are dealt with:

- Magnetoelastic materials, which can change their magnetisation curve when subjected to deformations or forces
- Piezomagnetic materials, which exhibit coupling between their magnetic polarisation and mechanical deformations
- Pyromagnetic materials, which are able to change their magnetic properties or acquire them in response to changes in temperature

Each material is accompanied by a written description of aspects connected with its composition and structure, synthesis and processing, characterisation and modelling, integration into devices or the main trends in current research, with a view to promoting the use of these materials in industry, particularly in health science-related applications. Their most outstanding properties will be analysed in greater detail, as they open up fields of application where other intelligent materials would not lead to such appropriate solutions.

It is important to point out that these magnetoactive materials have been grouped together in just one chapter as they do not yet have such a marked number of medical applications as those to which we have dedicated an entire chapter. Another reason is that they are all linked to magnetic phenomena.

10.2 Magnetorheological Fluids

10.2.1 Introduction: Basic Properties

Magnetorheological fluids (MR fluids) are able to change their rheology when subjected to a magnetic field. This property can be very accurately controlled by varying the magnetic field intensity, which provides a rapid and effective system to control the response of very diverse fluid-mechanical devices. These kinds of fluids are composed of magnetic particles suspended within a carrier fluid. Thus, they are typically composed of micrometer or nanometre-scale spheres distributed in a mineral oil or liquid synthetic polymer.

The response of the magnetorheological fluids is the result of the induced distribution of the magnetic suspension particles (usually in the 0.1–10 μm range) within the fluid when an external magnetic field is applied (usually about 100 mT in air). The microscopic particles align themselves along the lines of magnetic flux, as can be seen in Fig. 10.1.

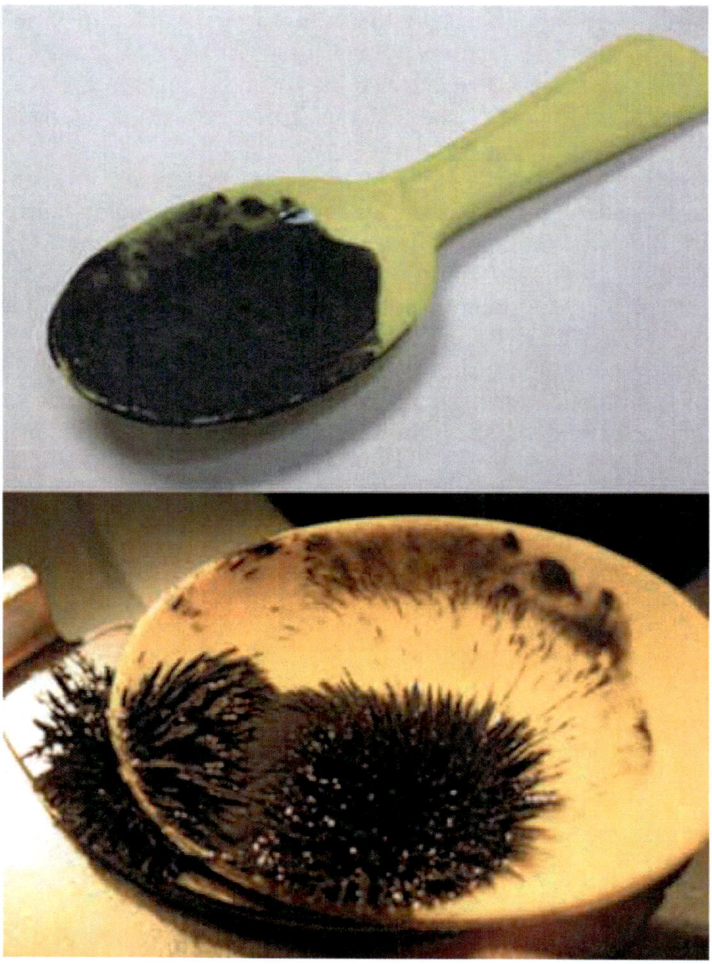

Figure 10.1 Magnetorhelogical fluid as purchased (upper image). Effect of a magnetic field on its structure and properties (lower image).

Thus, the resulting chains of particles restrict the movement perpendicular to the direction of the lines of flux, leading to an anisotropic behaviour and to an increase in the viscosity of the fluid (Torcuato, 2006). This phenomenon is considered completely reversible and almost instantaneous (response time is about 10 ms) for these fluids.

The magnetically controllable properties of magnetorheological fluids depend on the carrier fluid and its additives, the magnetic field applied, the working condition and the size, shape, concentration, density and distribution of the particles. The first patent related to MR technology was issued to the inventor Jacob Rabinow in the 1940s, though this technology had little practical use at the time. However, in the last 20 years there has been serious research in this field, especially when other technologies began to converge that made their use practical and a real possibility.

Numerous research efforts have been carried out in order to improve magneto-rheological fluids, in specialised companies like Lord, Repsol-YPF and in different universities. Although MR fluids have many potential applications, they are limited by aspects such as their high density and wear in materials due to the presence of iron, and their very high cost or precipitation of particles.

When attempting to provide a short introduction to the usual models for modelling the behaviour of this type of fluid, it is advisable to begin by remembering the difference between Newtonian and non-Newtonian fluids (such as MR fluids).

The behaviour of Newtonian fluids (with constant viscosity and a linear relationship between shear forces and their deformation rate) can be shown in an approximate form by the following expression:

$$\tau = \mu \frac{\partial v_x}{\partial y}$$

where

τ is the shear stress [Pa];

μ, the dynamic viscosity [Pa·s] constant in Newtonian fluids (but variable for MR fluids);

v_x, the velocity according to direction [m/s];

y, the axis perpendicular to the shear direction; and

$\frac{\partial v_x}{\partial y}$, the rate of deformation [s^{-1}].

However, MR fluids behave as non-Newtonian fluids and can be modelled in accordance with Bingham's plastic models, and also incorporate the effects of the magnetic field (or the associated electric field) into the fluid viscosity. The most commonly used method to reach an approximation of how these fluids behave is by using the following expressions, although it is always advisable to adjust them using the information from the characterisation tests for each specific type of MR fluid:

$$\tau = \tau_y + \mu \frac{\partial v_x}{\partial y} \quad \tau > \tau_y$$

$$\mu \approx \mu_a + (\mu_b - \mu_a) \cdot e^{-\alpha|B|} \approx \mu_a + (\mu_b - \mu_a) \cdot e^{-\beta|E|}$$

Although, on occasions, depending on the type of base fluid, the type of geometry and proportion of magnetic particles used, the viscosity of the MR fluid can also be approximated with expressions such as

$$\mu \approx \mu_a - k \cdot |\mathbf{E}|^2$$

where

τ_y is the shear stress limit at which the MR material begins to behave as a fluid [Pa];

$|\mathbf{E}|$, the electric field activation modulus [N/C];

$|\mathbf{B}|$, the magnetic induction field modulus resulting from the activation [T];

$\alpha, \beta, k,$ the fitting constants or those provided by each manufacturer; and

$\mu_a, \mu_b,$ the reference viscosity values [Pa· s].

10.2.2 Main Present and Potential Applications

Nowadays, the main manufacturers of magnetorheological fluids (Lord Corporation) offer specific solutions for many applications, mainly within the following sectors:

- Suspension systems and shock absorbers
- Fan clutches
- Crash-protection systems
- Buildings and bridges
- Medical applications

In the near future many other applications are expected to be available, because their possibilities are almost endless. The most extended application for the fluids developed is their use in a magnetorheological suspension, where a controllable fluid replaces traditional hydraulic oil in each shock absorber. As sensors monitor road and vehicle conditions, a controller modifies the intensity applied and therefore the damping characteristics are adjusted in real time. This enables remarkable improvements in both comfort and handling.

Magnetorheology has had an important role in recent advances in the military, aeronautic and automotive industries. So-called MR technology has been integrated not only into military tactical and combat vehicles but also into primary suspension systems of high performance vehicles designed by Cadillac, Audi, Ferrari, Honda and others. In addition, these new technologies are used in the seat and cab suspension designs of agricultural and other off-highway vehicles in order to improve their operating environment.

Apart from their use for suspension applications, there are a lot of patents concerning MR fluids for fan clutches. The main aims of these inventions are to provide smooth, efficient torque-transfer in clutch devices. The designs include a large range of applications for improving controllability and the high off-state drag. Another present application for MR fluids is obtained by combining variable control magnetorheology with advanced sensors in passenger protection systems. In these cases, the protection systems can be adjusted to provide the perfect resistance based on impact severity and passenger size. There is also a civil and structural application in skyscrapers and protecting long bridges which are susceptible to vibrations induced by high winds and seismic activity. In order to mitigate their effect, large dampers are built into their design, which protect against shocks through a continuously controllable and cost-effective solution.

Among medical applications, some of the most innovative and promising ones are explained below:

Haptic devices

Tactile and force feedback or haptic systems are used in computer-assisted surgery training, as well as for orthopaedic surgery and physiotherapy. Active dampers have been developed based on MR fluids and their utilisation in haptic systems provides a very precise control which enhances surgeons' skills (Bar-Cohen and Mavroidis, 2001; Neelakantan, 2002; Rizzo, 2007).

In particular, by using sensorised surgical instruments, suitable signals could be acquired and used for controlling the haptic device. The surgeons could use the surgical instruments to interact with biological tissues and organs during a simulated operation and test their compliance by touching the haptic device (Scilingo *et al.*, 2003).

Prosthetics and rehabilitation

The Lord company, in collaboration with Biedermann Motech, manufacturer of prosthetic components, has developed a device that improves the mobility of leg amputees. The new design is based on MR dampers and produces an increase in gait balance, stability and energy efficiency. Other medical systems based on similar active control elements are used in training devices for rehabilitation purposes which allow an adjustable resistance to movement according to the patient's progress (Dong, 2005).

Cancer therapy

Human and animal biocompatibility and tolerability to magnetorheological materials has been successfully tested in previous research (Sheng *et al.*, 1999). Some techniques developed for cancer therapies which target chemotherapeutic agents to the tumour sites by employing magnetic nanoparticles as carriers is a promising cancer treatment that reduces the side effects of conventional chemotherapy. Electron microscope research shows that the ferrofluids can be enriched in tumour tissue and tumour cells (Alexiou *et al.*, 2006).

Therefore, these studies show a remarkable improvement on conventional cancer therapy but still cause toxicity to the body. Other interesting studies are based on MR fluids introduced into the blood vessels supplying the tumour. When a magnetic field is applied a seal is formed which blocks the blood flow and cuts off the oxygen supply leading to tumour necrosis. There are interesting *in vitro* investigations of these therapies (Sheng *et al.*, 1999) concerning the study of the seal kinetics and pressure resistibility of the seal.

Braille readers/translators

Developing a panel with a surface whose stiffness could be subjected to local changes could be applied to the development of Braille reading and writing systems to assist the blind, without any need to store information in physical external supports (perforated or embossed cards).

The use of electro/magnetorheological fluid for this purpose has been demonstrated in the laboratory (Bansevicius and Virbali, 2007), although no commercial devices are yet available.

X-ray collimator

Prototype lenses have recently been developed that include magnetorheological fluid in their interior. These have been used to help collimate X-rays in dental radiology apparatus with some positive preliminary results (Dyszkiewicz *et al.*, 2009).

10.2.3 Present Capabilities and Recent Advances

Most studies conducted throughout the last few decades have focused on the synthesis and processing of these materials based on the dispersion of different magnetic particles in different organic and synthetic fluids.

Characterisation testing is therefore essential if a detailed knowledge of the properties of these materials is to be acquired to be able to compare the results of different formulations. As an example, we include below some details of the standard characterisation process used for these fluids (Echávarri *et al.*, 2009).

Our colleagues at the Machine Engineering Division (DIM) from the Universidad Politécnica de Madrid (UPM) have collaborated with the Repsol-YPF company and the Applied Physics Department of the University of Granada in the development and characterisation of new magnetorheological fluids for shock-absorbers used for different applications.

Two oils have been developed along with tests, in order to validate their possible industrial application: MR-Lub1 and MR-Lub2. The carrier fluid is the same for both of them but the second fluid includes a higher percentage of magnetic particles. The cited characterisation was carried out in a commercial damper mounted in an MTS damper test system shown in Fig. 10.2.

The first characterisation includes a quasi-static test (velocity of the damper below 1 mm/s) to determine the effect of the electric intensity (which produces a magnetic field) on the increase of the damping force in the damper. The results for MR-Lub1 are depicted as a brief example in Fig. 10.3, which clearly shows a non-linear behaviour.

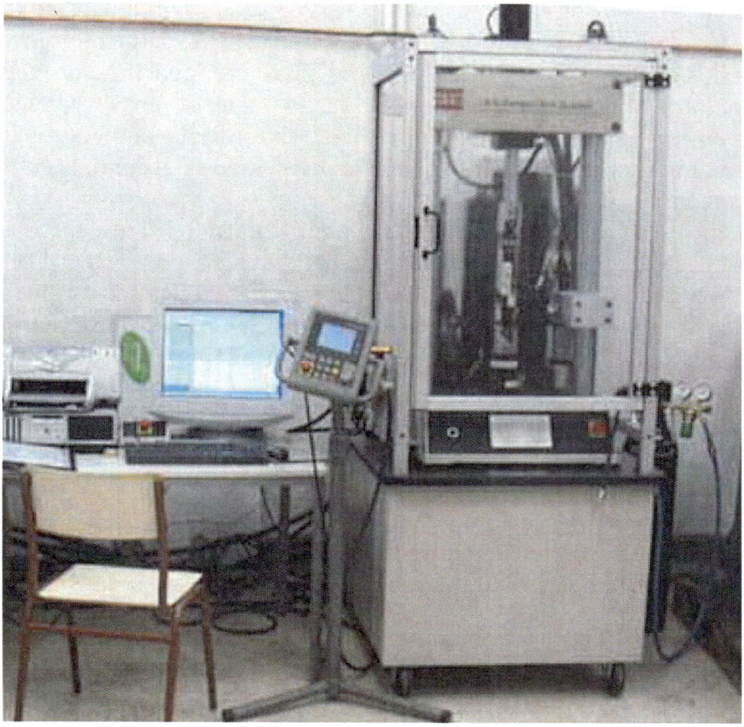

Figure 10.2 MTS damper test system.

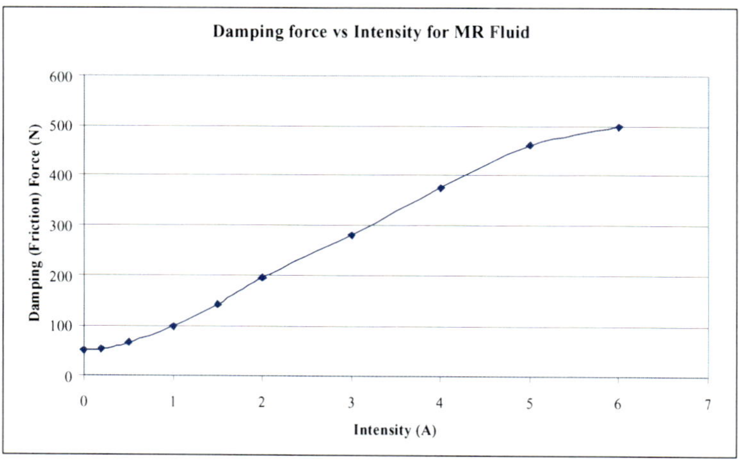

Figure 10.3 Damping force vs. intensity for MR fluid.

The reversible magnetorheological behaviour, obtained for the damper during dynamic tests, can be found in some of the references (Echavarri, 2008. The damping force obtained at each point when the intensity is growing is very similar to the force measured when intensity is decreasing. Nevertheless, the results show a slight remaining magnetisation when low intensities of around 1 A are applied.

Some comparisons between dynamic tests in the shock absorber with MR-Lub1, MR-Lub2 and two commercial fluids by Lord at a velocity of 1 m/s have also been included in such references, showing that the higher quantity of magnetic particles in MR-Lub1 than in MR-Lub2 leads to an increase in the sum of the traction (T) and compression (C) forces, although similar force-intensity behaviour is observed in all the tests performed.

10.2.4 Main Challenges and Research Trends

Magnetorheological current research related to the development of magnetorheological fluids is centred on resolving some of the main limitations mentioned, of which the major ones are

- To prevent the decanting of particles in the core of the fluid that lead to non-homogeneous properties, possibly by using electromechanical agitators or by reducing the size of the particles
- To examine aspects related to the corrosion that these fluids exert on other components of the machines and devices into which they are integrated
- To continue developing new formulations with properties that can be adjusted in line with the end application

If progress is to be made in all these areas, thorough characterisation tests need to be performed in order to gain deeper knowledge of how these fluids behave and their effects on the systems benefitting from their use.

On the other hand, and more closely related to the development of active medical devices, it is important to underline the possible benefits of using these fluids in combination with other intelligent transducer-based actuators (like shape-memory or piezoelectric ceramics). The response speed of these intelligent transducers can be controlled by magnetorheological actuators in series or in parallel, whose controlled damping can sometimes help delay a response in order to obtain a behaviour that is more suited to the body's needs.

MR fluid-based dampers, for example, have been introduced into active exoskeletons whose movement is brought about by other actuators, but in which the inclusion of MR dampers helps gain optimised control (Bar-Cohen, 2004). In this way, the development of haptic devices with ever more realistic teleoperation features is coming closer. Combining these haptic devices with other visual tools that form part of the so-called enhanced reality techniques could lead to high-quality surgical training tools.

Regarding the medical industry, it is also important to embark on very detailed studies to analyse the physiological effects of any MR fluid leakage from active medical devices, as well as detailing procedures for obtaining biocompatible end applications based on these materials.

On the other hand, integrating these fluids into the core of liquid-state monomers for subsequent polymerisation is enabling magnetorheological elastomers to be developed that have properties that fall between a fluid and a solid, whose controllable stiffness is of major scientific and industrial interest. For this reason, the following section has been devoted to these kinds of magnetoactive elastomers that have properties and uses in common with the fluids described here.

10.3 Magnetorheological Elastomers and Hydrogels

10.3.1 Introduction: Basic Properties

Very closely related to the magnetorheological fluids of the preceding section are magnetorheological elastomers and hydrogels. In this case, they are apparently solid materials (although all "solid" polymers are actually aggregates in a state of non-thermodynamic equilibrium that flow at very slow speeds, for which reason the term "sub-cooled liquid" is more appropriate). These magnetorheological elastomers and hydrogels are able to change their stiffness and damping according to the magnetic field around them (Borcea, 2001; Zhou, 2004; Kallio, 2005; Guerrero-Sánchez *et al.*, 2009).

In the last decade, magnetorheological elastomers (MREs) have been developed using polymer matrices (polyurethanes, natural rubber and various silicons) with magnetic powder or particles dispersed in them (the most used up to the present is carbonyl iron powder) to obtain magnetomechanical coupling. The variations in the external magnetic field change the alignment of the particles due to the flexibility of the elastomeric matrix. To a certain extent, this enables some of the properties of these composites to be controlled, such as the elasticity modulus, tensile stress or the damping coefficient.

Since the matrix is "solid" in this case, the magnetorheological elastomers do not exhibit the problems of sedimentation that are typical of magnetorheological fluids, which is a great advantage. However, these groups of active materials should not be perceived as mutually exclusive, but rather as complementary, since MRFs are more suitable for tasks where the viscosity of a component needs to be controlled, whereas MREs are more suitable for controlling the stiffness of certain system components.

Research has recently been carried out into solid magenetorheological composite materials in which a hydrogel acts as a matrix and the magnetic nano- and micrometric particles act as filling. This means that actuators can be produced with the coupling of additional properties that exhibit hydroactivity and magnetoactivity.

The concept has been successfully tested using poly(vinyl alcohols) or PVAs, although a whole range of hydrogels can benefit from having magnetic particles integrated to obtain additional functionalities (Vekas, 2008).

Immersing samples of these composite hydrogels in water generally leads to isotropic volume increases, although applying a magnetic field during the polymerisation process leads to privileged orientations and to actuators that have an isotropic response. On the other hand, the variations in the magnetic field affect the mechanical properties of these composite hydrogels, which means that components can be obtained with stiffness and controlled damping.

For further information on the advantages of hydrogels as active materials that can be designed to respond to multiple stimuli, Chapter 12 can be referred to. Some possible applications of these magnetoactive hydrogels as multilayer actuator components or "functionally gradient actuators" are detailed further on in this section. However, by combining them with the technologies described in Chapter 13, innovative possibilities could be discovered that are worth studying.

10.3.2 Main Present and Potential Applications

Main applications proposed for these new, innovative types of magnetorheological solids are related to the typical problems of

Mechanical Engineering, such as the active control of vibrations and noise, for which it is extremely useful to have elastomers whose elasticity and damping modulus can be modified in a controlled manner according to the operating conditions of a machine or installation.

The feasibility of developing adaptive tuned vibration absorbers or ATVAs has already been demonstrated, with promising results (Deng and Gong, 2007).

In the area of health sciences, the most immediate applications of these materials are maybe more related to specialisations, such as Orthopaedic Surgery, Physiotherapy and Sports Medicine than to Internal Medicine or Surgery (for which the other families of active materials analysed in this handbook are already providing very outstanding alternative solutions to those available up to present).

We believe their possibilities as active vibration absorbers have a clear application in the design of special footwear for rehabilitation or even for top sportsmen and women, for the design of shock-absorbing soles that can be adapted to the therapeutic progress of a specific patient or to the type of ground being used for training. Also, the different parts (backrest, headrest, seats, shock-absorbers and others) of rehabilitation machinery can be improved by using these materials that possess controllable stiffness and damping, which were dealt with in the previous section on "magnetorheological fluids".

The combined use of MRFs and MREs can help widen the range of applications for certain components (with MRFs taking care of the minor forces and MREs taking care of the strongest forces). Therefore, these materials should not be considered to be as loggerheads, but taken as potential collaborators.

Possibly more complex applications associated with the development of implantable devices may benefit from the use of these materials for fabricating active membranes that are able to regulate drug administration, as some researchers have already proposed (Csetneki, 2006).

10.3.3 Present Capabilities and Recent Advances

Most research undertaken throughout the last decade has focused on synthesising and processing these novel materials by dispersing different magnetic particles in different pre-polymer ionic liquids, which after polymerisation can be used to produce magnetorheological elastomer or magnetorheological hydrogel (Shen *et al.*, 2004; Guerrero-Sánchez *et al.*, 2009).

The synthesis of new materials makes characterisation and modelling essential. This has been carried out by various research groups that have analytically characterised and modelled the changes in the mechanical properties of these materials according to the magnetic field applied (Zhou, 2004; Shen *et al.*, 2004). Numerical models have also been proposed based on FEM techniques that can be used to analyse more complex designs and geometries (Szymczyk *et al.*, 2008), particularly when the main commercial CAE software is beginning to incorporate models for many types of active materials or a universal or adaptable finite element is finally developed to simulate "intelligent" or "multifunctional" materials.

The non-linearity of these materials and the influence of many factors on their mechanical response (magnetic field, temperature, humidity and others) means that an artificial neural network-based approach could be a suitable alternative for developing accurate simulators. Chapter 14 includes a section dedicated to the modelling of complex systems using artificial neural networks, with a detailed case study, by way of example.

10.3.4 Main Challenges and Research Trends

One major challenge of these magnetoactive elastomers and hydrogels consists in widening their range of application. Therefore, we think it important to propose using them not only as dampers with controllable properties (in a certain sense, the passive parts of a structure or machine, whose mission is to minimise the effects of the loads they have to bear), but also as actuators for medical tasks. They can be thus used to replace other types of active materials used in active surgical tweezers or in catheter ends for minimally invasive surgery.

To obtain optimised actuators, it is important to insist on the fact that multilayer structures or microstructured components must be obtained with these materials by using layer-by-layer fabrication techniques, like those put forward in Chapter 13. For example, dip-coating or spin-coating can be used, followed by polymerisation, sol-gel techniques or the use of vacuum casting to produce more complex geometries, as described in this chapter.

To summarise, the inclusion of magnetic particles in the core of the hydropolymers before starting in-mould polymerisation, enable samples to be produced with a higher particle concentration in the lower zone than the upper zone, through the decanting of these magnetic particles during the polymerisation process.

So, functionally gradient magnetoactive materials can be rapidly produced (see Chapter 13), capable of responding to magnetic stimuli with deformations so that magnetoactive actuators and microactuators can be produced to develop surgical tweezers and active catheter ends, for example. A higher concentration of particles can be encouraged at the ends of a sample with linear geometry in order to produce even larger deformations in the presence of variable magnetic fields (Figs. 10.4–10.6).

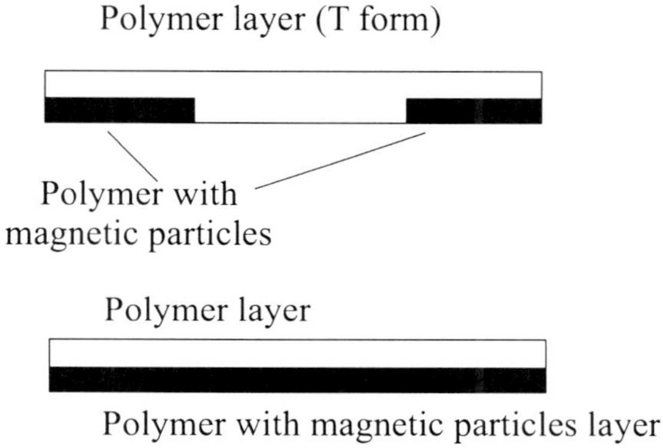

Figure 10.4 Scheme of microactuators composed of layered elastomers and elastomers with magnetic charge.

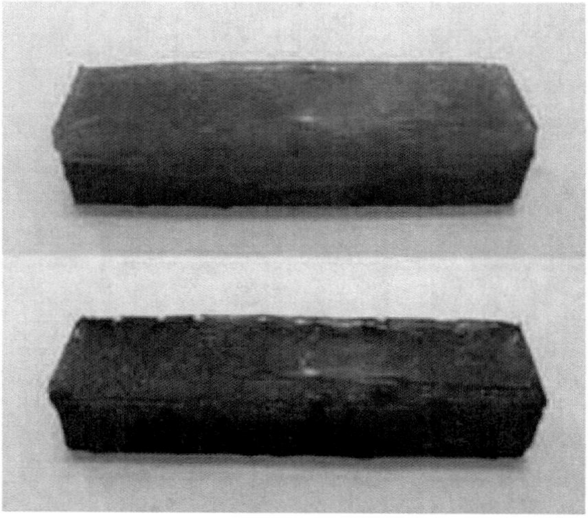

Figure 10.5 Example of microstructured actuators composed of layered elastomers and elastomers with magnetic charge.

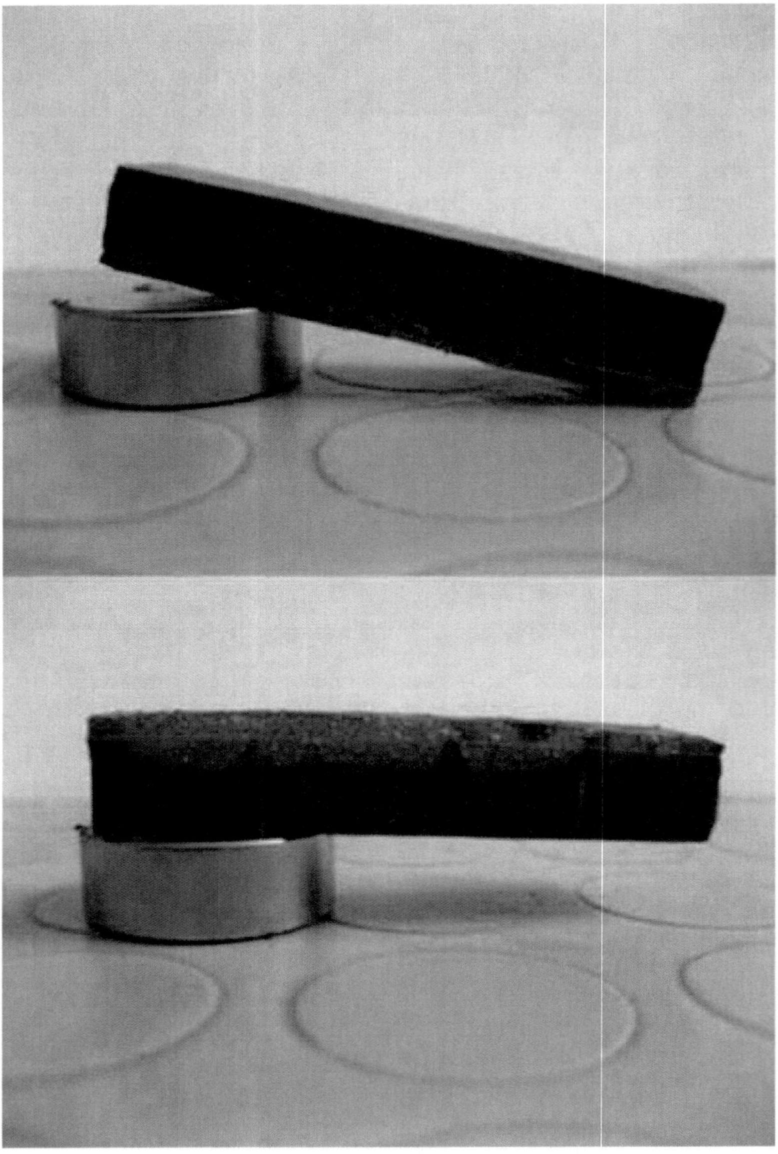

Figure 10.6 Example of actuation with MRE probe. Top image: Layer with low content of magnetic particles in contact with the magnet. Bottom image: Layer with high content of magnetic particles in contact with the magnet.

10.4 Magnetostrictive Materials

10.4.1 Introduction: Basic Properties

As we have seen from previous chapters on piezoelectric and pyroelectric ceramics and polymers when ferromagnetic materials are exposed to a magnetic field they are able to generate permanent magnets, as the magnetic moments of their particles become oriented in the direction of the field applied, reaching a saturation magnetisation in the direction of the field applied. When the external magnetic field is withdrawn, the orientation is maintained and the material becomes a permanent magnet with spontaneous magnetism. The application of an opposite magnetic field causes a rotation of the magnetisation vector following a hysteresis curve until a saturation magnetisation value opposite to the initial value is attained, although identical in modulus, which is described in excellent texts on "General Physics" and "Field and Wave Theory" ("Fundamental University Physics", Vol. II, Alonso, Finn, 1967; "Physics for Scientists and Engineers", Vol. II Tipler, 2003).

In order to model magnetostrictive materials an initial approach is to take the set of equations describing the behaviour of piezomagnetic materials, since to a certain extent they are linked phenomena. Just as changes in the surrounding magnetic field can cause deformations, the application of mechanical stress (and consequently, the imposition of deformations) leads to changes in the surrounding magnetic fields.

Magnetostriction is a typical property of ferromagnetic materials and consists of the appearance of shape changes when the materials are exposed to an external magnetic field. The effect was first described by James Joule when he observed the response of a piece of Ni when it was exposed to variations in the external magnetic field. Internally, ferromagnetic materials exhibit a division of domains, each with a magnetic polarisation. When a magnetic field is applied, the domains rotate, aligning with the field, but with a certain amount of friction between the interfaces between domains, which gives rise to losses in the form of heat (which is also responsible for part of the heat and noise from transformers). These domain rotations cause shape changes in the material, as can be seen in the schematics of Fig. 10.7. The stronger the field applied the more the domains that become oriented, for which reason the phenomenon exhibits a certain linearity until saturation is reached.

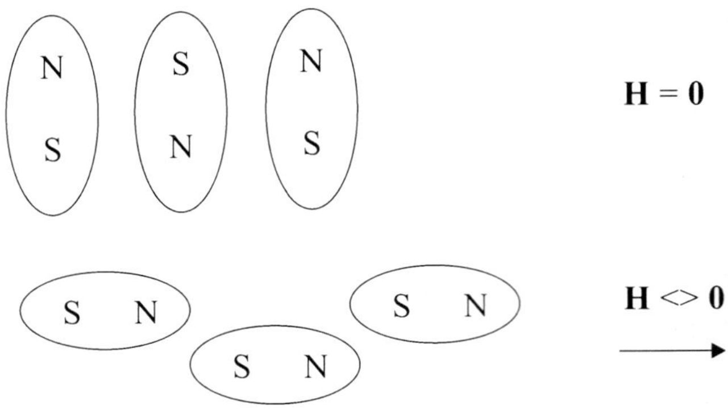

Figure 10.7 Outline of how magnetostrictive materials behave.

Magnetostrictive materials are usually used as actuators in applications required to convert magnetic energy into kinetic or potential energy and are beginning to be used to solve health sciences-related problems, as will be explained in the next subsection. This phenomenon is usually present in ferromagnetic materials but it is important to mention some materials that exhibit this phenomenon in a particularly pronounced or "gigantic" manner, like Terfenol-D (TbxDy1-xFe2), which is currently the most used material, as it shows the most outstanding magnetostriction of around 0.001 m/m when saturation is reached) or Galfenol (iron and gallium alloy).

These materials are normally supplied as bars or blocks so as to facilitate their being easily integrated as actuators into more complex devices. Among the major manufacturers are ETREMA Products Inc. and ZLX Tech, apart from those mentioned in the references at the end of the chapter. ETREMA Products Inc. specifically supplies different size actuators that range from 1 mm side cubes, to bars that are 200 mm long and 65 mm in diameter.

Actuators usually integrate a Terfenol-D bar or tube as the nucleus of the device, with a coil or solenoid around the material, through which an electric current is made to flow to generate the electrical field that triggers activation. To give a preliminary idea of the mechanical properties typical of actuators manufactured with Terfenol-D we can cite

- Maximum deformation: 0.1%–0.2%
- Developable force during activation: 40–70 MPa
- Young Modulus: 20–35 GPa

- Reaction time: < 1 s
- Curie temperature: 380°C

However, for more detailed properties it is important to consult the specific suppliers who usually provide characteristics sheets with the order.

10.4.2 Main Current and Potential Applications

These materials are capable of developing considerable forces during activation, which makes them one of the families of active materials with the highest energy density known. They can be used to design actuators that can displace high loads for use in robots, adaptable structures, transducers for a large number of industries (design of loud speakers, automobile injectors, among others) and even micro-electromechanical systems (MEMS). They have also been used as ultrasound generators whose medical application is direct when designing ultrasound image applications where generation is done by a magnetostrictive actuator (in a later chapter we will see how reception can sometimes be achieved by magnetoactive sensors). Magnetomechanical coupling can also be used for detection tasks, which is where recent advances in device miniaturisation acquires importance (MTS Temposonics® is one of the most important and combines activation with detection).

10.4.3 Main Challenges and Research Trends

More research must be done into the development of new materials that will boost the magnetostrictive properties of some ferromagnets. Property characterisation testing and response simulation are especially important for this purpose. As an aid to accurate characterisation and the ensuing comparison of the different formulations, speckle interferometry-based methodology is extremely useful, as other major research indicates (Chicharro Higuera, 2000).

On the other hand, recent patents have proposed developing composite artificial muscles as linear structures comprising electroactive polymers, shape memory alloys and magnetostrictive materials, to name but a few, that are then capable of responding to multiple stimuli according to the use to which they are put. Patent US6511508 specifically deals with the development of multiactive bands to correct refractive errors of the human eye. In whichever circumstance, the combined use of various materials can result in optimised responses for intelligent systems that have activation and detection capabilities.

10.5 Magnetoelastic Materials

10.5.1 Introduction: Basic Properties

Magnetoelastic transducers are based on the property typical of ferromagnetic materials, which is that they exhibit changes to their magnetisation curve (which relates the magnetic induction field **B** with the magnetic excitation field **H**) in response to the deformations produced in the material. This change in the material's magnetic properties can be detected, even remotely, which means they can be used as deformation (or mechanical stress) sensors to replace piezoresistive or piezoelectric sensors.

The phenomenon is closely linked to the Villari effect, which in one sense is the opposite of the magnetostrictive effects, as in this case the imposition of deformations generates variations in the magnetisation, while with other magnetostrictive materials the change in the magnetic field applied induces deformations.

These magnetoelastic sensors are usually manufactured in the form of strings or film. Some typical magnetoelastic materials have iron-rich alloys, the major ones being $Fe_{40}Ni_{38}Mo_4B_{18}$ (Metglas 2826MB) and $Fe_{81}B_{13.5}Si_{3.5}C_2$ (Metglas 2605SC), whose low cost (combined with their high mechanical strength of 1000–1800 MPa) make them ideal candidates for pressure sensors (Grimes *et al.*, 2002).

On the other hand, it must be pointed out that not only the deformations imposed on these materials bring about changes to their magnetic properties, but that also changes to the surrounding magnetic field bring about certain deformations accompanied by magnetostriction. This has an application in the development of resonance sensors (Ong, 2002; Chanu, 2008) which respond to the excitation of variable magnetic fields.

When these magnetoelastic sensors are inserted into a solenoid through which an oscillating current is flowing, the magnetoelastic material is subjected to a variable magnetic field that induces a change in the magnetisation of that material, apart from vibrations due to accompanying magnetostrictive effects. If the initial current in the solenoid is switched off, the vibration of the magnetoelastic material will alter the magnetic flux of its surroundings, inducing a current in the solenoid with a transitory response (a result of the damped vibration of the magnetoelastic material) in accordance with the expression:

$$i(t) = A \cdot e^{-\xi \cdot \omega_n \cdot t} \cdot \sin(\omega_r \cdot t - \alpha)$$

where

i is the induced current [A];

A, the signal amplitude [A];

ξ, the damping coefficient;

ω_n, the natural pulse of non-damped oscillation [rad/s];

ω_r, the oscillation pulse of the transitory response [rad/s]; and

α, the lag [rad].

It is advisable to excite these magnetoelastic materials by using oscillating fields with frequencies close to resonance. In this way, the vibratory response will show a lower damping coefficient and the current to be induced in the solenoid will have a wider amplitude and duration, which will increase the sensor's sensitivity and quality. For a typical magnetoelastic strip subjected to an oscillating current, this resonance frequency can be approximated with the aid of the following expression:

$$f_0 = \frac{1}{2L}\sqrt{\frac{E_m}{\rho_m}}$$

where

f_0 is the resonance frequency [Hz];

L, sensor length [m];

E_m, the Young modulus of the magnetoelastic material [N/m^2]; and

ρ_m, the magnetoelastic material density [kg/m^3].

A change in the sensor's mechanical properties such as an increase in mass or thickness, results in a change in its natural frequency. These natural frequency alterations can be characterised and monitored with the aid of a solenoid or an RF winding, even for very slight variations in its mechanical properties. Thanks to this technique various biomedical, biological and biochemical applications are being developed based on the use of magnetoelastic sensors for recording how certain reactions evolve.

Therefore, sometimes a thin layer of bioactive polymer is deposited on the surface of a magnetoelastic sensor. This polymer can expand or narrow in the presence of some reagents (whose evolution needs to be recorded) or as a response to changes in pH, which entails a change in the sensor's mechanical properties. In this case the following expression enables the resonance frequency of the system to be approximated and serves as a reference when these changes are being monitored in the course of a particular reaction.

$$f = f_0 \sqrt{\frac{m_0}{m_t} + \frac{E_c / \rho_c}{E_m / \rho_m} \cdot (1 - \frac{m_0}{m_t})}$$

where

f is the resonance frequency of the system [Hz];
f_0, the initial resonance frequency [Hz];
m_0, the magnetoelastic mass [kg];
m_t, the total mass of the sensor [kg];
E_m, the Young modulus of the magnetoelastic material [N/m^2];
E_c, the Young modulus of the coating [N/m^2];
ρ_m, the density of the magnetoelastic material [kg/m^3]; and
ρ_c, the coating density [kg/m^3].

In other cases the surface of a magnetoelastic transducer can be used as a substrate to assess the speed of growth of determined cells and micro-organisms, as this increase in the mass deposited on the sensor also involves a change in its resonance frequency. If the transducer is integrated into the measuring device of a microcantilever, increases in mass can be detected (and therefore the growth of cells and colonies of micro-organisms) and the mechanical response of the sensor and the change in resonance frequency can be recorded. Empirically adjustable expressions can be used like the one proposed by other researchers in the development of "cantilever MEMS-sensors" (Chen *et al.*, 1995; Nugaeva *et al.*, 2005):

$$\Delta m \approx \frac{\mathrm{k_c}}{4 \cdot n \cdot \pi^2} (\frac{1}{f^2} - \frac{1}{f_0^2})$$

where

Δm is the increase in mass [kg];
f, the resonance frequency of the system [Hz];
f_0 the initial resonance frequency [Hz];

k_c, the spring constant [N/m] generically defined as the ratio of the force applied to the end of the cantilever (perpendicular to the cantilever) and the deflection found; and

n, a correction factor depending on the geometry.

Although there are other ways of working with these kinds of sensors, the use of their resonance properties is currently the most widespread method and has given rise to applications like those detailed below. It is important to emphasise that the equations set out must be validated or re-adapted for each specific design, since the resonance frequency not only depends on the geometry and properties of the magnetoelastic material, but also on the boundary conditions resulting from their being integrated into complex devices. In whichever case, these equations can be used as initial approximations for a preliminary assessment of the size of the sensors and the range of excitation frequencies (and subsequent reading) that is applicable.

10.5.2 Main current and Potential Applications

The following may be mentioned as some of the most marked medical applications that could result in commercial devices in the coming years to provide innovative solutions for *in vitro* and *in vivo* diagnosis.

Measurement of cell growth and colonies of micro-organisms

Various researchers have developed devices for the *in vitro* assessment of the speed of growth of tumour tissue and fungal colonies, bacteria and other micro-organisms by using magnetoelastic materials as transducers that allow high precision monitoring of this growth, in line with the working principles described above (Xiao *et al.*, 2008).

Sensors for detecting changes in pH

By coating magnetoelastic sensors with layers of polymer that are bioactive or sensitive to different reagents, highly specific chemical sensors can be produced that can accurately detect changes in pH, among other values, based on the geometrical changes to the polymer layer as a result of the chemical reaction taking place, which changes the resonance properties of the polymer-magnetoelastic multilayer sensor (Ong, 2002; Chanu, 2008).

Splint for detecting occlusal conditions

In Chapter 7, we set out a case study of an intraoral splint for detecting intraoral pressures by using piezoelectric sensors wired to an extraoral monitoring device.

The use of magnetoelastic resonant wireless sensors (Grimes *et al.*, 2002) may also be suitable for developing intracorporeal pressure monitoring devices, particularly intraoral pressures, to replace other piezoelectric-based solutions (Lafont Morgado and Díaz Lantada, 2008).

Figures 10.8 to 10.12 depict the process for integrating an intraoral splint into a magnetoelastic sensor. Also included is a size comparison with an alternative solution, for recording bite pressure and wireless communication with the exterior, based on the use of piezoresistive sensors (González Bris and Díaz Lantada, 2009).

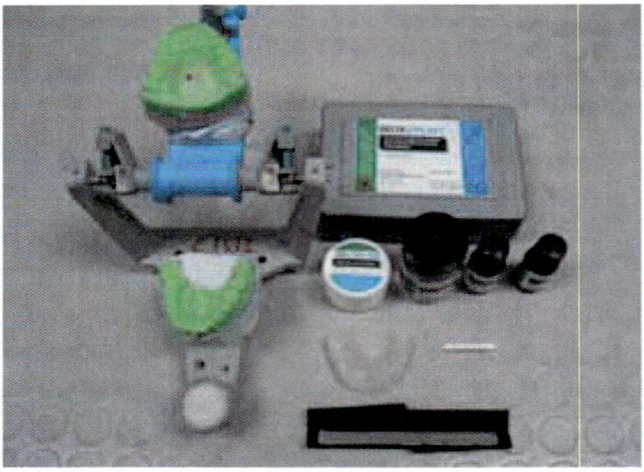

Figure 10.8 Components for producing an intraoral splint with a magnetoelastic sensor.

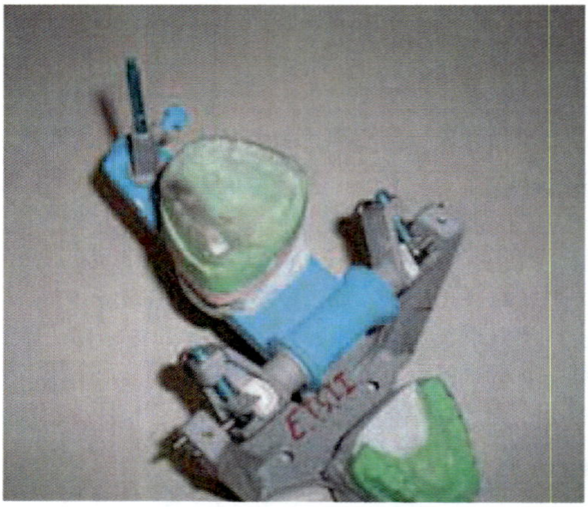

Figure 10.9 Magnetoelastic sensor attached to a thermoshaped plate with photopolymerisable resin.

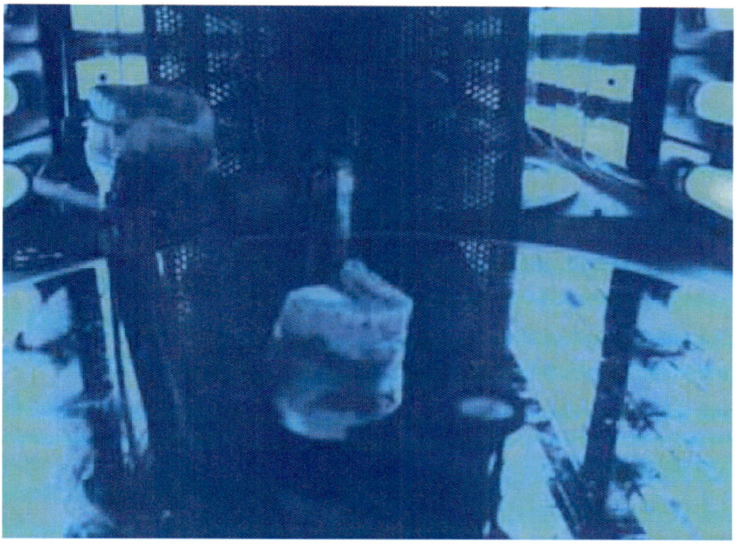

Figure 10.10 Photopolymerisation in a UV oven for stabilising encapsulation.

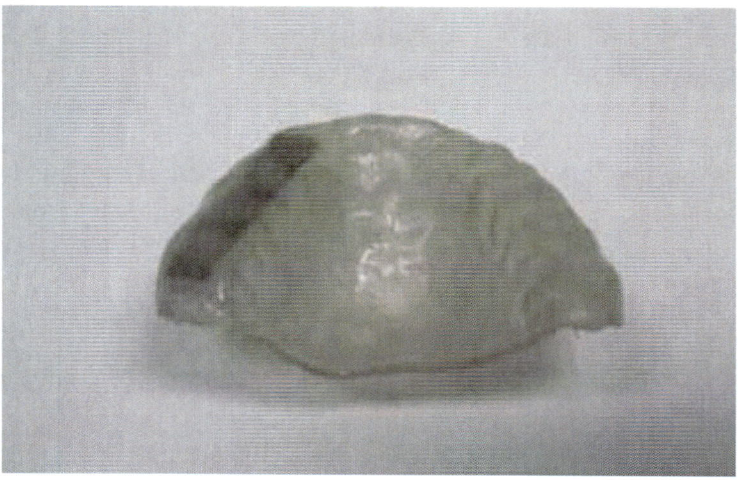

Figure 10.11 Intraoral splint with magnetoelectric sensor for detecting bite force.

The magnetoelastic solution does not require any intraoral electronics, which is a great advantage for optimising the comfort of the end devices.

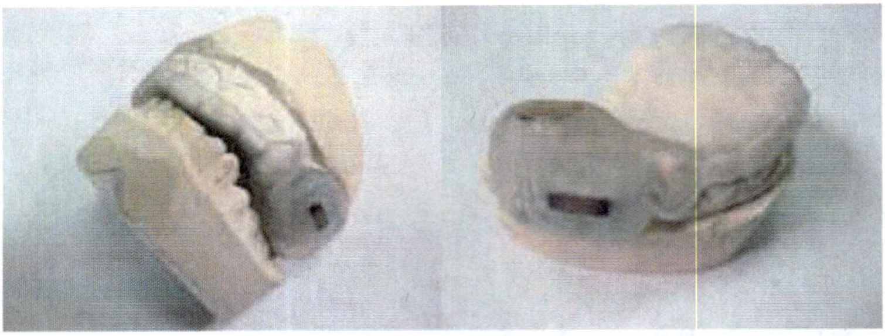

Figure 10.12 Intraoral splint with an alternative piezoresistive-based detection system next to intraoral electronics for outside communication. Patent: González Bris and Díaz Lantada, 2009.

10.5.3 Main Challenges and Study Trends

Some of the main research in the field of magnetoelastic materials is centred on finding new formulations to improve the properties of the materials as sensors as well as actuators by coupling them with magnetostrictive properties. This is done by systematically incorporating different dopants and performing a thorough characterisation testing using slightly different formulas. By so doing, the incorporation of Al to the CoAlxFe2-x04 system was successfully accomplished in order to enhance its properties as a force transducer (Nlebedim *et al.*, 2009).

The search for new applications for magnetoelastic materials for *in vitro* devices for biological or biochemical laboratory and *in vivo* studies and for implants with optimised diagnostic capabilities continues to be one of the main challenges for future years. Enormous benefits can be derived from using them in combination with other active materials or as component parts of multilayer structures to increase the number of variables the systems responds to (Pfützner *et al.*, 2006).

It is especially important to ensure the biocompatibility of the end devices through safe, functional encapsulation. To do this, fast rapid prototyping technologies are ideal for comparing the different design alternatives in a way that is especially fast and financially acceptable. Customised prosthetic designs can also be produced (this is dealt with in greater detail in Chapter 15).

10.6 Piezomagnetic Materials

10.6.1 Introduction: Basic Properties

Piezomagnetism is a material property that links magnetic fields to stress fields and deformations in these materials, and in many ways is similar to piezoelectricity (Busch-Vishniac, 1999). Actually, these phenomena almost always appear simultaneously and in conjunction with pyroelectric phenomena, although depending on the materials used as transducers, piezoelectric, pyroelectric or piezomagnetic phenomena will predominate.

For any materials that are used as sensors or actuators due to their piezomagnetic properties and assuming that their piezoelectric and thermal effects are small, their behaviour can be described by the following expressions (comparable to those described for piezoelectricity in the Chapters 8 and 9):

$$\{\mathbf{S}\} = [\mathbf{s}]\,\{\mathbf{T}\} + [\mathbf{d_m}]\,\{\mathbf{H}\}$$

$$\{\mathbf{B}\} = [\mathbf{d_m}]\,\{\mathbf{T}\} + [\mu]\,\{\mathbf{H}\}$$

where

- $\{\mathbf{S}\}$ is the deformation vector [m/m];
- $\{\mathbf{T}\}$, the stress vector [N/m^2];
- $\{\mathbf{H}\}$, the magnetic excitation vector or field [$m^{-1} \cdot s^{-1} \cdot C$];
- $\{\mathbf{B}\}$, the magnetic induction vector or field [T] ≡ [$kg \cdot s^{-1} \cdot C^{-1}$];
- $[\mathbf{s}]$, the matrix of elasticity or of elastic compliance of the material [m^2/N];
- $[\mathbf{d_m}]$, the vector of piezomagnetic coefficients [$m \cdot s \cdot C^{-1}$] ≡ [T/Pa]; and
- $[\propto]$, the vector of the material's magnetic permeability [$m \cdot kg \cdot C^{-2}$].

According to the above, magnetic moments can be induced by applying forces and the changes in the surrounding magnetic field cause deformations in the material. These expressions also provide an approximation for modelling magnetostrictive phenomena. Some authors (Busch-Vishniac, 1999) consider them as similar phenomena, while others maintain there are some differences (Cullity, 1971). However, it would appear to be commonly accepted that a magnetic moment can be produced in piezomagnetic materials by simply applying a mechanical force, the surrounding magnetic field being zero, but this does not coincide with the behaviour of magnetostrictive materials.

On the other hand, the response of magnetostrictive materials is not as linear as that shown by piezomagnetic models, although it is useful as an approximation to their behaviour.

These piezomagnetic phenomena were first observed in some antiferromagnetic crystals such as cobalt and manganese fluorides or silver and magnesium nitrides. Although this is also the case with some ferromagnetic materials, the phenomenon is usually found in asymmetrically structured materials (Dzialoshinskii, 1958; Borovik-Romanov, 1960). Whichever the case, it must be pointed out that there are some suppliers that can provide these materials ready for direct use as the component parts of a wide range of devices, for detection and activation tasks with medical applications like those proposed below.

10.6.2 Main Present and Potential Applications

Listed below are some of the most outstanding applications that may lead to commercial devices in future years, as innovative solutions to *in vitro* and *in vivo* diagnostic requirements and problems.

Transducers for ultrasound imaging

Piezomagnetic materials have been proposed to replace piezoelectric materials in different image and acoustic-related industrial applications. They therefore appear to be good candidates for acoustic transducers and for the medical industry as transducers for ultrasound imaging systems (Daga *et al.*, 2009). These systems send out high frequency sound waves that are reflected off the body structures and then received through the appropriate transducers by a computer that then converts them into images.

Pressure sensors in intelligent instrumented prostheses

In the same way that ceramic as well as polymer piezoelectric sensors have been successfully tested in various prostheses (Lafont Morgado *et al.*, 2007; Diaz Lantada, 2009), piezoelectric sensors may be a viable alternative. Remote reading with no need for wires is a particularly attractive possibility (Bian *et al.*, 2009). This is also the case with prostheses that incorporate magnetoelastic transducers, as mentioned in the previous section, with working principles that are similar to those found in piezomagnetic materials.

Magnetic Microsystems or "magMEMS"

Piezomagnetic micro-film is helping to promote the development of cantilever microsensors as the component parts of more complex

MEMS systems that bring major benefits such as "self-test", "self-calibration" and "remote sensing and activation", which makes the end devices safer and more versatile. Although most of the examples available are prototypes for performing "concept testing", their impact on the Microsystems industry in the coming years looks to be promising (Gibbs, 2005).

For further information on the different procedures and techniques regarding film structures and the use of thin layers, Chapter 13 can be referred to.

10.6.3 Main Challenges and Research Trends

Some of the leading research in the field of pyromagnetic materials is focused on producing new piezomagnetic materials that will have enhanced sensing properties through the systematic incorporation of different dopants and exhaustive characterisation tests using slightly different formulations.

The properties of the $Ba_{6-x}R_{2x}(Nb_{1-x}Fe_{2+x})O_3$ system possessing piezoelectric and piezomagnetic properties have been analysed. It has also been studied as a potential component part of magnetorheological fluids (Li, 2008, 2009). This team of researchers has also very recently examined the properties of the $Co_xFe_{3-x}O_4$, $Bi_{2-x}Fe_xO_3$ and $Ga_{2-x}Fe_xO_3$ systems concerning their applications as acoustic transducers (Li, 2008, 2009).

These kinds of sensors have microthreads or filled micro-films for epoxy resin matrices, with which complex geometries and parts can be obtained so that their stress fields (mechanical) can be continuously monitored. This may be very useful for producing safer "intelligent self-sensing implants" that can alert the patient or their doctor when forces or deformations are reaching inadmissible figures. Of all these materials, the $Tb_{1-x}Dy_xFe_{2-y}$ – epoxy and $Pb(Zr_{0.52}Ti_{0.48})O_3$ – epoxy systems are worth a special mention.

10.7 Pyromagnetic Materials

10.7.1 Introduction: Basic Properties

As we have learned from previous chapters, when ferromagnetic materials are heated above their Curie temperature, they become paramagnetic (due to phase change), losing their ferromagnetic properties and their spontaneous magnetisation, which is very common with metals (Fe, Co, Ni) and polymers (PVDF and its copolymers). In this sense these ferromagnetic materials exhibit a variation in magnetic properties with temperature, called pyromagnetic effects, which means they can be used to develop magnetothermal sensors.

Other materials possess even more pronounced pyromagnetic properties, like $YbFeO_3$, $Y_3Fe_5O_{12}$, $Gd_3Fe_5O_{12}$, FeRh or MnAs in which a rise in temperature produces a marked effect on their magnetisation curve. This means they can be used as temperature sensors in the same way that piezomagnetic materials can be uses as pressure sensors.

For any materials that are used as sensors for their pyromagnetic properties and assuming that their piezomagnetic and magnetoelectric effects are small, their behaviour can be described by the following expression (Fuentes, 1998; Newnham, 2005):

$$\{\mathbf{B}\} = [\mathbf{i}_m]\,\Delta T + [\propto]\,\{\mathbf{H}\}$$

where

- $\{\mathbf{B}\}$ is the magnetic induction vector or field [T];
- $\{\mathbf{H}\}$, the magnetic excitation vector or field $[m^{-1}\cdot s^{-1}\cdot C]$;
- ΔT, the rise in temperature of the material [K];
- $[\mathbf{i}_m]$, the pyromagnetic coefficient vector according to the three spatial directions [T/K]; and
- $[\propto]$, the material's magnetic permeability vector $[m\cdot kg\cdot C^{-2}]$.

10.7.2 Main Present and Potential Applications

Pyromagnetic materials have been an object of interest since the time of Edison when he put forward his idea of a pyromagnetic-based current generator. Recent possibilities for medical applications seem to have awoken new interest in this kind of material. Listed below are some of the most outstanding applications in health sciences. These could lead to commercial devices in future years as innovative solutions for both *in vitro* tests to back up biochemical and biological research as well as for the *in vivo* diagnosis and monitoring of different medical conditions.

Biomarkers development

It has been clearly demonstrated that pyromagnetic film can be successfully used to develop sensors capable of detecting specific enzymes to activate certain exothermic reactions in the presence of appropriate reagents, thereby generating a small amount of heat that can be detected by the change in the magnetisation of the pyromagnetic film. These sensors are therefore highly specific as they only detect the required enzyme and let it be accurately quantified, which paves the way to their being used in a wide range of biochemical research-linked activities (Yachi *et al.*, 2000).

Photodetector development

Pyromagnetic properties can be used to develop photodetectors as an alternative to other more commonly used principles that have been dealt with in other chapters (pyroelectric, photovoltaic, photoemissive and photoconductive principles, to name but a few). When a sufficiently intense light source falls on a pyromagnetic film, the material absorbs part of the light radiation and heats up. This has enabled pyromagnetic sensors to be used to detect visible and infrared radiation (Toyohiko *et al.*, 1999).

Other potential medical uses of this phenomenon are the use of safety sensors to alert to the danger of excessive light or thermal radiation, for example in cosmetic surgery operations (photoepilation) or when exposing tissue to different laser treatments, as well as other possible sources of radiation used for various therapies (Guzhva *et al.*, 1977; Walser, 2005). Their use as a possible substitute for the materials usually used in infrared thermography are also worthy of detailed study.

Temperature control in hypothermia treatment

The use of nanoparticles, remotely guided by magnetic fields to position them next to tumours and then expose them to alternate magnetic fields that induce high frequency vibrations in the nanoparticles, which results in very localised heating, could become an ideal mechanism for eliminating malignant cells.

The changes in magnetic properties brought about by changes in temperature in the pyrolelectric materials may be of major help for optimising these treatments. On the one hand, some magnetic particles can be designed to have a Curie temperature (which operates as a "safety switch") above which the material loses its ferromagnetic properties and stops heating up.

On the other hand, the pyromagnetic properties can be of help in monitoring the temperature during action on the tumour, allowing a better control over the process (Sharma, 2009).

10.7.3 Main Challenges and Research Trends

Some of the main research in the field of pyromagnetic materials is centred on finding new formulations to enhance their sensing properties by the systematic incorporation of different dopants and exhaustive characterisation tests using slightly different formulations. The outcomes of varying the composition of the CoS_2-*x*Se*x* system to enhance its properties as a radiation sensor were successfully tested in the past (Walser and Bene, 2005) and similar methodologies may well be successful for new materials.

It could be very worthwhile to make objective comparisons between the different active materials that can be used as temperature sensors (like pyroelectric, pyromagnetic, thermocouple materials etc.) in order to analyse factors such as precision, response speed, repeatability or the ranges of use, so as to be able to establish which thermoactive sensors are best for each field of application.

If the use of these materials is to become widespread in industry, not only does more effort needs to be put into enhancing their properties and synthesising new formulations, but also into mass production processes where geometries can be produced that will make it easier to integrate the sensors into complex devices (films, microthreads and others), as well as their being produced by suppliers who provide access to these materials.

10.8 Main Conclusions

This chapter has provided a detailed description of the different types of magnetoactive materials that are able to change their mechanical properties or geometry in response to changes in the magnetic field surrounding them (which usually makes them suitable for use as actuators) or which can change their magnetic properties as a consequence of changes to the variables surrounding them (which usually makes them suitable for use as sensors).

Regarding the development of actuators, three basic kinds of magnetoactive materials have been dealt with: magnetorheological fluids, elastomers and magnetorheological hydrogels and magnetostrictive materials.

Regarding the development of sensors, three particularly important kinds of magnetoactive materials have been dealt with (which respond to various stimuli such as the imposition of deformations, pressure changes or temperature changes):_ magnetoelastic, piezomagnetic and pyromagnetic materials.

The chapter has been structured to deal firstly with the materials that have the greatest number of applications as actuators and secondly, materials that have the greatest number of applications as sensors. We hope that this grouping will help shed light on the common denominators possessed by magnetoactive transducers in spite of their different ways of acting and detecting.

Various magnetoactive actuators can often be activated with the aid of similar "support" devices that can generate magnetic fields in a controlled manner (wound encapsulated coils together with electricity generators and others). On the other hand, the devices and excitation electronics and the subsequent reading of the various magnetoactive sensors often have properties in common, that facilitate solutions requiring the simultaneous monitoring of different stimuli.

For each material, we have described aspects connected with its composition and structure, synthesis and processing, characterisation and modelling, integration into devices or the main trends in current research related to its composition and structure, with a view to promoting the use of these materials in industry, particularly in health science-related applications. Materials having the most outstanding properties have been analysed in greater detail, as they open up fields of application where other intelligent materials would not lead to such appropriate solutions.

We have also attempted to analyse the major applications in medical device development for each of these magnetoactive materials, as well as including some more detailed case studies that may be of help to other researchers undertaking medical device development and who might benefit from using magnetoactive transducers as sensors or actuators as a means of improving the final diagnosis or therapy.

Additional information can be found in the following list of references, which includes results from some of the main researchers in this multidisciplinary field, as well as in the websites of the different suppliers included in the annexes of the handbook, some of them already mentioned within the chapter.

References

Alexiou, C.; Schmid R.; Jurgons R.; *et al.* "Targeting cancer cells: magnetic nanoparticles as drug carriers". European Biophysics Journal, 35(5), 446–450, 2006.

Bansevicius, R.M.; Virbalis, J.A. "Two-dimensional Braille readers based on electro-rheological fluid valves controlled by electric field". Mechatronics, 17(10), 570–577, 2007.

Bar-Cohen, J.; Mavroidis, C. "Virtual reality robotic telesurgery simulations using MEMICA haptic system". Proceedings of SPIE's 8th Annual International Symposium on Smart Structures and Materials, 2001.

Bar-Cohen, Y. "Electroactive polymer actuators as artificial muscles: Reality, potential and challenges". SPIE Press. Washington, 2004.

Bian, L.;Wen, Y.; Li, P.; Gao, Q.; Zheng, M. "Magnetoelectric transducer with high quality factor for wireless power receiving". Sensors and Actuators A: Physical, 150(2), 207–211, 2009.

Borcea, L.; Bruno, O. "On the magneto-elastic properties of elastomer-ferromagnet composites". Journal of the Mechanics and Physics of Solids, 49(12), 2877–2919, 2001.

Borovik-Romanov, A.S. "Piezomagnetism in the antiferromagnetic fluorides of cobalt and manganese". Soviet Physics JETP, 11, 786, 1960.

Busch-Vishniac, I.J. "Electromechanical sensors and actuators". Springer Verlag. New York, 1999.

Chanu, A.; Martel, S. "MRI controlled magnetoelastic nano biosensor for *in-vivo* pH monitoring: A preliminary approach". 7th IEEE International Conference on Nanotechnology, 166–170, 2008.

Chen, G.Y.; Thundat, T.; Wachter, A.; Warmack, J. "Adsorption-induced surface stress and its effect on resonance frequency of microcantilevers". Journal of Applied Physics, 77 (8), 3618–3622, 1995.

Chicharro Higuera, J.M. "Estudio de la magnetoestricción por interferometría de speckle". PhD Thesis, Universidad Politécnica de Madrid, 2000.

Csetneki, I.; Filipcsei, G.; Zrinyi, M. "Smart nanocomposite polymer membranes with on/off switching control". Macromolecules, 39, 1939–1942, 2006.

Cullity, B.D. "Fundamentals of magnetostriction". Journal of Metals 1, 323, 1971.

Daga, A.; Ganesan, N.; Shankar, K. "Harmonic response of three-phase magneto-electro-elastic beam under mechanical, electrical and magnetic environment". Journal of Intelligent Material Systems and Structures, 20(10), 1203–1220, 2009.

Deng, H.X.; Gong, X.L. "Adaptive tuned vibration absorber based on magnetorheological elastomer". Journal of Intelligent Material Systems and Structures, 18(12), 1205–1210, 2007.

Díaz Lantada, A. "Metodología para el desarrollo de dispositivos médicos activos basados en el empleo de polímeros activos como sensores y actuadores". PhD Thesis, Universidad Politécnica de Madrid, 2009.

Dong, S.; Lu, K.Q.; Sun, J.Q.; Rudolph, K. "Rehabilitation device with variable resistance and intelligent control". Medical Engineering and Physics, 27(3), 249–255, 2005.

Dyszkiewicz, A.; Polec, P.; Zajdel, J.; *et al.* "Collimation of X-Ray Diagnostic Bundle by Means of Steering Ferrofluid". Second International Conference on Biomedical Electronics and Devices, Special Session on Active Materials for Medical Devices (AMMD), Biodevices 2009, Porto, Portugal, 2009.

Dzialoshinskii, I.E. "The problem of piezomagnetism". Soviet Physics JETP 6, 621, 1958.

Echávarri Otero, J.; Díaz Lantada, A.; Lafont Morgado, P.; *et al.* "Characterisation and medical applications of magnetorheological fluids". Second International Conference on Biomedical Electronics and Devices, Special Session on Active Materials for Medical Devices (AMMD), Biodevices 2009, Porto, Portugal, 2009.

Flores, G., Sheng, R."Medical applications of magnetorheological fluids: A possible new cancer therapy". 7th International Conference on Electrorheological (ER) Fluids and Magnetorheological (MR) Suspensions, 1999.

Fuentes, L. "Magnetic-coupling properties in polycrystals". Textures and Microstructures, 30, 167–189, 1998.

Gibbs, M.R.J. "Applications of magmems". Journal of Magnetism and Magnetic Materials, 290-291, 1298–1303, April, 2005. Proceedings of the Joint European Magnetic Symposia (JEMS' 04).

González Bris, C.; Díaz Lantada, A. "A wearable passive force sensor/active interrogator intended for intra-splint use for the detection and recording of bruxism". 3rd International Conference on Pervasive Computing Technologies for Healthcare 2009. London, April 2009.

González Bris, C.; Lafont Morgado, P.; Díaz Lantada, A. *et al.* Sistema de telemetría mediante comunicación inalámbrica empleando campo magnético sensor-pasivo / interrogador-activo para diagnóstico y detección de episodios bruxistas". Spanish Patent Document, OEPM P200900875, 2009.

Grimes, C.A.; Mungle, C.S.; Zeng, K.; *et al.* "Wireless magnetoelastic resonance sensors: A critical review". Sensors, 2, 294–313, 2002.

Guerrero-Sánchez, C.; Corine, F.; Schubert, U.S. "Magnetorheological solid composites based on ionic liquids". Behavior and Mechanics of Multifunctional Materials and Composites, 2009.

Guzhva, V.G.; Koltok, Y.V.; Kuzmichev, V.M.; Latynin, Y.M. "Pyromagnetic detection of radiation pulses". Sovietic Journal of Quantum Electronics, 7, 384–385, 1977.

Kallio, M. "The elastic and damping properties of magnetorheological elastomers". VTT Publications, 2005.

Lafont Morgado, P.; Díaz Lantada, A.; Martínez Álvarez, A.; *et al.* "Instrumented splint for the diagnosis of bruxism". International Conference on Biomedical Electronics and Devices Biostec 2008 – Biodevices, 2, 216–222. IEEE Engineering in Medicine and Biology Society. Madeira, January, 2008. INSTICC Press, 2008.

Lafont Morgado, P.; Díaz Lantada, A.; Martínez Álvarez, A.; *et al.* "Dispositivos médicos basados en el empleo de polímeros electroactivos". 8° Congreso Iberoamericano de Ingeniería Mecánica. Pontificia Universidad Católica del Perú. 23–25 October 2007 in Cuzco.

Li, Q.; Li, Y.; Huang, Z. "Multifunctional piezomagnetic ferrite materials and their newly acoustical and vibration control devices". PIERS Proceedings, Hangzhou, China, March, 2008.

Li, Q.; Li, Y.; Huang, Z. "Investigation into new type piezomagnetic materials and acoustical transducers exhibiting piezoelectricity and piezomagnetic effect". Progress in Electromagnetics Research Symposium, Beijing, China, March, 2009.

Neelakantan, V. "Force feedback system using magneto-rheological fluids for telerobotic surgery". International Congress on Industrial and commercial applications of smart structures technologies, 2002.

Newnham, R.E. "Properties of materials: Anisotropy, symmetry, structure". Oxford University Press, 2005.

Nlebedim, I.C.; Ranvah, N.; Melikhov, Y.; *et al.* "Magnetic and magnetomechanical properties of CoAlxFe2-xO4 for stress sensor and actuator applications". IEEE Transactions on Magnetics, 45(10), 4120–4123, 2009.

Nugaeva, N.; Gfeller, K.Y.; Backmann, N.; *et al.* "Micromechanical cantilever array sensors for selective fungal immobilization and fast growth detection". Biosensors and Bioelectronics, 21, 849–856, 2005.

Ong, K.G.; Zeng, K.; Yang, X.; *et al.* "Quantification of multiple bioagents with wireless remote-query magnetoelastic microsensors". IEEE Sensors, 6, 514–523, 2006.

Pfützner, H.; Kaniusas, E.; Kosel, J.; *et al.* "Magnetostrictive bilayers for multi-functional sensor families". Sensors and Actuators A: Physical, 129(1–2), 154–158, 2006.

Rabinow, J. "The magnetic fluid Clutch", AIEE Trans 67, 1948.

Rizzo, R. "Electromagnetic Modeling and Design of Haptic Interface Prototypes Based on Magnetorheological Fluids". IEEE Transactions on Magnetics, 2007.

Scilingo E.P., Sgambelluri N., De Rossi D., Bicchi A. "Haptic displays based on MR fluids: design, realization and psychophysical validation", Proceedings of the11th Symposium on Haptic Interfaces for Virtual Environment and Teleoperator Systems, 2003.

Sharma, R.; Chen, C.J. "Newer nanoparticles in hyperthermia treatment and thermometry". Journal of Nanoparticle Research, 11(3), 2009.

Shen, Y.; Golnaraghi, M.F.; Heppler, G.F. "Experimental research and modelling of magnetorheological elastomers", J Intell Mater Syst. Struct , 15, 27–35, 2004.

Sheng, R.; Flores, G. "*In vitro* investigation of a novel cancer therapeutic method using embolizing properties of magnetorheological fluids", Journal of Magnetism and Magnetic Materials 194, 1999.

Szymczyk, W.; Boczkowska, A.; Niezgoda, T.; Zubko, K. "FEM simulations of a magnetorheological elastomer with consideration of magneto mechanical coupling". Poster at the E-MRS Fall Meeting 2008.

Torcuato M. "Estudio de suspensiones magnetorreológicas en medios no acuosos". Master Thesis, Universidad de Granada, 2006.

Toyohiko, Y.; Toyonao, O.; Shigeki, C.; Hirosi, O.; Kyoshiro, S. "Construction and characterization of pyromagnetic photosensor". Transactions of the Society of Instruments and Control Engineers, 35(4), 453–457, 1999.

Vekas, L. "Ferrofluids and magnetorheological fluids". CIMTEC, 2008.

Walser, R.M.; Bene, R.W.; Caruthers, R.E. "Radiation detection with the pyromagnetic effect". IEEE Transactions on Electron Devices, 18(5), 309–315, 2005.

Xiao, X.; Guo, M.; Li, Q.; *et al.* "*In-situ* monitoring of breast cancer cell (MCF-7) growth and quantification of the cytotoxicity of anticancer drugs fluorouracil and cisplatin". Biosensors and Bioelectronics, 24, 247–252, 2008.

Yachi, Y.; Chiba, S.; Osada, H.; *et al.* "Magnetic enzyme sensor utilizing pyro magnetic film". IEEE Transactions on Magnetics, 36(5), 3730–3732, 2000.

Zhou, G.Y. "Deformation in magnetorheological elastomer and elastomer–ferromagnet composite driven by a magnetic field". Smart Materials and Structures, 13(2), 309–316, 2004.

Chapter 11

Optoactive and Photoactive Materials for Biodevices

Andrés Díaz Lantada
Mechanical Engineering Department, E.T.S.I. Industriales, Universidad Politécnica de Madrid, c/ José Gutiérrez Abascal 2, 28006 Madrid, Spain
adiaz@etsii.upm.es

11.1 Introduction

This chapter is focused on the study of different chromoactive (or optoactive) materials that can change their colour or optical properties in response to different stimuli, and different photoactive materials that can emit light as a response to a range of stimuli or react to light stimuli. This opens up many possibilities for their being used to develop sensors, actuators and multifunctional devices.

Therefore, this chapter deals with a range of materials with different working principles but with some things in common that link optical properties and light effects to different thermal, electrical and mechanical stimuli, among other things. For these reasons we have grouped them together in one chapter (as we also did with Chapter 10).

Due to their current low impact on the medical sector only one chapter has been devoted to it, although an entire handbook could be devoted to the optically active materials we have dealt with as they have enormous future potential.

These materials are usually formed from combinations of ceramic and polymer materials that have generally been processed to obtain

Handbook of Active Materials for Medical Devices: Advances and Applications
Edited by Andrés Díaz Lantada

www.panstanford.com

multilayer structures possessing different functionalities, adapting the properties of the whole to specific requirements, which makes them attractive to different sectors of industry.

Regarding the family of chromoactive or optoactive materials that can change their colour or optical properties in response to different stimuli, the major medical applications of some of the main materials are detailed. Such materials are electrochromic or electrochromatic,thermochromicorthermochromatic,photochromic or photochromatic and piezochromatic and hydrochromatic.

Regarding the family of photoactive materials that can emit light as a response to a range of stimuli or react to light stimuli, the major medical applications of some of the main materials are detailed. Such materials are electroluminescent, fluorescent, photosensitive, photoelectric or phototropic. The materials in this family have numerous applications for the development of sensors and actuators.

We will also take a brief look at optical fibres as passive materials for transporting information but that can also be integrated into complex systems in order to produce active devices. The importance of these fibres in other sectors of industry, such as telecommunications or computing, has been fully demonstrated and also has an important place in the Medical Industry.

After describing the different aspects of the main families of materials that respond to light and colour, we will examine the different methods that can be used to synthesise, process and characterise the numerous materials belonging to these families.

Additionally we will describe the main challenges and research trends concerning these chromoactive and photoactive materials and briefly analyse how Nature is a continuous source of inspiration, as we have seen when dealing with other kinds of intelligent materials.

11.2 Optoactive Materials: Families and Applications

Optoactive and chromoactive materials can change their optical properties or colour in response to a range of stimuli. This has led to their being used as optical switches in the Electronics Industry and to produce "intelligent" windows in the area of architecture and to provide many solutions to interior decoration that change in response to the environment.

The increasing number of medical applications that have emerged over recent years is the reason for including this chapter and examining the main kinds of optoactive or chromoactive materials in this section.

11.2.1 Electrochromic or Electrochromatic Materials

Nanotubes are allotropic forms of carbon with a cylindrical structure, and are generally glass materials made up of ceramic and polymer multilayers. Applying a voltage between their sides leads to a change in the material's colour or its degree of transparency. There are many solutions to their construction and processing depending on the end device required, as will be analysed further on.

The usual way to manufacture electrochromic windows or panels is by using five or seven layers of different materials. The two outer layers are usually polymer (polycarbonate or PMMA) which endow the window or panel with its properties of strength and thermal and acoustic insulation. The following two layers are made of a transparent conductive material and are connected to the power supply. Between these two layers is the middle layer or the three middle layers, which is where the reaction takes place that causes the change in properties.

One of the three middle layers is usually manufactured using an electrochromic ceramic material, usually either WO_3, whose electrochromic properties have been known since the 1960s, or V_2O_5 and other oxides of molybdenum, iridium, titanium and manganese and metals from the VB, VIB and VIIIB groups. Another of the three middle layers is the counter electrode, which is a material that can store ions. This counter electrode is usually a conductive polymer or a metal oxide, like nickel oxide, which is the most widely used oxide. The layer right in the middle is sandwiched between the electrochromic layer and the counter electrode. This is made of an ionic conductive material, generally an electrolytic solution or a solid electrolyte.

Applying a voltage brings about a reduction of the electrochromic material and the migration of positive ions from the counter electrode to the electrochromic material where they become fixed, causing changes in the visible UV spectrum of this material. The situation remains stable until a voltage is applied in the opposite direction, which means that these kinds of solutions normally consume little energy. More detailed information on these reactions and the properties of these materials can be found by referring to Granqvist's excellent handbook on electrochromic materials (Granqvist, 2002).

If there is only one middle layer, liquid crystal polymer is usually used. If a voltage is applied to it the structure becomes reordered to let or impede the passage of light. A liquid middle layer is also often used into which particles in suspension can be injected according to the circumstances of the surroundings. This is done by an electronic control that receives information from different sensors that monitor the surroundings in order to attain a greater or lesser optical and thermal insulation.

All these alternatives are providing major energy management solutions in the building sector and contributing to greater comfort in homes. One of the medical applications for these kinds of windows and panels is in operating theatres and hospital wards where they act as screens or dividing panels to ensure patients' privacy. These electrochromic materials are also beginning to be used to design electrochromic fingernails and other cosmetic and aesthetic applications.

11.2.2 Thermochromic or Thermochromatic Materials

Thermochromism is a material's ability to change colour in response to thermal stimuli, such as changes in environmental temperature. Two families of thermochromic materials are normally used to develop devices possessing these properties. These are liquid crystals and leuco dyes, which have been used to produce dyes, paints, papers and rigid, flexible and elastic supports with thermochromatic capabilities for a whole range of applications.

Due to thermal effects, thermochromatic liquid crystals exhibit glass transitions (structural changes) which have a strong influence on their optical properties and change their colour (due to a change in the distance between their molecules and their relative orientation). At low temperature, they exhibit a crystalline phase but if the temperature is increased up to the isotropic liquid phase that is typical of high temperatures, these materials pass through one or more nematic, choleristic or smectic phases with the ensuing changes in transparency and colour.

They are usually used in applications where a change in colour is precisely produced at a specific temperature. However, it is a more costly alternative than using thermochromatic dyes.

Problems also arise at high temperatures or under prolonged exposure to ultraviolet radiation, which cause these materials to age prematurely as is also the case if they are exposed to certain solvents.

Thermochromatic dyes usually comprise a basic transparent dye or leuco dye (usually water or some kind of oil), to which various thermosensitive chemical compounds have been added, causing them to change colour with temperature but without requiring large amounts of thermosensitive material. These dyes are not usually directly applied to the material of the end device but use transparent protective microcapsules as containers.

The most widely used dyes are weak acids (parabens, bisphenol-A, lactones and others) that are in equilibrium with their environment but this equilibrium is disturbed by changes in temperature or pH and leads to colour changes.

Other materials like some metal and iodine oxides (Cu_2HgI_4, Ag_2HgI_4, VO_2 with some dopants, $Cd_xZn_{1-x}S_ySe_{1-y}$ (x = 0.5...1, y = 0.5...1 and others) exhibit phase transitions at temperatures close to atmospheric temperature together with a colour change, thereby providing some new alternatives for the manufacture of thermochromic devices.

Thermochromic materials are already used on many food and health product labels to detect any failure in the cold chain (which can cause serious anomalies and deterioration) during the transportation or storage of these products. One of their most direct medical applications is their use as easy-to-read thermometers or for textiles with thermochromatic dyes for making children's pyjamas (and for hospital patients) that automatically alert to fever to help the early detection of infections. Figure 11.1 shows an example of activation by body contact of a typical thermochromic band.

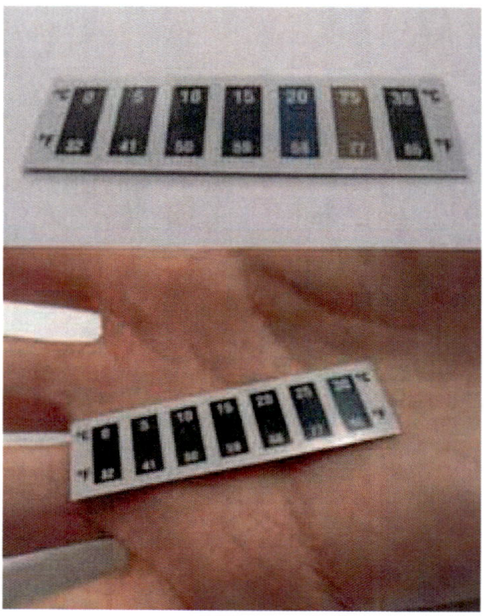

Figure 11.1 Example of temperature activation through a calibrated (0–30°C) thermochromatic band.

Various firms like B&H Colour Change Ltd., Color Change Line Corp., GEM INNOV and Liquid Crystal Resources among others, are devoted to manufacturing these kinds of materials. If it is wished to develop a specific application, it is a good idea to contact these suppliers stating the range of activation temperatures required or even the colour changes sought, to find an initial technical support that can then be compared to one's own characterisation tests.

11.2.3 Photochromic or Photochromatic Materials

Photochromism or change in colour (or optical properties) through the effect of light or to be more exact, UV radiation, occurs in materials that are capable of reversible chemical transformations (and catalysed by this UV radiation) between two states with different absorption spectra. It is really a specific case of photochemical reactions but is called photochromism when the change in the absorption spectrum occurs in the visible range.

Therefore, of all the reactions likely to generate photochromic processes, it is worth mentioning cis-trans isomerisations, dissociation processes and electron-transfer reactions (oxidation-reduction) among others.

Photochromism can take place in both organic and inorganic compounds, and also appear in some biological processes and systems (as occurs with retinaldehyde in the vision process). Some photochromic materials worth mentioning are spiropyrans, spiro-oxacynes, azobenzenes, some quinones and silver chloride (a key component in the development of photography).

The use of photochromic polymers is well-known in the production of glass for glasses that adapt to the light, like those shown in Fig. 11.2. There is therefore nothing strange in thinking that these materials could also be used for contact lenses or active intraocular implants. Some of them (with delayed reversibility) can also be used to detect if certain food or health products that can be negatively affected by exposure to UV radiation are being exposed to such during transportation or storage. Their use has also been suggested as a support for optical devices, and as fibre optic sensors where the photochromatic material acts as a safety switch for excess radiation or helps adjust the optical signal crossing through the device.

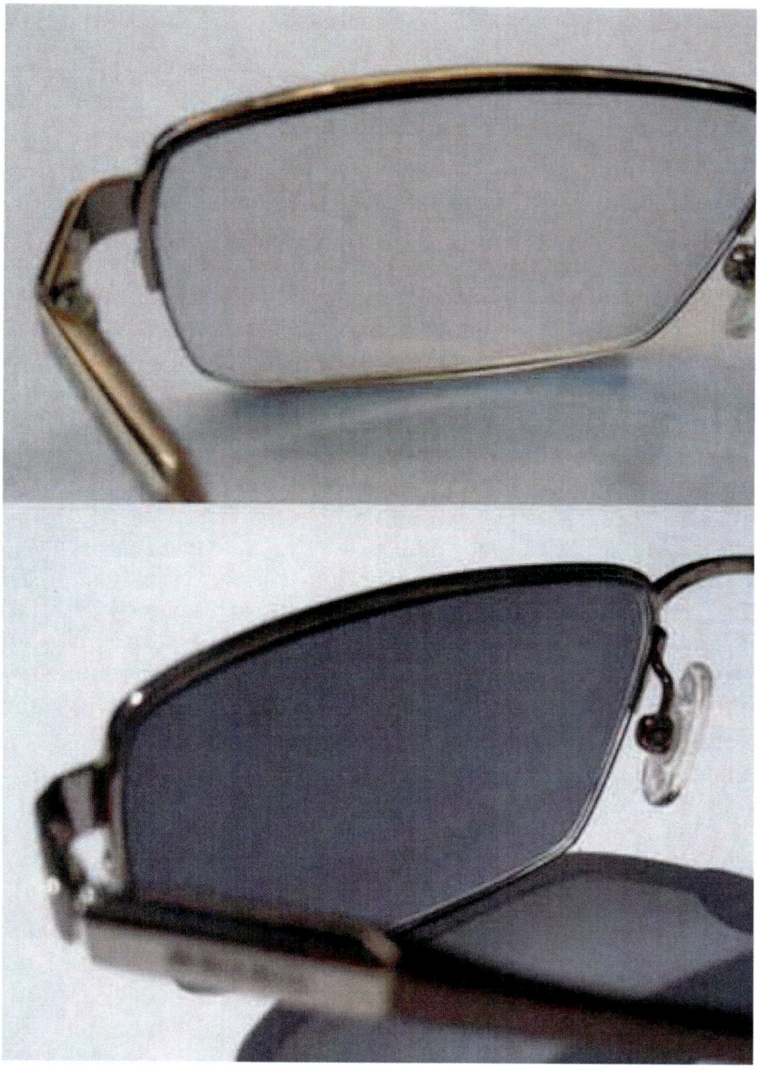

Figure 11.2 Example of photochromatic lens activation through exposure to UV radiation.

More exact information on the properties of these materials can be found by referring to the excellent text on photochromism by Dürr and Bouas-Laurent (Dürr and Bouas-Laurent, 2006).

11.2.4 Piezochromatic Materials

Piezochromism is the ability of some materials to change their colour or optical properties in response to the application of external pressures or deformations. These effects are usually found in polymers such as polythiophenes or poly(alkylsylanes), as well as in many polymers incorporating metal particles at their core. High pressures deform the polymer structure and change the frequency at which the material's maximum absorption spectrum is reached and hence its colour. Its main limitation is connected with sensitivity since significant colour changes are only attained at high pressures, although new synthesis and manufacturing processes are contributing more and more effective solutions at low pressures.

Some of the uses put forward by manufacturers are piezochromatic carpets as an aid for evaluating the performance of high ranking athletes by measuring step imbalances, to supplement other more conventional piezoresistant or piezoelectric-based systems. They can also be used to study bite pressures and to analyse devices to counteract temperomandibular joint disorders in persons, in combination with the other measuring systems previously described (Lafont *et al.*, 2007, 2008). The piezochromatic sensors supplied by firms like Sensor Products Inc. (Tactile Pressure Experts, Bentley and Mayers, 2003) and Color Change Line Corp. (which also supplies thermochromatic sensors), could be a suitable choice for conceptual validations and prototype testing, as well as for the future mass manufacture of devices.

Some polymers commonly known as photoelastic polymers also need mentioning (epoxy resins, some polystyrenes and other birefringent resins) which, when pressed, change their refractive index, which means they can also be considered as piezochromatic. If a part manufactured in these materials is carefully examined (e.g., using stereolithography) lines can be discerned, usually coloured ones, which according to their relative proximity allow a qualitative evaluation to be made of the areas subjected to the greatest forces and deformations. This has been proven to be of use in combination with rapid prototyping technologies and using simple test benches (Ros *et al.*, 2007), to assess the goodness of different prosthesis designs and select the right ones without any need to invest in the manufacture of prototypes using final materials.

Other alternative operating principles for producing piezochromatic materials are based on dye microcapsules being integrated into the core of the polymer or cellulose material, which, when pressed, causes the microcapsules to break and the material is marked. Another instance is the graphite strips used by dentists to adjust unload splints, fillings and other oral implants.

11.2.5 Hydrochromatic Materials

It can sometimes be of interest to use materials that can change colour in the presence of water, which can usually activate reversible oxidation-reduction reactions in these materials (a role previously exerted by UV radiation on photochromatic materials).

At present, proposals for applications are limited. One of the few commercial uses is for umbrella textiles that can change colour in the rain. On the other hand, they could turn out to be of use for visually marking water leakage in certain containers, tanks and even fluid medical devices.

Most suggestions for these materials that change colour have come from the textile, decoration or consumer product industries (Iqbal, 2009). The impact on the Medical Industry is expected to take longer due to the high responsibility of the devices involved.

Many other materials also have optical reactions when exposed to different stimuli, which for reasons of space cannot be described here. That is, a whole range of materials with colour changes in response to stimuli that give rise to chemical reactions, like the well-known litmus paper that is sensitive to changes in pH, among many others. There are also tribochromic materials that show an optical response to contact phenomena, with a certain similarity to piezochromatic phenomena. Optical phenomena in magnetorheological fluids and elastomers when exposed to magnetic stimuli have also been described. These are used to develop X-ray collimeters for better quality medical imaging (Dyszkiewicz *et al.*, 2009).

11.3 Photoactive Materials: Types and Applications

Photoactive materials can react to light stimuli or emit light in response to different external stimuli. This has led to their being used as light generators as well as sensors and actuators that are activated by the intensity of the light captured. In recent years, the number of medical applications has been growing little by little. For this reason we have decided to include this chapter and deal with the main kinds of photoactive materials as described below.

11.3.1 Electroluminescent Materials

Electroluminescence is an electro-optical phenomenon consisting of the emission of light by a material as a response to an electric current passing through it. Applying a current usually excites the electrons in the material and this additional energy is released in the form of photons. It therefore differs from other light-emitting mechanisms like heating up to incandescence, sonoluminescence or the emission of light in response to a sound-pressure wave, mechanoluminescence or the emission of light in response to mechanical phenomena and the emission of light from chemical reactions (Fink and Beaty, 1978).

The phenomenon of electroluminescence is particularly marked in semi-conductors and the devices are usually constructed by superimposing layers of inorganic or organic materials (LEDs and OLEDs). This superposition of layers enables optimal size devices to be produced (thin-film electroluminescent devices or TFELs), which are supplied with the required voltage. A standard structure consists of one or more semi-conductive inorganic or organic layers located between the negative electrode, usually a thin metal layer, and the positive electrode, usually an optically transparent conductor (that allows the circuit to be closed and let the light generated pass through).

Some of the materials usually used are zinc sulphide (doped with manganese, copper or silver to obtain different colours), natural blue diamond (diamond with borium inclusions), standard semi-conductors like InP, GaAs or GaN, as well as organic semi-conductors (polyanylene, some polycyclic aromatic hydrocarbons, and the composite PEDOT: PSS, etc.), to name but a few.

For the negative electrode, highly reflective metals or alloys coated with a reflective metal layer are usually used. For the positive electrode, which lets the light pass through, glass with an indium oxide or pewter coating is usually used, as well as other polymer materials like PEDOT and even carbon nanotubes, to obtain optimised surface features.

The Medical Industry has benefited from these materials by their use in many displays and screens used to control numerous devices. This has become the standard application of electroluminescence in most industries as well as for use in interior and exterior decoration. We should also consider the use of these materials as an aid to the design of multipurpose intelligent catheters where the luminescent material would carry the light to the target area of the operation in minimally invasive surgery as an alternative to fibre optic illumination.

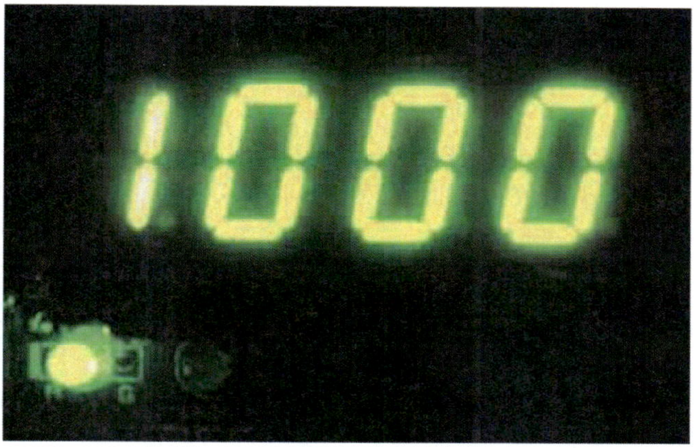

Figure 11.3 Example of an electroluminescent display.

11.3.2 Fluorescent Materials

Fluoresence is the emission of luminous electromagnetic radiation by a material that has previously absorbed electromagnetic radiation from another wavelength (an electron absorbs a photon reaching a higher state of energy, and then reemits it at a lower frequency). Emission is usually performed at a higher wavelength (therefore it is lower energy radiation) than that received. The difference in energy is due to thermal losses (the material heats up). However, particularly when high radiation is being absorbed, an electron may absorb two photons and the ensuing emission can have a shorter wavelength. In whichever case, the phenomenon is especially attractive when the absorbed photon is in the ultraviolet (invisible) region of the spectrum. This usually causes a re-emission in the visible region and the material appears to "shine" of its own accord.

The first research into the phenomenon at the end of the 19th century was conducted on fluorite (calcium difluoride), which on occasions reveals traces of europium, which serves to activate the fluorescence. Quinine salts and sulphates are currently used as a standard for comparing the intensity of different fluorescent materials. However, if more detailed information is required on this type of material and molecules that are susceptible to generating this kind of effect it is advisable to refer to more specific texts (Invitrogen Corporation, 2010).

Once again, the first industrial applications of these photoactive materials came from interior decoration and design as well as from the world of art. However, they are being increasingly used in health sciences, especially biology, biochemistry and medicine.

For example, fluorophores or extrinsic fluorescent markers, such as small molecules or proteins, are being used as a non-destructive method for marking and monitoring certain biological systems, usually proteins, microorganisms, cells and tissue, with the aid of spectrofluorometers. In this way controlled cell separation can be performed as well as procedures for detecting DNA or specific nucleic acid sequences and for other works in immunology consisting in attaching a fluorophore to an antibody in order to trace its path and evaluate its behaviour (Guilbault, 1990; Valeur, 2001). New applications are constantly emerging that may also be strengthened if they are combined with the capabilities possessed by other intelligent materials.

11.3.3 Phosphorescent Materials

Phosphoresence is an optoluminesent phenomenon related to fluorescence but where the re-emission of the light radiation received does not occur immediately, but is delayed in time and is slower. Most photoluminescent effects (fluorescence among them), in which a substrate absorbs and re-emits a photon occur very rapidly (around 10 ns). However, in the special case of phosphorescent materials this re-emission can be delayed for minutes or even hours.

Some typical phosphorescent pigments and materials are zinc sulphide and strontium aluminate. These have been widely used in decoration, jewellery and watch-making, to produce diverse elements that glow in the dark.

In various health sciences, mainly biochemistry and biology, but more recently in sport medicine and other medical disciplines, fluorescent markers (in solution) have been used for the *in vitro* assessment and distribution of oxygen in intact and damaged tissue, since oxygen is a good reducer of the phosphorescent intensity of these composites (Rumsey *et al.*, 1988; Vinogradov and Wilson, 1994; Hogan, 1999). Combining these detection principles with the activation capabilities of other intelligent materials may lead to the production of minimally invasive devices for performing *in vivo* gasometry.

11.3.4 Photoelectric Materials

The photoelectric effect consists of the emission of electrons by a material as a result of it being exposed to a source of electromagnetic radiation, usually of a very short wavelength (visible or ultraviolet). The effect was first described by Heinrich Hertz in 1887 and then satisfactorily explained by Albert Einstein in 1905, a work for which he received the Nobel Prize for Physics in 1921.

Elements like rubidium, cesium and antimonium are particularly outstanding photolelectric elements, although current applications based on this and other related effects use other materials, mainly semi-conductors for the production of photodiodes, phototransistors and a whole range of optical sensors for different imaging technologies, many of which have applications in the Medical Industry.

However, some biological materials like chlorophyll *a*, with a coupling of photoelectrochemical or optoelectrochemical properties are beginning to be used in the development of biosensors that work on a molecular level but can nonetheless detect certain composites very quickly using very small amounts of reagent, which is a bonus for laboratory work (Tugulea, 2000; Nam *et al.*, 2004). This kind of device can also be considered for optical sensors or for energy-to-light conversion systems (biological photovoltaic cells), although their response and efficiency need to be optimised.

11.3.5 Phototropic Materials

Phototropisms are the typical movements made by plants and some microorganisms (usually fungi and algae) with a tendency to grow or move towards light sources. Auxines (plant hormones) are responsible for this type of phenomena as they react to light by emitting protons towards the area of the plant that is in the dark, which increases the cell pH in this area. The acidification of the cell wall activates some enzymes known as expansins whose mission is to break some of the bonds of the cell wall to make the area more flexible while also breaking some hydrogen links in the cellulose making up the cell wall. In this way, the cells in the dark region expand and the plant bends towards the light.

Living plants could obviously be considered as phototropic systems, but it would be interesting to develop synthetic materials with marked phototropic properties, maybe based on a combination of multilayers of different inorganic and organic materials or even by integrating live microorganisms at the core of the material (that react to light). Maybe we could also imitate other biological principles like photo-orientation which occurs in plant cells when the chloroplasts change their position according to the light intensity.

Some photochromic materials have occasionally been wrongly designated as phototropic (when these materials simply undergo a colour change but no appreciable movement through the photo-optical effect).

Phototropic activation, as outlined in Figs. 11.4 and 11.5, is always linked to the proposals for future action described at the end of the chapter. These underline the countless action lines that emerge from adopting biomimetic approaches and from a combined use of intelligent "synthetic" and "biological" materials including integrated living microorganisms (diatoms, algae and fungi are some), as sensors or actuators for multifunctional devices, particularly for tasks that fall within the scope of health sciences.

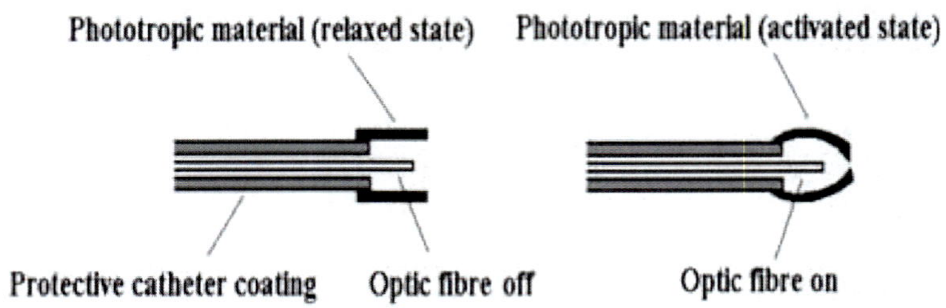

Figure 11.4 Diagram of a phototropic microactuator.

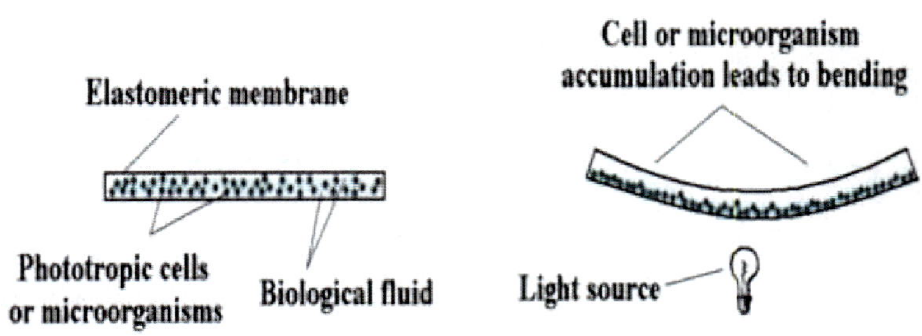

Figure 11.5 Proposal for phototropic material to produce light-controllable actuators. Possible use of the positive and negative phototropisms of specific microorganisms.

Many other materials are able to react to light stimuli (some, like photochromatic materials also belong to the family of chromoactive materials, as we have already seen) or emit light when faced with different stimuli. There are mechanoluminescent or sonoluminescent materials like those already mentioned and other much brighter ones like triboluminescent materials (which emit light through contact phenomena like flint) or fractoluminescent materials (which emit light when they break). They have not been described here as up to date no marked medical applications have appeared and so they remain somewhat outside the scope of this handbook.

11.4 Present Capabilities and Recent Advances

This section deals with some current capabilities concerning the processing of a wide range of polymer and ceramic materials that are fundamental for gradually increasing the complexity of chromoactive and photoactive materials, as well as for enhancing the capabilities of active medical devices based on these "intelligent" materials.

11.4.1 Laminated Glass Production

Many optically active materials can be produced using standard multilayer laminated glass manufacturing processes. The process for producing laminated glass basically consists in bonding several sheets of glass by using an intermediate polymer adhesive. Many elements can be laminated between the glass, such as printed, coloured, safety, anti-theft/bullet-proof plastic films, paper with designs, LED diodes, cloth, soundproof materials, solar-controlled materials, photovoltaic glass and others.

The most standard process for laminated glass production (which can basically be included in the families of multilayer structures and also microstructured materials) usually comprises the following stages:

- Washing the sheets of glass to be bonded
- Placing the adhesive on the sheets of glass to be bonded
- Pressing the sheets to achieve bonding
- Curing and thermal processing in a furnace
- Use of after-processes like UV curing

A very convenient alternative to pressing and then furnace-curing is to stack the sheets of glass to be bonded and then put them in vacuum bags and process them in an autoclave at a high temperature, using pumps to create a vacuum in the bags. This will obtain more outstanding end properties.

On an international level the following companies are devoted to laminated glass production or to enhancing the processes or machinery involved, particularly autoclaves as an aid to processing different materials, especially multilayer glass: ASC Process Systems, Bond Tech Corporation and Symtech with their "flexlam" lamination system.

Other even more innovative systems carry out the laminating process without the need for an autoclave. This is the case with the lamination carried out by companies such as Gyrotron Technology Inc. with their GTitechnology protected under patent (www.gyrotrontech.com), which increases productivity and cuts the energy consumed in the process, although it would be important to compare the achievable quality of the different processes.

The progress made by some companies is worth mentioning. DreamGlass (www.dreamglass.es), ProDisplay^{TM}, Saint-Gobain Recherche among others, include a middle layer electroactive (electrochromic) liquid crystal whose transparency can be controlled by applying a voltage that can change the orientation of the polymer molecules. An outline of the activation process is shown in Fig. 11.6 together with the example of Fig. 11.7.

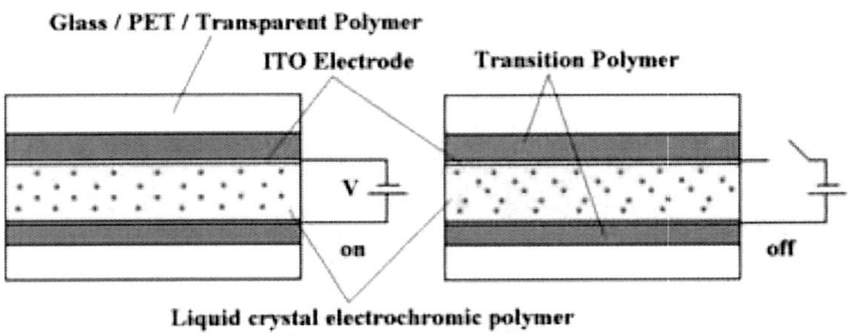

Figure 11.6 Schematics of the activation of an electrochromic liquid crystal layer integrated into multilayer glass for "intelligent" windows and panels with controllable opacity.

The final material is similar to that in conventional devices but the size of the sheets is larger and the final mechanical properties are also enhanced. This is because transition polymer layers are used (EVA, EHB) with properties that fall between those of the outer glass and those of the liquid crystal core, in addition to the use of transparent ITO (indium-tin oxide) coatings that act as electrodes.

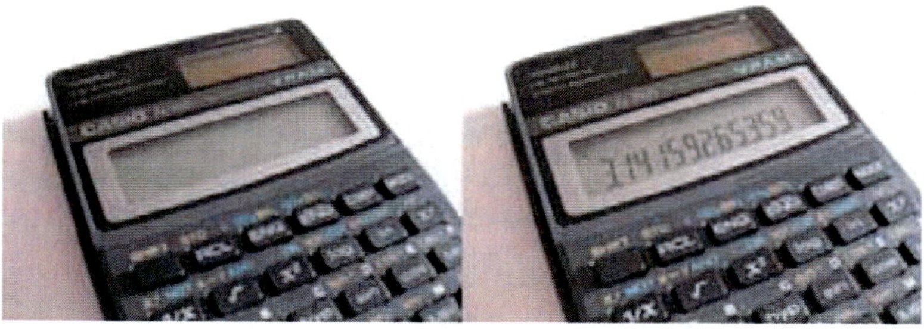

Figure 11.7 An example of electrochromic liquid crystal panel activation.

Instead of using intermediate sheets of electroactive liquid crystal to control transparency, other proposals use a layer of water flowing between two outer layers of glass. The water helps control the temperature of the rooms where the glass is fitted and its transparency can be controlled at will by injecting pigments that temporarily colour the water in the middle layer. One of the companies currently doing research into this kind of system is Intelliglass, a spin-off of Madrid Polytechnic University.

Systems based on similar but miniaturised operating principles can be of use for developing different active medical devices that require integrated optical switches and other subsystems that are standard in the micro-electromechanical systems (MEMS and opto-MEMS) industry. They can also provide better privacy in waiting rooms, operating theatres, and be used for bath screens and other uses.

However, the gradual increase in the number of laminated layers, usually glass or polymer, enable additional functionalities to be added to increasingly complex applications. In this way, different optical or chromic actions can be combined in a single material. This is in addition to the contribution of the materials dealt with in other chapters, which can be used as active fibres or as sensors that respond to a range of stimuli.

We believe it is important to include some texts on the use of "intelligent" materials and glass in the references. Many of these materials are optoactive or electro-optical and are providing a range of solutions to many industries like the building industry (ergonomics and energy saving), biomedicine (active implant development) and other industries connected with the development of MEMS, particularly in the field of opto-MEMS (Gad-el-Hak, 2002; Yoder, 2006).

11.4.2 Fibre Production

Optical fibre is a glass or polymer fibre that can transport light in its interior. This has led to enormous improvements in telecommunications, like increased data-transfer capacity and the distance over which data can be transferred, the reduction in information loss and the likelihood of electromagnetic interference, compared to traditional systems. The light entering the fibre is kept inside it by the total internal reflection phenomenon, which means these fibres act as waveguides (Hecht, 2002).

Although the total internal reflection phenomenon and wave guiding have been known since the 19th century through the works of Colladon, Babinet and Tyndall, among others, it was not until the 1920s that practical applications were discovered for some lighting processes linked to Surgery and Dentistry. However, modern optical fibre did not appear until the 1950s when glass fibre with a transparent coating to enhance its refractive index began to be used. Its application to medicine was almost immediate with the invention in 1956 of the first flexible gastroscope.

Since then, progress in synthesis and processing together with a continuous search for new uses have made it popular for developing a range of medical devices, many of which could be called "active", since they assist a number of procedures for early diagnosis as well as for ever less invasive surgery, for which reason fibre optic endoscopes are currently in common use.

Optical fibres change their light-transport properties in response to a range of external stimuli such as temperature, pressure, deformation, acceleration etc., which bring about changes in the intensity, phase, frequency or polarisation of the light transported. These effects have led to these fibres being used as transducers in the development of a whole new family of "fibre optic sensors". Although it is not really an "active" material in the sense that it plays a passive role, since it is used to transport light, we have thought it important to include optical fibre due to its particularly outstanding medical applications and its interest as a support material for developing sensors, actuators and multifunctional systems, often in combination with other active, multifunctional or "intelligent" materials. Described below are some points concerning its synthesis and processing.

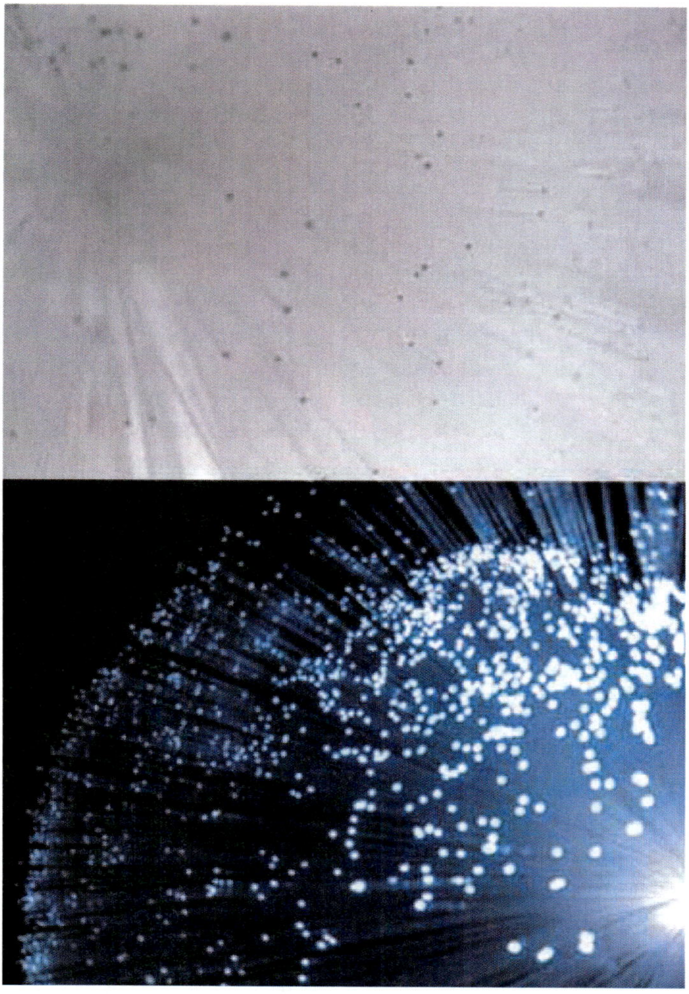

Figure 11.8 Example of a set of optical fibres switched off and on.

Optical fibres are usually made of silicon dioxide, although other materials like fluoraluminate, fluorozirconate and some metaphosphates are also used in specific cases (Fig. 11.8). They are sometimes manufactured in polymer materials but they are more difficult to soften than silicon dioxide glass fibres, which gives them a limited use in telecommunications.

The production process usually begins with a pre-form with a controlled refractive index that is subjected to stretching to produce the thin fibre. "Internal vapour deposition" is a standard method in which silicon dioxide or germanium dioxide vapours are deposited on the inside of a glass tube that is gradually filled. In this process, the vapours to be deposited are obtained by injecting a gaseous mixture of silicon tetrafluoride, germanium tetrafluoride and oxygen on the inside and heating the mixture to around 1900 K. The considerable thermal difference between the gas and the tube walls (much colder) cause the particles in the gas to adhere to the walls.

Another standard method is "external vapour deposition", in which silicon dioxide or germanium dioxide vapours are deposited on the outside of an initial bar. In this case, the vapours to be deposited are obtained by the oxidation (using water in an oxyhydrogen flame) of a gaseous mixture of silicon tetrafluoride and germanium fluoride.

Having produced the pre-form, it is placed on the stretching tower where the end of the pre-form is heated and is then subjected to stretching to form a kind of rope whose diameter and stress is continuously monitored to control the end properties and dimensions (mainly mechanical and optical) of the fibre produced. Moreover, during stretching, urethane acrylates are applied to the outside of the fibre which then undergoes UV curing (usually once or twice) so as to produce a coated fibre with enhanced properties.

11.4.3 Other Outstanding Technologies

Of the other technologies for producing multilayer glass and different kinds of optoactive materials in general, some thin layer deposition technologies must be mentioned besides the physical deposition or chemical vapour ("PVD" and "CVD") technologies referred to in other chapters, such as

- **Sol-gel deposition processes.** These sol-gel processes are characterised by their transition from a sol phase to a gel phase, usually by various hydrolysis and polycondensation reactions, and are used to produce vitreous and ceramic materials. The sol is made up of solid particles (usually around 0.1 to 1 μmin diameter) dispersed in a liquid, while the gel comprises a solid network of macromolecules immersed in a solvent.
- **Langmiur-Blodgett deposition technologies.** This is a very exact deposition technology (performed by the superimposition of monolayers) using different organic

coatings, such as fatty acids, phospholipids and polymers with long lateral hydrophobic chains. Nanostructures can be produced with molecular alignment and controllable roughness and thickness and are widely used for producing biosensors. Their high precision means that the materials obtained can be either microstructured or nanostructured.

- **Self-assembled monolayers technology.** Layers can be deposited on a substrate by consecutively alternating the adsorption of catatonic and ionic species. It is a relatively cheap and simple technology for controlling the molecular structure of materials and influencing their macroscopic properties. It has recently been used to obtain multilayer structures by bonding very different materials like polyelectrolytes, metal colloids, biological molecules, conductive polymers and light emitting polymers.

These are laboratory processes that are particularly suited to producing samples in research projects for comparing the properties of the many formulations. These are examined in greater detail in Chapter 13, which deals with the different thin-layer and multilayer active structure manufacturing technologies.

11.5 Main Challenges and Research Trends

11.5.1 Biomimesis as a Source of Inspiration

Biomimesis is the application of natural systems and methods to solve problems of engineering and technological sciences, and we must once again underline its importance. During its evolution Nature has designed a number of innovations far superior to what the human mind alone would have conceived, due to the fact that Nature has been contributing effective solutions to real-world problems over millions of years of trial and error (Dawkins, 2006, 2009). By observing Nature, new chromoactive or photoactive materials can be found that will be based on the structure and activation principles of biological materials that possess these qualities.

In fact, there are many remarkable examples of chromoactive and photoactive materials being used in both the animal and vegetable world in order for them to adapt better to the environment, usually to assist in finding food or strengthening defence mechanisms. Most of these systems can be used as conceptual designs for the design of active synthetic devices that can reproduce certain biological actions in a controlled way.

There are many well-known examples of chromoactive biomaterials or biostructures in the animal world. For example, chameleons and some amphibians mimic their surroundings by changing colour to go unnoticed. This ability is due to their dermis having a multilayer structure that layer by layer has different coloured pigment cells (chromatophores, guanophores and melanophores) that can be used to regulate the tonality, shininess and design of their skin (in the same way as a LED television). A chameleon's skin can therefore be considered to be a biomaterial or a photochromatic biostructure. Various synthetic multilayer structure designs follow similar solutions or at least combine layers with different actions to optimise their response to different stimuli.

As an additional example of a biomaterial or chromoactive biostructure, we can cite recent studies regarding the colour change undergone by a beetle's shell when it comes into contact with water, which means we are dealing with a hydrochromatic biomaterial. Under normal conditions, the light interferes with the structure to produce the green colour of the shell. When water penetrates the wide-open porous layers, it destroys the phenomenon of interference which makes the shell turn black. It is thought that this change is linked to defence strategies. Synthetic materials designed in line with these principles could be used to control food and drug quality by detecting any unwanted moisture.

A familiar example of living organisms being used to produce chromoactive sensors is litmus paper, which reacts to changes of pH. It is usually produced from various species of lichens, nowadays mainly *Roccella montagnei* (Mozambique) and *Dendrographa leucophoea* (California).

There are also many varied examples of biomaterials or photoactive biostructures capable of either generating light or reacting to light stimuli. Many creatures that live in the abyssal zone exhibit phenomena of electroluminescence, fluorescence and phosphorescence and can generate their own light to find food or a mate and even to ward off possible predators.

Fireflies are another familiar example of bioluminescence. They belong to a species of insects in which the females are able to oxidise luciferin in the presence of the enzyme luciferase. This is a very fast reaction that generates light to make the insect shine and attract the males for reproduction. In the face of danger the light immediately goes out. It could be of use to use similar reactions or a hypothetical training of these bioluminescent cells to develop biodevices for teleoperated inspection in environments lacking in light.

As an additional curiosity we would like to refer to the fur of polar bears. This exhibits total internal reflection phenomenon that behaves similarly to optical fibre by making a large amount of the light radiation received go directly to the skin. This is of enormous help in combating the low temperatures of their environment.

Regarding the vegetable world, we have already mentioned the importance of phototropisms in plants and in some organisms that are halfway between the animal and vegetable world, like algae and fungi. Therefore, auxines, which are vegetable hormones, can be considered as "intelligent" materials as they show a variety of responses to a range of stimuli. This could be put to use in the development of new multifunctional materials and devices for detection or actuation procedures.

Many other proteins and enzymes can also be described as "intelligent", as on a molecular scale they exhibit dynamic behaviour. Some photoreceptive proteins are able to convert sunlight directly into electrical signals, which leads us to think of biological solar microcell development as a possible aid to powering other microdevices. Information and microelectronic technologies could also be strengthened by the use of "intelligent" proteins and enzymes.

Financing strategies to foster collaboration between the university and industry combined with a more interdisciplinary education could promote these promising multidisciplinary technologies for the production of biosensors, bioactuators, biodevices, biomachines or biocomputers (Choi *et al.*, 2004).

11.5.2 Combining Materials for Optimised Optoactive Devices

When multilayer structures are subjected to mechanical forces, particularly when the layers are ceramic, peeling is produced due to the fragility of these materials, their high stiffness and problems of adhesion. This is why more and more flexible polymer materials are being used to produce photoactive materials with enhanced mechanical properties.

Continuous research is also being carried out into deposition techniques in order to obtain thin layers and to develop the middle or transition layers that help bond materials that possess very different mechanical properties. The progress made in the last decades in adhesives technology has also been very positive for the production of more flexible, stronger and long-lasting multilayers, while for medical device development, encapsulations and bonds using biocompatible adhesives are especially promising.

The optimisation of energy consumption in active biodevices and active medical devices in the near future may be related to the use of photoactive materials, above all, photoelectric and photoelectrochemical materials that are suitable for powering microdevices that work with nothing more than a light source but without the need for batteries (which will not only help minimise consumption but also size). Although the idea is not exactly new (Seibert and Janzen, 1980), recent research is confirming the feasibility of these proposals and the future looks promising (Das, *et al.*, 2004; Jefryes *et al.*, 2008; Enviro-News, 2010).

Again, the use of biological materials are of major importance in assisting the discovery of new functionalities in complex systems, many of which will be based on "intelligent" synthetic materials that can be strengthened by technological solutions that are taken from Nature or "borrowed" from other living creatures.

11.5.3 Optical Tweezers as Actuators for the "Nanoworld"

Recent decades have seen the development of new microscopy technologies that have helped evaluate and monitor the *in vivo* behaviour of a wide range of proteins, enzymes and other macromolecules, as well as the response of many microorganisms (cells, viruses and bacteria, among others) to a variety of stimuli. The stimuli normally used for these studies are mechanical (using atomic force microscopes), magnetic and optical. In 1986, Ashkin and his team described the first three-dimensional, stable optical trap (or optical tweezers), made by using the electromagnetic radiation pressure of a single laser beam. A few years later, Block and his collaborators demonstrated the use of optical traps to manipulate organisms, which opened up the way to new forms of nanoscale manipulation (by applying forces in the range of a few piconewtons to objects of around 10–100 nm) (Block, 1989, 1992, 1995).

These tweezers or optical traps are gradually becoming excellent tools for minimally invasive micro-and macromanipulation in many areas of health science and biomedical engineering (Neuman and Block, 2004; Shaevitz, 2006). The activation ranges (in terms of force and distance) of optical tweezers or traps make them especially suited to the study of biochemical and biological phenomena. In recent years they have made possible such complex work as the mechanical and structural characterisation of biological polymers like DNA, cell membranes and even complete cells.

Using chromoactive materials to construct lenses with optical properties that can be controlled at will, may help optimise optical trapping systems and encourage new applications for them, particularly in the development of nanoengines, nanomotors and biological nanomechanisms. For this purpose it is extremely important to design behaviour models of these tools and use simulation programs based on these models in order to be able to analyse such complex phenomena.

11.6 Improving Results and Main Conclusions

This chapter has provided a detailed description of different chromoactive (or optoactive) materials that can change their colour or optical properties in response to different stimuli, and different photoactive materials that can emit light in response to a range of stimuli or react to light stimuli. We have focused on their fundamental properties and major current and potential applications.

Regarding optoactive or chromoactive materials, we have looked at a wide range of subtypes, specifically electrochromic or electrochromatic, thermochromic or thermochromatic, photochromic or photochromatic and piezochromatic and hydrochromatic materials. Regarding photoactive materials, we have provided a detailed description of the following types: electroluminescent, fluorescent, phosphorescent, photosensitive, photoelectric or phototropic materials.

We have also examined the different processing methods for producing photoactive and chromoactive materials, generally in the form of multilayer structures and we have described some future proposals for a combined use of biological and synthetic materials to optimise the working of multifunctional devices and systems.

Many of these materials have already proved to be highly suitable for developing low-cost, low-consumption sensors and actuators, mainly for the electronics and telecommunications industries, although many medical applications or applications linked to other health sciences like biochemistry or biology have also been described.

However, the important thing is to continue thorough research into specific aspects like searching for medical applications for these materials, possibly by encouraging more direct relations between universities, research centres and business. Another way could be to set up coordinated action groups on a large scale to seek out technological supply and link it to specific medical needs. If this is to be promoted, it is important to gradually integrate these kinds of topics or even subjects on the Science and Technology of "intelligent" materials into the syllabuses of technology degree courses and other biomedically linked courses.

Additional information can be found in the following list of references, which includes results from some of the main researchers in this multidisciplinary field, as well as in the websites of the different suppliers included in the annexes of the handbook, some of them already mentioned within the chapter. We hope that researchers interested in these materials and their applications will have found this useful, as well as being of help for setting up future contacts between research centres.

References

Ashkin, A.; Dziedzic, J.M.; Bjorkholm, J.E.; Chu, S. "Observation of a single-beam gradient force optical trap for dielectric particles". Optics Letters, 11(5), 288, 1986.

Bar-Cohen, Y. "Electroactive polymers as artificial muscles". SPIE Press, 2004.

Bentley, D.J.; Mayers, G.E. "Measure pressure with thin film". Paper, Film & Foil Converter, May 1, 2003.

Block, S.M. "Making light work with optical tweezers". Nature, 360(6403), 493–5, 1992.

Block, S.M. "Nanometres and piconewtons: The macromolecular mechanics of kinesin". Trends in Cell Biology, 5, 169–175, 1995.

Block, S.M.; Blair, D.F.; Berg, H.C. "Compliance of bacterial flagella measured with optical tweezers". Nature, 338(6215), 514–518, 1989.

Choi, J.W.; Nam, Y.S.; Fujihira, M. "Nanoscale fabrication of biomolecular layer and its application to biodevices". Biotechnology and Bioprocess Engineering, 9(2), 76-85, 2004.

Das, R.; Kiley, P.J.; Segal, M.; *et al.* "Integration of photosynthetic protein molecular complexes in solid-state electronic devices". Nanoletters, 4, 1079–1083, 2004.

Dawkins, R. "The blind watchmaker". Penguin Books, 1986, reissue 2006.

Dawkins, R. "The greatest show on earth, the evidence for Evolution". Spanish Edition, Espasa Calpe, S.A., 2009.

Díaz Lantada, A. "Metodología para el desarrollo de dispositivos médicos activos basados en el empleo de polímeros activos como sensores y actuadores". PhD Thesis, Universidad Politécnica de Madrid, 2009.

Dürr, H.; Bouas-Laurent, H. "Photochromism: Molecules and systems". Elsevier, 1st Edition 2003, 2nd Edition, 2006.

Dyszkiewicz, A.; Polec, P.; Zajdel, J.; *et al.* "Collimation of X-Ray Diagnostic Bundle by Means of Steering Ferrofluid". Second International Conference on Biomedical Electronics and Devices, Special Session on Active Materials for Medical Devices (AMMD), Biodevices 2009, Porto, Portugal, 2009.

Environmental News Technologies Expert. "From pea plants to bio solar cells". (www.enviro-news.com), March, 2010.

Fink, D.G.; Beaty, H.W. "Standard handbook for electrical engineers". McGraw Hill, 11th Edition, New York, 1978.

Gad-el-Hak, M. "The MEMS handbook". CRC Press. Florida, 2002.

Granqvist, C.G. "Handbook of inorganic electrochromic materials". Elsevier, 1st Edition 1995. 2nd Edition, 2002.

Guilbault, G.G. "Practical fluorescence". Marcel Dekker, New York, 1st Edition 1973, 2nd Edition, 1990.

Hecht, E. "Óptica". Addison-Wesley Iberoamericana España, S.A., 1999.

Hecht, J. "Understanding fiber optics". Prentice Hall, 4th Edition, 2002.

Hogan, M.C. "Calibration of a phosphorescence quenching method for measurement of intracellular PO2 in isolated single skeletal muscle fibers". Medicine & Science in Sports & Exercise, 31(5), 278, 1999.

Invitrogen Corporation. "Molecular probes: The Handbook – Fluorescence fundamentals". 2010.

Iqbal, M. "Textile dyes". Rehbar Publishers Karachi, 2009.

Jefryes, C.; Gutu, T.; Jiao, J.; Rorrer, G.L. "Metabolic insertion of nanostructured TiO2 into the patterned biosilica of the diatom Pinnularia sp. by a two-stage bioreactor cultivation process". ACS Nano 2(10), 2103–2112, 2008.

Lafont Morgado, P.; Díaz Lantada, A.; Martínez Álvarez, A.; *et al.* "Dispositivos médicos basados en el empleo de polímeros electroactivos". Actas del 8° Congreso Iberoamericano de Ingeniería Mecánica. Pontificia Universidad Católica del Perú. Cuzco, 2007.

Lafont Morgado, P.; Díaz Lantada, A.; Martínez Álvarez, A.; *et al.* "Instrumented splint for the diagnosis of bruxism". International Conference on Biomedical Electronics and Devices Biostec 2008 – Biodevices, 2, 216–222. IEEE Engineering in Medicine and Biology Society. 28–31 January, 2008, Madeira, Portugal.

Nam, Y.S.; Choi, J.W.; Lee, W.H. "Photoswitching characteristics of biodevice consisting of chlorophyll a Langmuir-Blodgett film". Journal of microbiology and biotechnology, 14(5), 1038–1042, 2004.

Neuman, K.C.; Block, S.M. "Optical trapping". Review of Scientific Instruments, 75(9), 2787–2809, 2004.

Ros, A.; Claramunt, R.; Sánchez Alejo, F.J. "Equipo de congelación de tensiones para ensayos fotoelásticos". Spanish Patent Document, OEPM 2285966, 2007.

Rumsey, W.L.; Vanderkooi, J.M.; Wilson, D.F. "Imaging of phosphorescence: a novel method for measuring oxygen distribution in perfused tissue". Science, 241(4873), 1649–1651, 1988.

Schwartz, M. "New materials, processes and methods technology". CRC Press, 2006.

Seibert, M.; Janzen, A.F. "Biological solar cell". American Section of the International Solar Energy Society Conference. Phoenix, 1980.

Shaevitz, J.W. "A Practical Guide to Optical Trapping". (genomics.princeton.edu), 2006.

Tugulea, L. "Photoelectrochemical behavior of chlorophylla in thin films". In "Nanostructured Films and Coatings", Chow, G.M. *et al.* (Editors), 347–354, Kluwer Academic Publishers, 2000.

Valeur, B. "Molecular fluorescence: Principles and applications". Wiley-VCH Verlag GmbH, 2001.

Vinogradov, S.A.; Wilson, D.F. "Phosphorescence lifetime analysis with a quadratic programming algorithm for determining quencher distributions in heterogeneous systems". Biophysical Journal, 67(5), 2048–2059, 1994.

Yoder, P.R. "Opto-mechanical systems design". CRC Press, Taylor & Francis Group. 3rd Edition, 2006.

Chapter 12

Hydroactive Materials for Biodevices

Andrés Díaz Lantada
Mechanical Engineering Department, E.T.S.I. Industriales,
Universidad Politécnica de Madrid, c/ José Gutiérrez Abascal 2,
28006 Madrid, Spain
adiaz@etsii.upm.es

12.1 Brief Introduction to Hydroactive Materials

The concept of hydroactive materials can refer to a whole range of materials that change one or more of their properties in the presence of water or as a response to moisture. So, when some materials rust they change colour, others change their volume when they absorb water, others change their electrical conductivity.

These are just some of the possible responses. However, in this chapter, we shall focus on the hydromechanical aspect, which is linked to the change in geometry that certain materials undergo, usually polymers ("hydropolymers"), in the presence of water.

Previous chapters have dealt with certain optical and electrical effects resulting from immersion in aqueous solutions, and we believe it is worthwhile to devote an entire chapter to hydroactive polymers, due to the large number of present and potential medical applications.

These hydropolymers also let us approach the concept of "environmentally multi-reactive materials", since their sensitivity to atmospheric stimuli (temperature, pressure, pH, electric current or UV radiation) is especially high and appears in a multi-coupled form,

Handbook of Active Materials for Medical Devices: Advances and Applications
Edited by Andrés Díaz Lantada

www.panstanford.com

as will be seen at the end of the chapter. This boosts their medical applications, not only as hydromechanical actuators, but also as sensors that can respond to a whole range of stimuli to monitor different physiological magnitudes.

Also included at the end of the chapter are some proposals for sensors and hydroactive actuators based on other intelligent materials combined in new ways or based on new principles of detection or actuation.

However, the main part of the chapter is focussed on the study of hydropolymers and their capability for hydromechanical activation.

Generally speaking, hydropolymers (also called hydrogels or super absorbent polymers, SAPs, which will be used as synonyms in the chapter) are cross-linked polymers in the form of a three-dimensional network of natural or synthetic origin that swell on contact with water to form soft, elastic materials and retain a significant fraction of the water in their structure without dissolving (Gerlach and Arndt, 2009).

The hydrated form is called hydrogel (swollen, viscous and elastic) and the non-hydrated form is called xerogel (compact and stiff). Xerogels have high porosity (around 25%) and a high surface/mass and surface/volume ratio (around 100–1000 m^2/g), with pore sizes usually ranging from 1 to 100 nm.

Polymer solids are particularly suited to forming gels due to their long-chain structure. The flexibility of these chains means they can deform to allow molecules of dissolvent to enter their three-dimensional structure. These hydropolymers can be classified into two types, depending on the nature of the bonds of the three-dimensional network of which they are comprised:

- Physical hydropolymers exhibit a three-dimensional network made up of bonds that are not entirely stable. They are usually van der Waals type bonds, much weaker than covalent bonds. They give rise to non-cross-linked meshes.
- Chemical hydropolymers, which are polymers where the network is formed through covalent bonds. This type of bond is very strong and its breaking causes the gel to become degraded. This gives rise to cross-linked meshes.

With cross-linked meshes, the molecular lattice is determined by the covalent nodes of the mesh. With non-cross-linked polymers, the lattice has physical origins (non-permanent), since the chains become intertwined with one another in a three-dimensional tangle that can store and retain liquid molecules.

Regarding swelling, the main difference between cross-linked and non-cross-linked polymers is that with the former, the entry of liquid cannot separate the chains since they are covalently bonded, while with the latter, the entry of liquid can untangle the chains and separate them, as the forces keeping them bonded are of physical origin and less magnitude.

There is, however, no radical difference between them, as in most cases the cross-linking in the hydropolymers is not only due to covalent bonds (σ bonds), typical of any cross-linked material, but also due to intermolecular van der Waals forces and the hydrogen bonds.

There are also other types of interactions, such as electrostatic forces, both attractive and repellent, intermolecular bonds of hydrophobic components and ionic interactions.

Hydropolymers have a set of general characteristics of which the most significant are

- They are of a hydrophilic nature due to the presence of water-soluble groups in the structure (-OH, -COOH, $-CONH_2$, -CONH, $-HSO_3$).
- They are insoluble in water due to the existence of a three-dimensional polymer network that gives the structure consistency.
- They have a smooth elastic consistency that is easily adaptable to human tissue. This is determined by the initial hydrophilic monomer and the low density of the polymer cross-linking.
- They swell up in water and considerably increase their volume until a physical-chemical balance is reached, while, in principle, keeping their original geometric proportions.
- They are thixotropic materials; that is, they become more fluid on being agitated or when subjected to alternate mechanical stress, and become more solid when they are in a state of rest (e.g., a typical effect that can be seen in plastic paint).

On the other hand, since hydropolymers were introduced into the field of Health Sciences (mainly Biology and Medicine), they have been shown to have a great potential as biomaterials, due to their good response when in contact with biological tissue. This usually leads to devices that are suitably biocompatible and endorses their use.

This remarkable feature is because the physical properties of hydrogels are more similar to those of living tissue than any other kind of synthetic biomaterial, particularly with regard to their relatively high water content, their soft, elastic consistency and their low surface tension.

Of the typical polymers possessing these properties that are finding the largest number of applications in medical device and application development, it is worth mentioning the following: poly(vinyl alcohols) or PVAs, poly(acrylic acids) or PAAs, silicon hydrogels, gelatine hydrogels, poly(glutamic acid), polyacrylamides, poly(HEMA), N-vinylipyrolidone among others.

The following section contains a brief summary of the existing applications and the most recent proposals for use for these materials as integral parts of medical devices, both passive and active.

12.2 Potential for Biodevices

The medical applications of these materials can be divided into active or passive according to their role in a specific device. Their passive applications in "passive devices" are based on the excellent properties of these materials (in their hydrated phase) when in contact with human tissue. Their active applications in "active devices" are usually based on making use of the super absorbent properties of these materials or based on the changes in geometry that occur when in contact with water so that hydroactive sensors and actuators can be produced. We shall now examine some of the main applications of some of the most highly developed materials to date.

After undergoing *in vitro* and animal *in vivo* testing and meeting the requirements for official approval, in some cases their commercialisation is subject to their attaining the goals described at the end of this chapter.

12.2.1 Passive Devices

Contact lenses

The good hydration capability of hydrogels and the possibility of producing devices with mechanical properties similar to those of many body tissues have led to hydrogels becoming standard materials for medical devices. A specific example is contact lenses where silicone hydrogel lenses are in general use. Their porosity allows oxygen to pass through specifically produced membranes, for which reason they are being used for disposable contact lenses (with a useful life that ranges from 12 to 14 h up to one month) with ever better optical and ergonomic properties, compared to more traditional materials like PMMA and others.

Prostheses in plastic surgery

Plastic surgery is a major area of application for these materials. Mammary implants have been filled with silicone gels for decades, although in some countries, like the United States, they are not permitted. This is due to their having been linked, on occasions, to the appearance of certain pathologies after leakage of the filling, as well as other problems (Berthe, 2001). In approximately 60 countries where this material is still available, it is used in 90% of plastic surgery. Nonetheless, objective critical studies need to be carried out to assess any potential damage resulting from their use and rigorous comparisons made with possible alternative materials.

Vertebral implants

Certain poly(vinyl alcohol) or PVA hydrogels have led to prostheses of intervertebral discs being obtained with properties very similar to those of the original tissue. After an exhaustive *in vitro* chemical and mechanical characterisation, they have been tested with promising results in animal models as well as in human patients (Biodevices, Ku, 2008).

Sutures

Certain sutures and surgical patches made of hydrogels are now replacing swabs, surgical staples and conventional stitches, due to the advantages of these polymers when in contact with body tissue. Worth mentioning are the TIELLETM series of dressings from Systagenix, made of hydrogel membranes with biocompatible adhesive for a faster healing of wounds. This is because the hydrogel absorbs exudates letting the damaged zone be well-oxygenated through its pores. It is also coming into generalised use in numerous areas associated with plastic surgery (Liew, 2001).

Pericardial patch

Certain hydrogel dressings like poly(2-hydroxyethyl methacrylate) are now being occasionally tested on patients who are about to undergo successive heart surgery. This is reinforced with an ethylene tetrafluoroethylene (ETFE) mesh which is implanted in the tissue that to be subjected to the operation, thereby conferring greater strength and reducing the chances of catastrophic post-operative ruptures of the tissue (Allder, 1990).

Sealants

Some gelatine and poly(glutamic acid) hydrogels and others, such as CorgelTM BioHydrogel from Lifecore Biomedical LLC, based on hyaluronic acid, are beginning to be used in some surgical operations to seal tissues damaged in standard thorax and lung operations.

Tissue growth substrate

Hydrogels have been used for some time as materials in tissue engineering. The traditional procedure consists in obtaining a biodegradable hydrogel substrate with an adequate surface texture, to which cells are incorporated in a second stage for them to then grow and form tissue (Langer, 1993).

As will be explained further on in Sec. 12.3.5, when dealing with the additional properties of hydroactive polymers, one of the most outstanding features of some hydropolymers is that they can be polymerised by the action of UV radiation. This is leading to new single-step approaches towards the obtaining of two-dimensional and even three-dimensional biological structures by using hydroplymers mixed with living cells (Mironov, 2009).

12.2.2 Active Devices

Super absorbent pads

One of the most successful industrial applications of hydropolymers is to be found in super absorbent pads. These have some hydrogel "pearls" on their inside that quickly absorb any excess fluid, improving user comfort and reducing any skin problems caused by a prolonged contact with an excess of moisture.

There are dozens of patents related to the design of sanitary towels and pads based on the use of super absorbent polymers (US 4950264, US 5922565, WO/1991/018573, WO/1994/027538, WO/1998/043584, etc.).

This property had already been used in the design of some models of super absorbent tampons. However, in some cases they were thought to be the cause of toxic shock, for which reason they were withdrawn from the market, with alternative functional principles being sought.

Pumps and capsules for drug administration

The porosity of these materials means that drugs can be injected inside them so they can be used to design micropumps combining different kinds of activation. In some cases, the hydrogel itself becomes deformed as it absorbs body fluids, which triggers the pumping of the drug into the body. Sometimes the hydrogel can be combined with other electroactive materials that subject the hydrogel to pressure, thereby causing the drug to be expelled. Some devices based on these principles are explained in Sections 12.3.5 and 12.4.

Some biodegradable hydrogels have also been used for a gradual administration of drugs through the manufacture of hydrogel spheres with micro-drops of drug injected inside.

The progressive degradation of the outer surface of these hydrogel spheres permits the gradual release of the drugs inside them.

Gastric balloons for obesity

In the treatment of especially complex cases of morbid obesity that fail to respond to dieting and little-invasive pharmacological treatments, gastric or gastroplasty bypass operations sometimes have to be resorted to. These are high-risk operations for patients, which, moreover, are irreversible. For this reason, in the last two decades some remarkable devices have been developed like those shown in Fig. 12.1, which shows the two most conventional alternatives.

On the one hand, there are various models of adjustable, inflatable intragastric balloons that fill part of the patient's stomach to prevent them from eating so much food. On the other hand, there are percutaneous bands that compress the stomach to reduce its volume and obtain similar results to those using gastroplasty.

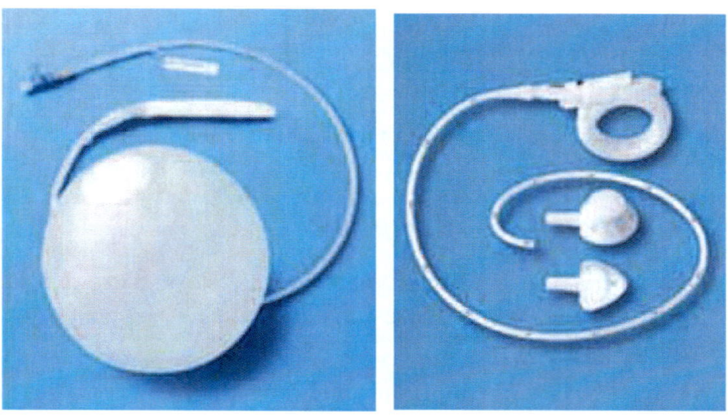

Figure 12.1 Inflatable intragastric balloon Heliosphere Bag® & Heliogast Band®. Helioscopie Medical Implants' remarkable solutions for severe obesity.

Both solutions are less aggressive than conventional gastroplasty (Trande, 2008). However, the use of gastric balloons made of cellulose-based hydropolymers that expand inside the stomach provides an even less aggressive solution. In fact, recent advances have led to pills whose effects last a few hours until they dissolve, which has the advantage of the solution not being "forever" (Ambrosio, 1998, 2006; Sannino, 2009).

Once again, it is important to emphasise how the use of active materials leads to devices with a smaller number of components and optimised functionality and results.

Actuators

These SAP hydropolymers or hydrogels can also be used as an active component that contributes additional functionalities to conventional surgical devices. Thus, properly integrated into pincer-type structures, they can react in the presence of water and cause changes in the geometry of the pincers (which were passive, in principle) in order to obtain active ends for catheters, as will be described as a case study further on in the chapter.

Electrodes in medical devices

The ability of some hydropolymers to respond to electrical stimuli makes them good candidates for sensors intended for measuring the electrical activity of certain body tissues, in accordance with the procedure laid down in patent US 7419486 (Kampa, 2005).

Further information on the behaviour of these materials and their response to different stimuli is detailed in the following section, before we go on to analyse the main current lines of research and the future possibilities of these complex hydroactive polymers.

12.3 Current Capabilities and Recent Advances

12.3.1 Synthesis and Processing

When a hydrogel or hydropolymer is synthesised there is a large number of polymers to choose from, which can be put into three categories:

- Monomers with non-ionisable lateral substituents, such as acrylamide, N-vinylpirrolydone, dihydro-ethyl-methacrylate and others.

- Monomers with ionisable functional groups, such as acrylic, methacrylic, sulphonic and amino acids, usually to obtain very absorbent hydropolymers, but with not very remarkable mechanical properties.
- Zwitterionic monomers with total null charge, but which, having atoms with opposite charges, are polar and especially reactive. They exhibit greater changes of volume in saline solutions than in water.

To prepare cross-linked hydrogels and hydropolymers, methods like radiation cross-linking can be used that use X-rays or UV radiation or copolymerisation reactions using cross-linking agents that unite with high molecular-weight chains through their functional groups. Moreover, in both cases triggering or initiating agents need to be used for the polymerisation reactions (free radicals, radiation, gamma radiation etc.).

In their commercial versions, these polymer materials are usually purchased in dual-component form; the monomers are separated from the initiator and the cross-linking agent which provoke the polymerisation reaction. After mixing, they are usually cast in moulds and kept there until cured to get the required shape (curing times usually take from 10 min up to several hours).

The use of rapid prototyping technologies to obtain models that can then be used to produce rapid moulds by shape copying is usually sufficient to achieve complex geometries with these hydroactive polymers.

The materials used to produce the samples shown in this chapter (with the trade names of "Hydromorph – Hydrospan", in their "Expanding" and "Contracting" versions) were purchased from the English firm "MUTR Teaching Resources" (www.mutr.co.uk), a spin-off of Middlesex University, which supplies different kinds of materials and accessories for laboratory teaching activities.

With this example, we have aimed for a fast, cheap manufacture of samples for carrying out the characterisation tests necessary to assess the speed of response, the capacity for successive activations, the deformations and forces that can be attained during activation, the minimum thresholds in size variation for uses as sensors and other aspects of interest.

To accomplish this, "LEGO" pieces were used to make ultra-rapid laboratory frames that could be adapted to the required sample sizes. This way, industrial frames are not necessary and material is not wasted when producing the samples, as shown in Figs. 12.2 and 12.3.

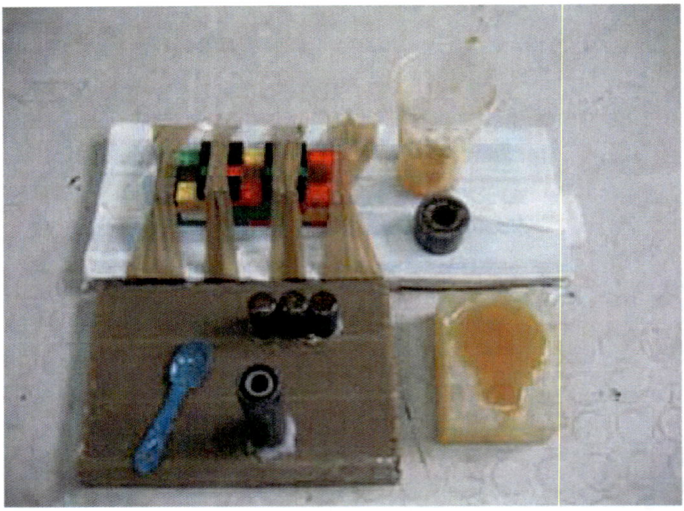

Figure 12.2 Rapid moulds for casting and obtaining samples.

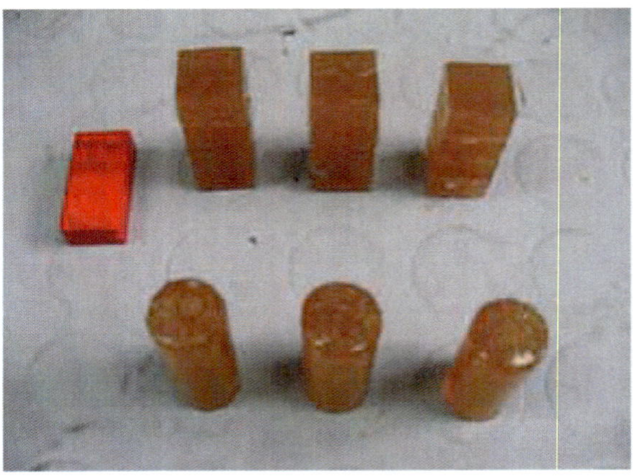

Figure 12.3 Samples obtained (non-hydrated form or "xerogel").

Sometimes, in addition to the monomers, the initiator and the cross-linking agent, water is added during processing in order to achieve hydrated geometries by mould casting. In these cases, after extraction from the mould, the water present in the hydropolymer slowly evaporates and the geometry gradually contracts.

Other more novel and more complex alternative processes that involve more stages are detailed in the section towards the end of the chapter on the challenges and trends of current studies.

12.3.2 Characterisation and Modelling

As already stated, a three-dimensional polymer network can absorb a large amount of the water or fluid with which it comes into contact. During swelling, the chains making up the network take on an elongated form and this dilation is accompanied by the appearance of a retractile force in opposition to the swelling process, which acts as a pressure exerted on the solvent in the mesh chains. As the mesh gradually swells with the solvent, this elastic pressure increases and the swelling reaches its maximum or equilibrium value when equilibrium between both forces is attained.

Highly cross-linked hydropolymers have a very compact structure and swell much less than the same hydropolymer with less cross-linking. However, hydropolymers that contain hydrophilic groups in their structure swell to a larger extent than those containing hydrophobic groups, which minimise the interaction of the material with the water molecules, resulting in much less swollen hydropolymers.

Nonetheless, with a view to developing devices based on these remarkable abilities to change their geometry or hydromechanical activation, it is a good idea to conduct systematic characterisation tests to be able to have a detailed understanding of how the hydropolymer behaves and the main factors influencing its response.

For the characterisation tests detailed below in Figs. 12.4 and 12.5, the samples manufactured using the rapid moulds described earlier were used, and the hydroactive material (expandable on contact with water) was supplied by MUTR, under the trade name of "Hydromorph - Hydrospan".

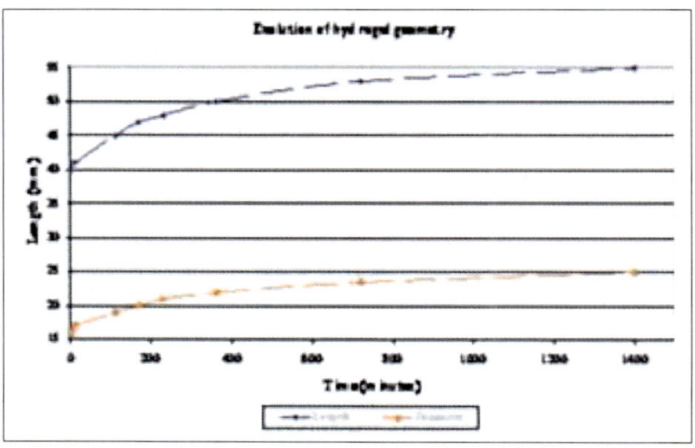

Figure 12.4 Geometric evolution of the hydropolymer samples on immersion in water.

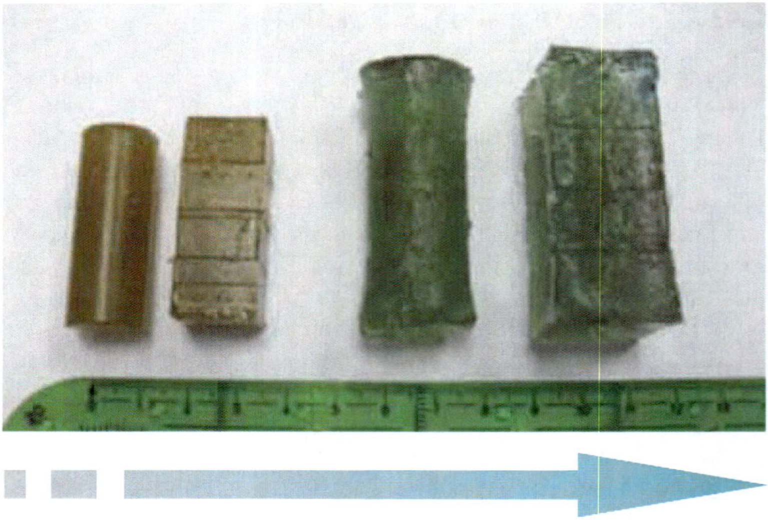

Figure 12.5 Geometric evolution of the hydropolymer samples on immersion in water. Total time: 24 h for the geometric change shown (which leads to a certain amount of oxidation).

A slower response can be observed than for other families of active materials (like piezoelectric materials, alloys and shape-memory polymers, electroactive polymers in general and others). This is a major issue to be improved upon as some surgical operations that could benefit from the use of these materials may be limited for this reason.

However, the deformations that can be attained are outstanding, going way beyond what can be achieved by the other families of intelligent materials mentioned, even if the geometric change is not completely homogeneous. However, this aspect can be optimised by more repetitive manufacturing processes (intended for mass production instead of for prototype production).

It must be emphasised that the characterisation test results are necessary in order to know how the material responds in the presence of body fluids and to analyse its characteristics as a sensor/actuator.

Therefore, similar characterisation test results have been used to fit analytical and numerical models to simulate the response of these materials after being integrated into the devices. It is worth pointing out the advances in simulation using the finite-element method that have enabled us to analyse and design different hydrogel-based actuators (PVA-PAA), that take account of the attainable deformations as well as the forces that can be developed during activation, by using our own codes entered in "ABAQUS" (Marra *et al.*, 2003; Westbrook, 2008).

Although, standard commercial software still does not include ad hoc elements to simulate these materials, it is to be hoped that in the coming years, different elements will be included in these programs for various families of active materials, as is already the case with piezoelectric materials in programs like "ANSYS Multiphysics".

One possible alternative for assessing the behaviour of these materials as actuators in a specific device is to take finite elements with another type of coupling to imitate the behaviour of the hydropolymer in accordance with the characterisation test results.

We will, therefore, now show an example of an active pincer design that integrates a hydroactive actuator at its end. It was modelled and simulated with NX-6, which does not have any specific finite elements for hydrogels. The program, however, does allow the use of elements with thermo-mechanical coupling (where thermal loads induce deformations). According to the test data in Fig. 12.4, in the presence of water the actuator expands, increasing its principal dimensions by up to 35%.

To emulate this effect, a polymer material was applied to the FEM model in the actuator zone, with a known thermal expansion coefficient, and a temperature increase was used in the actuator to lead to a 35% increase in length in the principal directions. A "surface contact" boundary condition also had to be applied to the zone where the actuator was adhered to the pincer, in order to simulate the situation in the actual device, shown in Fig. 12.8.

It can be seen in Figs. 12.6 and 12.7 how the results of the FEM simulations and the behaviour of the prototype device more or less coincide. This is a proof that the information obtained from the simulations may of great use as an aid to design work for optimising device and actuator geometry so that the deformations required for a correct activation will be produced.

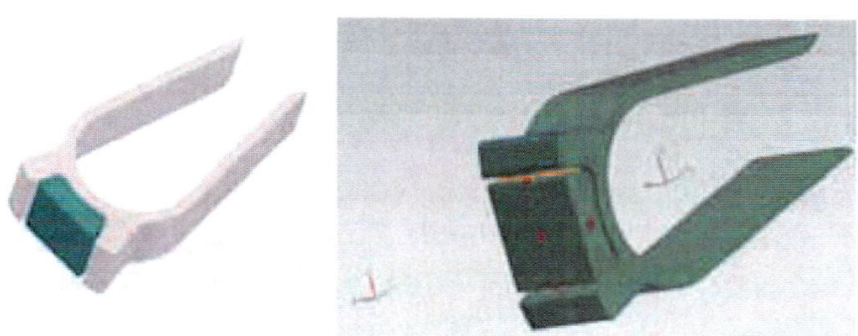

Figure 12.6 Design (solid edge) and FEM (NX-6) hydroactive pincer model.

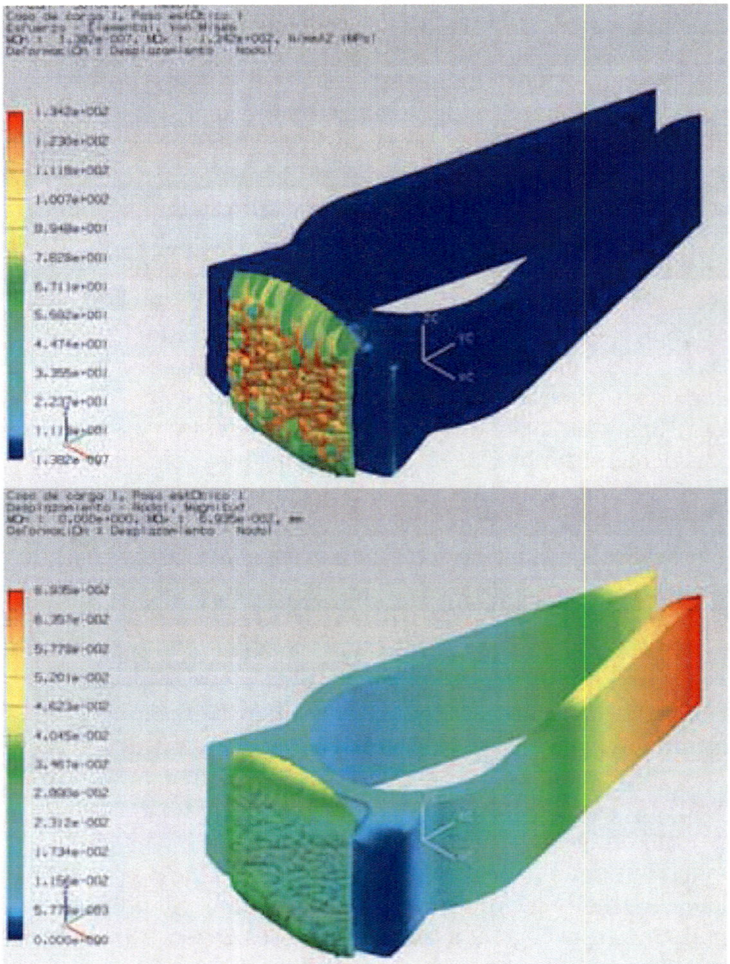

Figure 12.7 FEM simulation of activation (and closure): Results of forces and deformations.

12.3.3 Integration into Biodevices

Medical devices based on hydropolymers as actuators or sensors are sometimes surprisingly simple. This is the case with expandable gastric balloons as they are simply based on a part with a specific geometry wholly manufactured using a hydropolymer with no additional components.

However, many proposals for use are based on inserting a hydropolymer mini-probe (sensor or actuator) into a pre-existing device or a sensing or actuating subsystem inside a more complex device. To achieve this, the use of CAD-CAE-CAM technology together with rapid manufacturing tools must again be highlighted as a method for producing prototypes to verify an activation or detection principle for therapeutic or diagnostic work. So-called reverse engineering, consisting in designing new improved products from more conventional ones, can benefit enormously from this approach and can be useful for developing all kinds of active medical devices that can be innovated and enhanced by the use of active materials.

Dual-layer "elastic polymer-hydropolymer layer" or "superelastic alloy film" hydroactive pincers can open up new perspectives in minimally invasive surgery as active catheter ends, as will be seen in the following example.

In this case study, a surgical pincer was manufactured in epoxy resin using the stereolithography process with the aid of CAD files. The pincer had a housing at its end for the hydroactive material. The "actuator pill" to be integrated into the pincer, using epoxy-based "Araldite"-type adhesive, was made from the hydropolymer samples. However, for commercial applications, body-compatible adhesives must be used. Relevant information can be found in the help manuals and catalogues of the various suppliers (www.loctite.com/www.henkel.com/www.araldite.com and others).

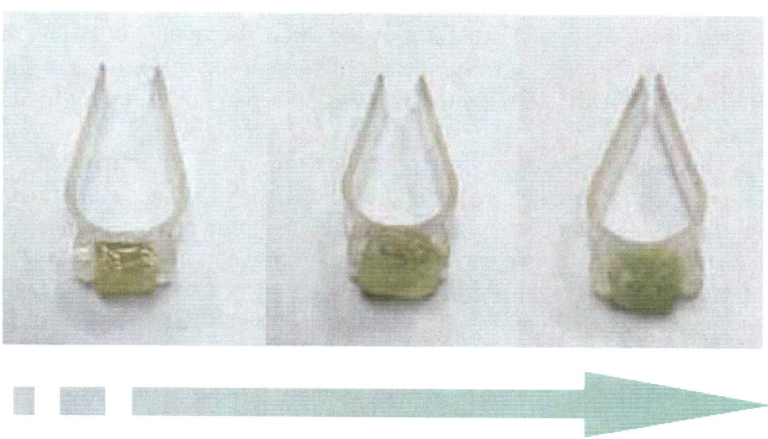

Figure 12.8 Hydroactive pincer for surgical catheter end (activation on immersion in water). Structure that integrates a hydropolymer pill as active component.

Design must be done in line with the properties of the material and the activation time required. This must be specified if the product reaches the production stage, since a longer immersion in an aqueous environment may lead to inadmissible deformations for the structure on which it is acting. The importance of properly characterising the hydroactive material must once again be emphasised if accurate behaviour models are to be attained for simulations to assist design work.

Design encapsulations to stop the polymer from moving in certain directions during activation can boost response speed and activation capability (developable forces and attainable deformation) in a specific direction.

12.3.4 Other Important Properties

The properties of a hydrogel and its structure are directly related (as is the case with polymers in general) in such a way that neither characteristic can be considered on its own since the method of synthesis has a direct influence on them. So, when stating the properties of hydrogels, reference must be made to the structural parameters conditioning them.

The volume of hydrogels depends on the equilibrium between the specific repellent and attractive interactions in the network. The combination of molecular interactions such as van der Waals forces, hydrophobic interactions, hydrogen links and electrostatic interactions, determine the extent to which the hydrogel swells in equilibrium. On the other hand, any effect leading to changes in the equilibrated hydrogel's water content will lead to changes in its structure.

Therefore, effects like the application of mechanical stress, changes in temperature, pH or electric field, the presence of chemical agents or solvents and exposure to radiation, have an influence on the geometry and dimensional stability of these materials.

A property of these materials that is giving rise to a wide range of industrial and medical applications is its selective ionic permeability (fundamental for ion exchange membranes in combustion cells, in haemodialysis equipment etc.). It has been observed how the amount of water absorbed by the hydrogel determines the size of its pores and the ions that can cross the membranes made of these materials. Thus membranes with different pore sizes can be designed that selectively let different ions pass through.

Detailed below are some property changes that take place in these materials as a response to different physical or chemical stimuli, which makes them better suited to being integrated into active medical devices for detection or activation procedures.

12.3.5 Response to Other Stimuli: New Ideas for Sensors and Actuators

As we stated in the introduction, apart from the hydromechanical coupling already described, these hydropolymers possess a whole range of possibilities due to their interrelated mechanical, thermal, chemical, optical and electrical properties (Westbrook, 2008; Gerlach, 2009).

These mostly non-linear couplings obviously make characterising and modelling of these materials more difficult for simulating applications where they will be subjected to various external stimuli. For this reason, it may be interesting to look more closely at simulating these hydropolymers by using artificial neural networks. These are a particularly appropriate tool for modelling systems with spectacular non-linearities and numerous coupled properties, as explained in Chap. 15, which presents a case study.

We will now detail the different phenomena and responses of these materials in the hope that other researchers will be encouraged to examine them in greater depth and discover new medical applications that will benefit from their use.

Response to changes in pH

Gels with ionisable groups are sensitive to pH since ionisation is determined by the pH in terms of equilibrium ionisation. The variation in environmental pH induces changes in the degree of ionisation of the electrolytes, and, therefore, a change in the extent to which the hydrogel swells.

Among the cationic groups sensitive to changes in pH are: $-N^+-$, $-NH^+-$, $-NH_2{}^+-$, $-NH_3{}^+-$ $-S^+$, and among the ionic groups, we can cite: $-COO^-$, $-PO_3{}^-$, $-SO_3{}^-$, to name but a few.

When hydropolymers with these groups have been properly characterised and tested, they can be useful for monitoring certain physiological magnitudes; for example, controlling the local evolution of organs and tissue after a surgical operation or for monitoring prostheses and detecting any possible corrosion that might occur on their surface (Kim, 2005).

Response to changes in environmental salinity

By using mechanisms similar to those mentioned above, some hydrogels also show a response to changes in environmental salinity. They are able to absorb greater or lesser amounts of water depending on the concentration of salt present, which enables them to be used as sensors for certain ions that can be found in physiological fluids (Dulong, 2007).

Among other biological applications, these materials have shown good results when treating water contaminated by an excess of salts. They are particularly suitable in arid zones and for desalinating sea water in islands with water shortages (Shawky, 2006).

Response to temperature changes

Temperature is one of the parameters that have the most impact on hydrogel properties, with drastic changes being brought about to some properties in specific cases with temperature changes of only 2 to 3 °C.

At standard laboratory temperature, the higher the temperature, the higher the evaporation rate of the hydrogel's water content, and the greater the reduction in volume, passing from hydrogel to xerogel more quickly.

However, its temperature sensing properties are not as remarkable as those mentioned in other chapters dealing with pyroelectric polymers or dual-layer microsensors and actuators.

On the other hand, it is important to point out that temperature changes can alter the surface behaviour of hydrogels and produce transitions from hydrophilic characteristics to hydrophobic characteristics. This is giving rise to many proposals for use in biotribology, microfluidics and biofabrication (Tanaka and Sato, 2007; Mironov, 2009).

Response to electric current

The so-called electroactive hydrogels are intelligent materials that can be compressed, expanded or bent in response to electrical stimuli. The most common mechanism consists in moving the ions at the core of the hydrogel by applying a voltage at their ends. This causes deformations in their structure, as is the case with ionic electroactive polymers.

Different formulations have already been successfully tested [chitosan-based, polyacrylamide, copolymers of polyacrylic acid and poly(vinyl sulphonic acid)], that allow considerable deformations to be attained in the activation process (Kim, 2005; Shamsudeen, 2006).

Recent research has shown that an increase in the porosity of electroactive hydrogels allows greater deformations to be attained during activation, and even bending angles of more than 90°, even though the response speed (tens or hundreds of a second) is less than that of other families of electroactive polymers (O' Grady, 2009).

On the other hand, an increase in the degree of cross-linking usually leads to reductions in the attainable deformations, as research shows (Ali, 2007). The research also proposes using these materials as drug reservoirs to ensure an electrically controlled and programmed supply.

Response to UV radiation

Many hydrogels react to UV radiation, which activates primary and secondary polymerisations in them. Apart from being used to obtain cross-linked hydrogels, this property is beginning to bring a wide range of solutions to problems of biofabrication and tissue engineering.

In fact, using photosensitive hydrogels with live cells at their core is being put forward as an alternative material for manufacturing technologies that have a similar approach to that of stereolithography, aimed at achieving a single-step layer-by-layer fabrication of three-dimensional biological structures (Dhariwala, 2004; Mironov, 2009; Hannachi, Yamato and Okano, 2009).

The initial results of this research are very promising, with a view to replacing the most traditional tissue engineering procedures using two steps; the first step being based on the fabrication of a biocompatible substrate on which to deposit the cells during the second step so they will grow to form the required tissue (see Chap. 15).

In the case of hydrogels intended for implantable devices, the influence of UV radiation must be characterised and taken into account if the device using this process is to be sterilised. If the hydrogel is unsuited to this, it is important to point out that sterilisation using water vapour or humid environments may also have a major impact on the device's geometry and properties, for which reason the successful use of CO_2 cold processes has been proposed (Jiménez and Zhang, 2008). Other processes like sterilisation by means of ethylene oxide, hydrogen peroxide and gamma radiation, have also been subjected to a detailed analysis (Kanjickal, 2008) and may be of use for certain applications.

12.4 Current Challenges and Future Possibilities

12.4.1 Ultra-Thin Film Production

Improvements in adapting these materials to the surfaces of the end devices, as well as greater elasticity and better mechanical performance in the long term, can be had by producing hydropolymers in the form of very thin films. These thin thicknesses can also lead to more compact sensing and actuating devices with greater sensitivity and numerous fluid and biological applications (Harmon, 2003; Heo, 2005; Peppas, 2007).

In this respect a gradual optimisation of sol-gel processes might be a step in the right direction (with which other active materials can also be obtained, such as electrochromic materials with electro-optical coupling, as described in the chapter on "Optically Active Materials"). These sol-gel processes are characterised by their transition from a sol phase to a gel phase, usually by various hydrolysis and poly-condensation reactions, and are used for producing vitreous and ceramic materials.

The sol is made up of solid particles (usually around 0.1 to 1 μmin diameter) dispersed in a liquid, while gel comprises a solid network of macromolecules immersed in a solvent. The conventional stages of the process (Brinker, 1990, Hench, 1998, Albella, 2006) include:

(a) Dispersion of particles in a liquid to form the sol material comprising the initial chemical solution. Metal alkoxides are usually used as precursor particles (R-O-M, where R is a radical, O an oxygen atom and M a metal atom) and metal chlorides. Using particles of materials like SiO_2 as precursors and organic additive, modified silica glass with multiple applications can be produced.

(b) Deposition of a thin layer of sol on the substrate to be coated, normally by centrifuging or spin-coating, immersion-extraction or "dip-coating" or by spraying.

Different technologies, such as Langmuir–Blodgett deposition and other methods to prepare self-assembled monolayers are enabling even thinner thicknesses to be attained and more flexible films that can adapt to the geometries of more complex devices.

(c) Polymerisation of sol particles by volatilisation of the stabilisers and the formation of the three-dimensional solid network that constitutes the gel. The alkoxides react rapidly in the presence of water (hydrolysis) to form R-OH and M-OH species molecules that can be then linked together by polycondensation to form OR-M-O-M-OR species three-dimensional networks with M-O-M bonds and remnants of H_2O and R-OH. The vaporisation of these H_2O and R-OH sub-products results in the required gel.

(d) Final thermal processing to obtain an amorphous or crystalline coating that is stable over time.

Of the different addition stages that can be achieved by sol-gel processes, depending on processing conditions and the end properties sought, we can cite the following:

- Xerogel: By gelation of the sol and conventional drying of the gel.
- Aerogel: By gelation of the sol and superdrying of the gel. Very porous solids are thus produced with an extremely high volume/mass ratio and are very useful for packaging.
- Dense ceramic: By sintering the dust from a milled xerogel or aerogel.
- Thin compact layer: By deposition of a thin layer of the sol on a substrate and subsequent polymerisation and drying.
- Fibres: By stretching the sol, followed by polymerisation and drying.

It should be mentioned that supercritical drying to obtain aerogels causes the fluid to reach supercritical conditions and a subsequent quasi-isothermal depressurisation is produced, thereby preventing the effects of contraction on crossing the gas-liquid interface. It also prevents the effects of the surface tension produced on the surrounding solid structures by the appearance of liquid, which endows this supercritical process with numerous applications for the manufacture of MEMS and NEMS, many of which are based on the use of active materials like those described in this handbook.

Some of the many advantages of sol-gel processes for thin layer deposition are the wide ranges of attainable thicknesses (from tens of nm to several mm), the excellent adhesion between the substrate and the coating, low operating temperatures and the economical process.

From a research point of view, what is exceptional is the ability to widely vary the end properties by making simple changes to parameters like initial concentration, precursor size, working temperature and sol viscosity.

12.4.2 Deposition with a Specific Pattern

Some recent research has benefitted from the use of thin-film hydrogels. Okano and his collaborators, for example, used poly-N-isopropylacrylamide (pNIPAm) as substrate for cell growth and easily managed to separate the tissues formed by simply changing the temperature from 37 °C to 32 °C.

This thermal stimulus leads to a change in the properties of the polymer substrate, which goes from hydrophobic to hydrophilic, allowing the tissue to be more easily separated (Kikuchi, Okano, 2005).

These possibilities combined with technologies that allow depositing materials with specific patterns can be highly useful as a support for different fluid devices, particularly in the lab-on-a-chip field in applications intended for handling very small quantities of fluid for optimising clinical analysis procedures.

With the aid of different sol-gel processes in combination with photolithography tools and other micro-manufacturing technologies, textured surfaces can be obtained or ones with surface patterns and hydrophilic and hydrophobic zones that can be independently controlled and made reversible using simple thermal stimuli. This can be used as a support for other already used lab-on-a-chip control systems, magnetic stimuli, vibratory piezoelectric impulses, capillarity and others) (Cardoso, 2008).

Some studies have already detailed the use of polymerisation processes induced electrically from hydropolymers to form patterns by the superposition of micro-drops of around 10 μm in diameter deposited on conducting substrates (Buttry, 1992, Baute, 2001, Cram, 2003, Reuber, 2006).

Any research trends channelled towards improving the precision, speed of detection and speed of activation of these materials are decisive if devices are to be produced to replace those based on other families of active materials with a long-standing tradition in industry (mainly shape memory alloys and piezoelectric ceramics, which, after being successfully used since the 60s, constitute mature technologies compared to other more recently discovered or studied families).

12.4.3 Encapsulation of Specific Receptors for Biosensors

Biosensors have undergone enormous changes since their beginnings 40 years ago. Nowadays, biological sensors are applied to environmental studies, toxic component detection, and monitoring illnesses, in all of which the success of the biosensor depends on its speed of response and sensitivity.

Due to their highly specific nature and sensitivity, natural bioreceptors are usually used as sensing components. Some of these are antibodies/antigens, nucleic acids, enzymes and cell structures.

In recent years, special emphasis has been placed on developing biosensors that are based on the encapsulation of bioreceptors at the core of the hydropolymer to assess the behaviour of living organs and tissues from the reactions observed (evolution, transformation or disappearance of the receptor) after being inserted and then extracted from an organ for examination (Pierre, 2004, Weber, 2005). The use of polymer networks as encapsulation material allows antibiotic agents to be used simultaneously and provides the bioreceptors greater protection and stability in aggressive environments.

The use of hydrogels is decisive as they allow the passage of fluid for the reactions needed for a subsequent assessment. Positive results have been demonstrated using PEG or pHEMA species platforms (Hasbullah, 2006, Peppas, 2007), even though there are very many possible combinations of hydrogel and receptors and more thorough studies are required to determine which combinations are optimum for each application.

- ***Hydroactive actuators based on other materials***

  Since they are related to the topics dealt with in the chapter, we will now include other hydroactive actuators based on different operating principles from those examined up to now for hydropolymers or hydrogels.

  The Fig. 12.9 shows an example of a hydroactive actuator [with patent (Chen *et al.*, 2008)]. It essentially depicts an electro-osmotic pump that forces fluid to pass between two chambers through a polymer membrane. The chambers are filled with a hydroactive material, usually a hydrogel capable of absorbing the fluid and considerably increasing its volume, thereby causing the actuator to bend, with the enormous advantage that it is reversible.

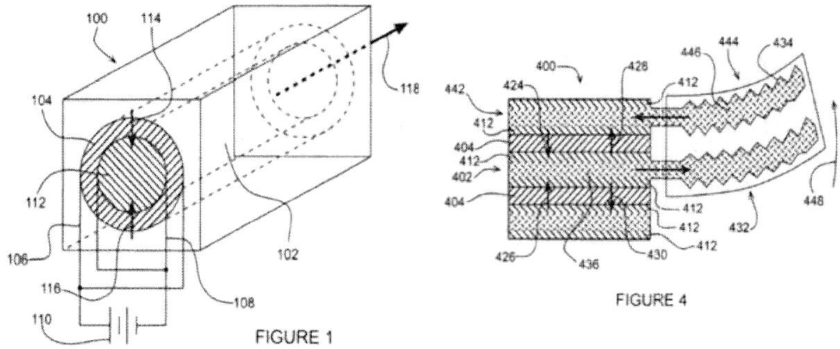

Figure 12.9 Schematic diagram of a hydroactive actuator. Chen *et al.* (2008).

By way of an additional example, we have included the nastic device illustrated in Fig. 12.10 [(Piyasena *et al.*, 2009; Carpi and Smela, 2009) with patent (Shapiro and Smela, 2006)], that has two chambers connected by micro-channels where activation is performed by pumping fluid between the stiff chamber (with a fluid reservoir) and the flexible chamber, by electro-osmotic effect. An alterative is to use an electroactive polymer as a pumping device in the reservoir chamber, which, on receiving an electrical stimulus pumps the fluid into the flexible chamber which becomes noticeably deformed.

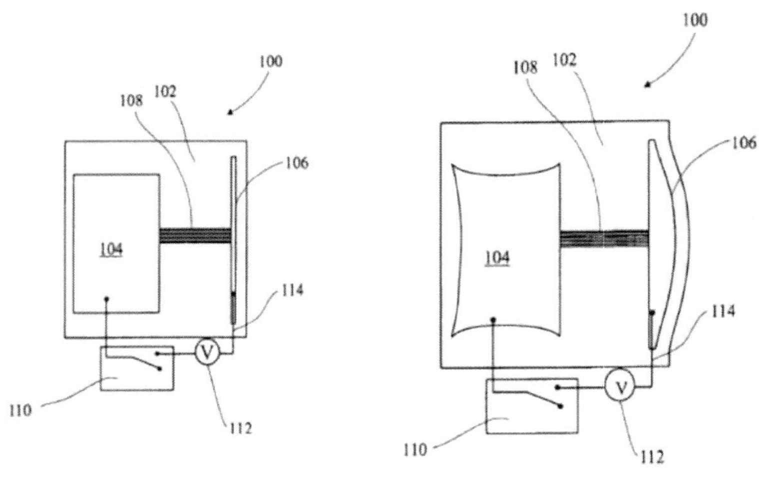

Figure 12.10 Schematic diagram of a hydroactive actuator (Shapiro and Smela, 2006; Piyasena *et al.*, 2009).

These devices are clear examples of the benefits of using different activation principles or different active materials in combination, to produce devices with optimised functionalities without the need for excessive complexity or difficult final sizes.

- o Combined use of synthetic and biological materials

  Recent research has been channelled towards producing hydroactive-related device mechanisms to handle fluids by using polymer substrates combined with living cells that are able to expand and contract in response to electrical stimuli. These solutions combine or synthesise the advantages of electroactive and hydroactive transducers and also offer a promising combination of biological and synthetic materials.

  To be exact, a small pump-device has been developed that can spontaneously produce pulsations. It is only 5 mm in diameter and is made with heart cells to generate its energy. To implement it, a set of these kinds of cells needs to be wrapped around a hollow polymer sphere that will then be filled with liquid. The contractions make the device act as a micropump (Tanaka *et al*,, 2007; Hornyak, 2007).

12.5 Main Conclusions

The chapter has focused on an analysis of hydropolymers or hydroacative polymers as possible medical device components. Generally speaking, these hydropolymers (also known as hydrogels or superabsorbent polymers - SAPs) are three-dimensional network cross-linked polymer materials of natural or synthetic origin that swell on contact with water to form soft, elastic materials that retain a significant undissolved fraction of that water in their structure.

Their geometric changes in the presence of water or humidity make them excellent candidates as sensors and actuators for a whole range of active devices. This is particularly so in the medical industry since their good properties in aqueous environments means that their response is often suited to living organisms.

On the other hand, their sensitivity to environmental stimuli (temperature, pressure, ph, electric current or UV radiation) is especially acute and takes on a multicoupled form. This favours their medical applications, not only as hydromechanical actuators but also as sensors that respond to numerous stimuli to monitor different physiological magnitudes.

Although facets such as slowness of response (compared to other families of active materials) may limit some applications, their remarkable coupling ability to combine a wide range of properties may lead to cause-effect relationships that have not yet been studied. However, an in-depth study of such relationships may well result in the development of active devices.

Numerous present and future applications have been detailed, as well as issues concerning synthesis, processing, characterisation, and the modelling and integration of these materials into medical devices. Reference has also been made to the main trends in research in the hope that other researchers will be motivated to look more closely into the different aspects regarding these complex materials.

Additional information can be found in the following list of references, which includes results from some of the main researchers in this field, as well as in the websites of the different suppliers included in the annexes of the handbook.

References

Albella, J.M. "Preparación y caracterización de recubrimientos y láminas delgadas". Programa de Doctorado en Ciencias Físicas de la Universidad Autónoma de Madrid – Instituto de Ciencia de los Materiales de Madrid (CSIC), Material Docente. Madrid, 2006.

Ali, A.E.H.; Rehiem, H.A.E.; Hegazy, E.S.A.; Ghobashy, M.M. "Characterization and potential application of electro-active acrylamido-2-methyl propane sulfonic acid/acrylic acid copolymer prepared by ionizing radiation". Journal of Macromolecular Science, Part A, 44(1), 91–98, 2007

Allder, M.A.; Guilbeau, E.J.; Brandon, T.A.; *et al.* "A hydrogel pericardial patch". ASAIO Transactions, 36(3), 574, 575, 1990.

Ambrosio, L.; De Santis, R.; Nicolais, L. "Composite hydrogels for implants". Proceedings of the Institution of Mechanical Engineers, Part H: Journal of Engineering in Medicine, 212(2), 1998.

Ambrosio, L.; Nicolais, L.; Sannino, A. "Biodegradable super absorbent polymer hydrogels and method for their preparation". Patent WO/2006/070337.

Berthe, J.; Van Geertruyden, J. "Osmotic instability of hydrogel-filled breast implants". British Journal of Plastic Surgery, 54(5), 465–466, 2001.

Brinker, C.J.; Scherer, G.W. "Sol-Gel Science: The Physics and Chemistry of Sol-Gel Processing". Academic Press, 1990.

Cardoso, V.F.; Rocha, J.G.; Soares, F.O.; *et al.* "Lab-on-a-chip fluid acoustic microagitation: Piezoelectric polymer beta-PVDF used as ultrasonic transducer". International Conference on Biomedical Electronics and Devices Biostec 2008 - Biodevices, 2, 262–267. IEEE Engineering in Medicine and Biology Society. INSTICC Press, 2008.

Carpi, F.; Smela, E. "Biomedical applications of electroactive polymer actuators". Wiley & Sons Ltd., 2009.

Chen, R.L.; Chen, B.C.; Chen, C.L.; Chen, C.H. "High energy density electroosmotic pump and actuator". US Patent 2008210559(A1), Teledyne Licensing LLC., 2008.

Dhariwala, B.; Hunt, E.; Boland, T. "Rapid prototyping of tissue engineering constructs, using photopolymerizables hydrogels and stereolithography". Tissue Engineering, 10, 1316–1322, 2004.

Dulong, V.; Mocanu, G.; Le Cerf, D. "A novel amphiphilic pH-sensitive hydrogel based on pullulan". Colloid and Polymer Science, 285(10), 1085–1091, 2007.

Gerlach, G.; Arndt, K.F. "Hydrogel sensors and actuators". Engineering and Technology (Springer Series on Chemical Sensors and Biosensors) Summary, 2009.

Hannachi, I.E.; Yamato, M.; Okano, T. "Cell sheet technology and cell patterning for biofabrication". Biofabrication, 1, 1–13, 2009.

Harmon, M.E.; Kuckling, D.; Frank, C.W. "Photo-cross-linkable PNIPA Am copolymers. Mechanical Properties of hydrogel layers". Langmuir, 19, 10660–10665, 2003.

Hench, L.L. "Sol-Gel Silica: Properties, Processing and Technology Transfer". William Andrew, 1998.

Heo, J.; Crooks, R.M. "Microfluidic biosensor based on an array of hydrogel-entrapped enzymes". Analytical Chemistry, 21, 68436851, 2005.

Horie, K.; *et al.* "IUPAC Recommendations of terms relating to reactions of polymers and to multifunctional polymeric materials". IUPAC Recommendations 2003. Pure and Applied Chemistry, 74(4), 889–906, 2004.

Hornyak, T. "Microchips with heart". Scientific American Magazine, May, 2007.

Jiménez, A.; Zhang, J.; Matthews, M.A. "Evaluation of CO_2 based cold sterilization of a model hydrogel". Biotechnology and Bioengineering, 101(6), 1344–1352, 2008.

Kampa, G.J. "Treatment and diagnostic catheters with hydrogel electrodes". US Patent 7419486, 2005.

Kanjickal, D.; Lopina, S.; Evancho-Chapman, M.M.; Schmidt, S.; Donovan, S. "Effects of sterilization on poly(ethylene glycol) hydrogels". Journal of biomedical materials research. Part A, 87 (3), 608–617, 2008.

Kim, I.S.; Oh, I.J. "Drug release from the enzyme-degradable and pH-sensitive hydrogel composed of glycidyl methacrylate dextran and poly(acrylic acid)". Archives of *Pharmaceutical* Research, 28(8), 983–987, 2005.

Ku, D.N.; Fan, J.W. "Biomaterial for soft tissue replacements". International Conference on Biomedical Electronics and Devices Biostec 2008 – Biodevices, 1, 23–29. IEEE Engineering in Medicine and Biology Society. INSTICC Press, 2008.

Langer, R.; Vacanti, J.P. "Tissue Engineering". Science, 260, 920–926, 1993.

Liew, S.; Disa, J.; Cordeiro, P.G. "Nipple-areolar reconstruction: A different approach to skin graft fixation and dressing". Annals of Plastic Surgery, 47(6), 608–611, 2001.

Marra, S.P.; Ramesh, K.T.; Douglas, A.S. "Characterization and modeling of compliant active materials". Journal of the Mechanics and Physics of Solids, 51(9), 1723–1743, 2003.

Mironov, V.; Trusk, T.; Kasyanov, V.; *et al.* "Biofabrication: A 21st century manufacturing paradigm". Biofabrication, 1, 1–16, 2009.

O´Grady, M.L.; Kuo, P.L.; Parker, K. "Optimization of electroactive hydrogel actuators". ACS Applied Materials and Interfaces, December 23, 2009.

Peppas, N.A.; Hilt, J.Z. "Intelligent polymeric networks in biomolecular sensing". In "BioMEMS and Biomedical Nanotechnology". Springer US, 2007.

Pierre, A.C. "The sol-gel encapsulation of enzymes". Biocatalysis and Biotransformation, 22(3), 145–170, 2004.

Piyasena, M.E.; Newby, R.; Miller, T.J.; Shapiro, B.; Smela, E. "Nastic actuators: electroosmotically driven microfluidic cells", Sensors and Actuators B, 141, 263–69, 2009.

Sanchez, C.; Molina, M.J. "Los plásticos aplicados en Medicina". Editorial UNED.

Sannino, A.; Demitri, C.; Madaghiele, M. "Biodegradable cellulose-based hydrogels: Design and applications". Materials, 2, 353–373, 2009.

Shamsudeen, R.K.; Fair, S.; Jayakumari, V.G. "Equilibrium swelling, conductivity and electroactive characteristics of polyacrylamide hydrogels". Indian journal of engineering & materials sciences, 13(1), 62–68, 2006.

Shapiro, B.; Smela, E. "Electrically driven microfluidic pumping for actuation". US Patent 7523608, 2009.

Shawky, H.A.; Shayed, E.; Ali, A.E.H.; Mottaleb, M.S.A. "Treatment of polluted water resources using reactive polymeric hydrogel". Journal of Applied Polymer Science, 100(5), 3966–3973, 2006.

Tanaka, Y.; Sato, K.; Shimizu, T.; *et al.* "A micro-spherical heart pump powered by cultured cardiomyocytes". Lab on a Chip, 7, 207–212, 2007.

Trande, P.; Mussetto, A.; Mirante, V.G; De Martinis, E.; Olivetti, G.; Conigliaro, R.L.; De Micheli, E.A. "Efficacy, tolerance and safety of new intragastric air-filled balloon (Heliosphere BAG) for obesity: The experience of 17 cases". Obesity Surgery, 1–4, 2008.

Weber, L.M.; He, J.; Bradley, B.; Haskins, K.; Anseth, S. "PEG-based hydrogels as an *in vitro* encapsulation platform for testing controlled β-cell microenvironments". Acta Biomaterialia, 2(1), 1–8, 2006.

Westbrook, K.K.; Qi, H.J. "Actuator designs using environmental responsive hydrogels". Journal of Intelligent Material Systems and Structures, 19(5), 597–607, 2008.

Chapter 13

Microstructured Active Materials in Biodevices

Andrés Díaz Lantada
Mechanical Engineering Department, E.T.S.I. Industriales, Universidad Politécnica de Madrid, c/ José Gutiérrez Abascal 2, 28006 Madrid, Spain
adiaz@etsii.upm.es

13.1 Introduction

The properties of materials are very closely linked to their chemical composition and internal structure, as we have seen from numerous examples in the handbook. Throughout history, human beings have learnt to use the materials that were available and process them to improve their properties by changing their composition and structure. Therefore, the gradual progress from Antiquity to the Middle Ages in processes like sharpening, hardening or forging led to better tools. However, the most outstanding progress in materials science and engineering was seen throughout the 20th century as a consequence of a better understanding of matter on a micrometric and nanometric level. By way of example, we can point to the spectacular rise of the polymer materials industry in the last 50 years or the notable expansion since the 1980s of superalloys that combine multiple components, apart from the new horizons opened up by the active or multifunctional materials to which this handbook is dedicated.

Handbook of Active Materials for Medical Devices: Advances and Applications
Edited by Andrés Díaz Lantada

www.panstanford.com

The advances in microfabrication technologies of the last four decades has led to new approaches being used for synthesising, shaping and processing materials that make it possible to operate on the their microstructure with greater precision in order to obtain mechanical, electrical, chemical and thermal properties that are ever more outstanding and controlled.

Microstructured materials are usually made up of the superposition of layers of different ceramic, metallic and polymer materials (multilayered materials), that succeed in combining the properties of mechanical, thermal and chemical strength in a particularly effective manner and can even be used to design materials intended for a specific application with "a la carte" properties.

For example, combining a hard core with very hard micrometric surface coatings has many applications in tribology for minimising the wear resulting from contact phenomena. On other occasions, when there is contact between parts, surface coverings are sought that have small friction coefficients or certain self-lubricating properties as a way of minimising wear and optimising the useful life of machine parts.

Another common and increasingly widely used example of microstructured materials is composite materials with a polymer matrix and reinforcement fibre, which have become essential for the aeronautic and automobile industry, among others. They will not be dealt with in this chapter due to the many excellent texts available that deal exclusively with composite materials and also because their main application is to obtain passive structural elements, whereas this handbook is focused on active devices intended for sensors or actuators.

One specific example of microstructured materials is functionally gradient materials or FGMs, where the variation in properties is not as abrupt as with multilayers comprising different materials, since their composition and structure change gradually throughout their volume. This is a result of their being manufactured using complex processes such as laser, physical, chemical or electrolytic deposition, powder metallurgy, plasma spray among others (Schwartz, 2006).

When microstructured materials are designed to act as transducers in a role as sensors or actuators, we can refer to them by the more specific term of "microstructured active materials". The fact that they are made up by bonding materials with different properties makes them able to respond, usually mechanically (by deforming), to different external thermal, electrical, magnetic or mechanical stimuli, which means they can be used for detection or activation requirements.

These microstructured synthetic materials have numerous applications in the field of health sciences. This will be clearly seen in the chapter, as on many occasions the marked mechanical properties of the biological tissue (which is replaced or complemented) is based on a very specifically ordered microstructure and on the combination of different materials that mutually strengthen one another.

Bone tissue, for example, combines compact zones that contribute stiffness and mechanical strength, with other porous or spongy zones that help absorb impact and vibrations. Teeth have an enamel surface coating with an extremely high surface hardness that protects against wear on a dentine core that is remarkably strong. The phenomenon also occurs in soft tissue, as with heart valves and the surrounding tissue which reveals additional deposits of collagen in the areas that are subjected to higher circumferential stress.

These kinds of examples can be appreciated in all types of living organisms, and by careful observation new innovative biomimetic microstructured materials are being developed. Using these materials to fabricate implants will bring better results as they are able to behave in the same way as the materials comprising the original tissue.

It should be pointed out that the considerable advantages of these innovative materials are not only confined to developing passive devices to replace body structures and tissue. Their ability to combine materials that respond in different ways to electrical, thermal, mechanical or magnetic stimuli in a multilayer structure or a structure that gradually varies its properties means that some responses can be given a wider range in order to produce more effective sensors or actuators than those previously analysed.

Their major applications are to be found in the medical industry and in the development of micro-electromechanical systems (MEMS), that include all kinds of micromachines, microactuators, and microsensors whose precision and speed benefits from acting on a microscale (Gad-el-Hak, 2003).

This chapter deals with all these aspects and describes certain limitations that can be resolved by structuring the materials on an even tinier scale, as we will see in the Chapter 14, that can also be used for developing nano-electromechanical systems (NEMS). As an additional introduction to macro-, micro- and nanoscale dimensions, Fig. 13.1 shows a diagram with some examples and standard measurements.

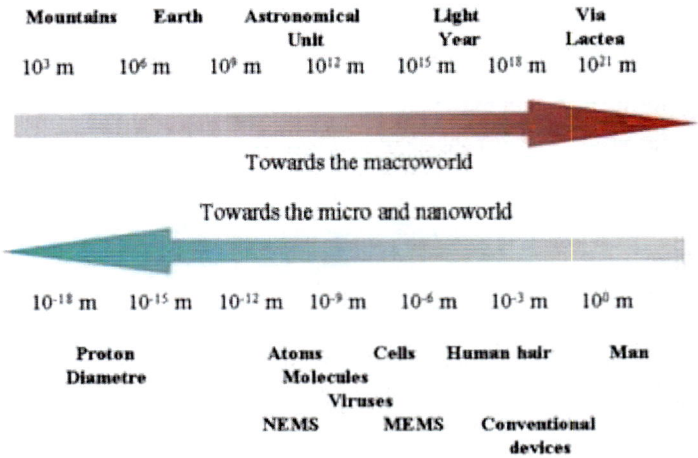

Figure 13.1 The journey to the macroscale and the journey to the micro- and nanoscale.

13.2 Types of Microstructured Active Materials and Their Basic Properties

13.2.1 Metal–Metal Composites

The best known and most widespread multilayer materials in industry are probably bimetals, comprising a welded joint made up of two films of different metals. Choosing metals with different thermal expansion coefficients means that as the temperature rises one of the films increases in length more than the other, causing the bimetal strip to bend.

This response is ideal for developing thermoactive actuators for a wide range of applications, the major ones being thermal switches, bimetallic thermometers and many thermal sensors and actuators for cantilever-based micro-electromechanical microsystems (MEMS) (Puchades and Fuller, 2008; Biodevices, 2010).

Figure 13.2 illustrates a typical example of linear geometry bimetal simulated using the finite-element method with the aid of Siemens PLM Solutions "NX-6" program. The bimetal was subjected to a rise in temperature to produce a mechanical response (bending). These tools are a great aid to designing actuators based on these principles, particularly when the actuator possesses complex geometry, as will be analysed further on.

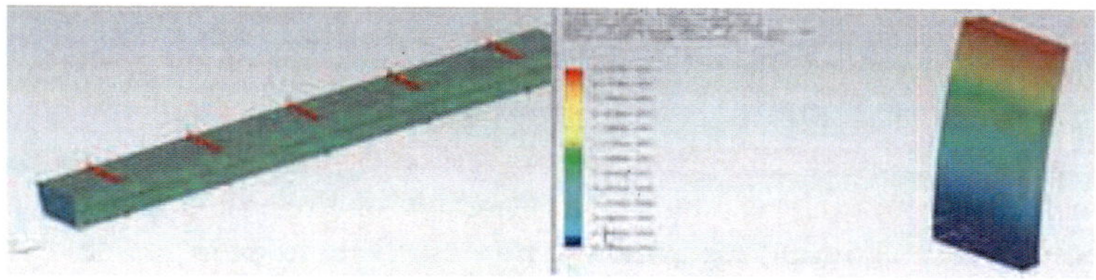

Figure 13.2 Example of a bimetallic actuator. FEM model and the result of displacements.

13.2.2 Ceramic–Ceramic Composites

As multilayer ceramics can now be produced, these piezoelectrics can usually be made more suitable as actuators by increasing the deformations and forces that can be developed and reducing the power supply required for activation. Therefore, the usual way to enhance their response or adapt it to a specific use is by using several layers of a specific piezoelectric material. The same applies to multilayer piezoelectric polymers, although in the case of actuators, ceramics are usually used, as previously stated.

Nonetheless, combining layers of piezoelectric materials also has advantages for the development of actuators. The use of dual layer structures comprising materials with different piezoelectric coefficients causes controllable deformations to appear (bending in the structure) depending on the applied voltage, due to the different deformations induced by the piezoelectric effect. Behaviour is similar to that of a bimetal although in this case coupling is electro-mechanical, whereas with bimetals coupling is thermo-mechanical.

Various actuators have been designed in line with this principle by using different compositions generally based on the PZT-PNN system (Zhu *et al.*, 2000; Bove *et al.*, 2001). These have enabled marked properties to be tested, both in activation mode and in detection mode. For structures made of these materials, in which the final material must exhibit a progressive variation in properties (FGM), powder metallurgy-based manufacturing processes are usually used. For dual-layer structures made of different materials pressure is usually applied first and then sintering.

13.2.3 Polymer–Polymer Composites

Some conductive polymers (polypyrrole or PPy, polyaniline, polythiophine, and others) can be subjected to reversible oxidation/

reduction processes by passing the right voltage between the opposite zones of the material. These processes induce variations in the electrical, optical and mechanical properties of the materials. These transitions from oxidated to reduced state involve changes to the volume of the polymer as a result of the exchange of ions between the conductive polymer film and the adjacent electrolyte (either in the form of a solution or as an adhered dry film), which has led to the development of multilayer electroactive actuators (Díaz *et al.*, 1988).

These actuators usually have a layer of conductive polymer (CP) that changes volume and a layer of flexible polymer that does not change volume (NVC), both joined together, thereby giving rise to structures that are capable of bending one way or another depending on the direction of the reaction. Triple layer actuators have also been described, with a conventional polymer middle layer and external layers of conductive polymer to achieve greater activation forces (Sansiñena and Olazábal, 2004; Bar-Cohen, 2004).

When dealing with dual-layer polymer microactuators and sensors it is especially important to bear in mind the thermomechanical effects of the system. The influence of more complex phenomena must also be considered, such as non-homogeneous heating, surface tension effects or the consequences of humidity on the final response. The geometry plays a key role when these phenomena are being analysed as other research has shown (Begley, 2005).

13.2.4 Metal–Ceramic Composites

The use of dual-layer metal-piezoelectric ceramic or semi-metal–piezoelectric ceramic materials can be used to make similar actuators to those mentioned above when dealing with ceramic–ceramic composites. Metallic film offers a much faster response due to its being more flexible while at the same time helping to optimise the transfer of forces (Ngernchucklin and Safari, 2009).

The bond between layers of these materials is usually performed by "diffusion bonding", a process that has some things in common with both liquid-state and solid-state welding. In this process, the bond is achieved by joining two flat surfaces at a high temperature (at around 50% to 90% of fusion temperature) and applying pressure for a few minutes or even hours. This leads to an interdiffusion of atoms across the interface which gives rise to the formation of bonds between the two materials on an atomic level. This type of bonding through "diffusion bonding" has the following advantages (Shirzadi *et al.*, 2001, 2004):

- It produces high quality bonds, without discontinuities at the interface or the presence of pores or defects that lower the mechanical strength of the bond.
- It enables materials of a different nature to be bonded (metal–ceramic, metal semi-metal, ceramic–ceramic and others).
- It enables parts with complex geometries and good dimensional tolerance to be obtained.

However, the initial investment in equipment is high and the process must be done in very controlled conditions using surfaces that have been meticulously prepared in advance, all of which imposes limits to their use in large-scale mass production.

13.2.5 Polymer–Metal and Polymer–Ceramic Composites

Using polymer–metal dual-layer actuators leads to more remarkable deformations than by using bimetals (due to the greater difference in the thermal expansion coefficients between polymers and metals), even though the range of applications is smaller due to the lower temperature glass transitions and fusions of polymers.

This aspect also influences the bonding method that can be used, since high temperature welding is discarded as it would lead to fusion of the polymer, for which reason adhesive bonds are preferable. Choosing the adhesive can be done with the aid of the online utilities of the various manufacturers (Henkel - Loctite®), bearing in mind that if the final application is medical there will be a restricted number of feasible adhesives.

Since, as a general rule, adhesive bonds are not as strong as fusion welding, soft welding or strong welding bonds, the design of this kind of bond must be given special thought and the following general recommendations followed:

- The contact area of the bonding surface must be as large as possible.
- The bonds must be designed to be worked with shears, avoiding the appearance of any load stress at the ends that may cause the adhesive to peel or crack.
- The surfaces to be bonded must not have any major fissures or roughness that will lead to properties lacking in homogeneity after curing.

As an aid to designing actuators with special thermal properties, it is important to mention the combined use of structures formed by shape-memory polymers (SMPs) with shape-memory alloy (SMA) filaments embedded in their interior, together with other heating elements that activate the alloy as well as the polymer. With this type of actuator the polymer behaves as a structural element and the shape-memory alloy is responsible for activation, while heating the polymer above its T_g enables the structure to bend without any loss of integrity (Manzo and Garcia, 2008).On the other hand, the use of metal and ceramic particles as additives when shaping polymer materials can change the conductivity of the polymers (usually from values of 10^{-8} S/cm to 10^{2} S/cm) and lead to polymer–metal and polymer–ceramic composites that have numerous commercial, aerospace, military and medical applications.

By using nanocharges that have a higher surface/volume ratio than microcharges more notable results can be achieved since the percolation threshold is reduced in a ratio of 1% to 2 % by volume, as described in Chapter 14.

These combinations have also led to electrically conductive shape-memory polymers and the appearance of new applications for these materials based on the thermo-electromechanical coupling of their properties. Thus, geometrical changes to the material can be activated simply by applying a voltage between its ends without any need for internal heating elements that inevitably mean that the end product will be larger (as explained in Chapter 5).

13.3 Medical Applications of Microstructured Materials

This section sets out the main medical applications proposed for these microstructured materials. In principle, these proposals are related to the development of passive structures with optimised properties (mechanical strength, resistance to corrosion and wear etc.), but currently these materials are coming to the fore for various applications that use these materials as active components.

Very strong hard core implants

Various microstructured materials and FGMs (functional gradient materials) are finding a use in biometric implant development. They behave more like the body's bone structures and reduce the problems arising from classic metal implants.

Solid implants made of titanium, nickel-titanium and some super alloys usually show a very high stiffness that does not correspond either to the original bone or the bone tissue into which they are integrated. With the passage of time different problems arise as this stiffness causes some of the body areas adjacent to the implant to be subjected to larger forces while other forces are hardly called upon. Therefore, stress-shielding phenomena appear together with osteoporosis (according to Wolff's law), that cause the tissue supporting the prosthesis to fail.

Microstructured materials and FGMs are among the design tendencies that are giving the best results in the fight against these problems. They enable implants to be produced that have variable porosity so as to obtain more flexible cores, marked strength and a high surface hardness. These implants behave more like real bone tissue (with a spongy interior and a compact exterior). Moreover, the use of microlayers as surface coating (usually hydroxyapatite) provides a satisfactory compatibility and facilitates the osseointegration of the implant (Ojeda, 2009).

Thus, various metal dental implants (like those initially developed by the Tokyo Medical and Dental University) are made of microstructured materials with pure titanium cores whose ceramic content gradually increases towards the outside, with around 10% ceramic content (apatite and ZrO_2) on the outer surface. They are usually produced by sintering (high frequency induction heating to reach temperatures of around 1100 to 1400°C) from controlled powder mixtures.

Bimetal microactuators: Surgical tweezers

By taking advantage of the progress in microfabrication over the last decades, bimetal microactuators can be produced with "tweezer" geometries to be coupled to active catheter ends to assist minimally invasive surgical operations.

By properly designing the geometry and carefully choosing the materials, the required activations can be achieved (usually displacements of 0.5 to 2 mm of the actuator ends) without any need to apply high temperatures. Temperature differences of 2 to 3°C are sufficient, which is particularly important when designing intracorporeal microactuators.

Piezoelectric microactuators: Response enhancement through multilayers As previously stated, using piezoelectric materials stacked in layers that are connected in parallel helps enhance the response by maximising the forces that can be developed as well as the displacements that can be attained. In the first approximation, the displacement is proportional to the load that the piezoelectric actuator can store and this stored load increases with the number of layers. Therefore, most piezoelectric actuator suppliers offer "stacks" with different numbers of layers for different applications.

As, in principle, the capacity of the actuator *C* can be approximated according to the expression shown below, the capacity increases with the square of the number of layers *n*. This is why there is such an interest in researching into the manufacture and processing of piezoelectric materials (both ceramic and polymer) with thicknesses *e* that are ever smaller for a determined area *A* (Hafez, 2006). For further information concerning the fundamentals of operation, conditioning and control of piezoelectrics, we recommend looking back to Chapters 7 and 9.

$$C \approx n\ \varepsilon_{33}\ \frac{A}{e}$$

Cantilever sensors

The so-called "microcantilever-based sensors" have led to simple solutions to various physical, chemical and biological problems over the last decade that are associated with the monitoring of multiple properties and effects, in the liquid as well as in the gas domain (for sensing the presence of gas, measuring viscosity, detecting cell growth and others). They usually comprise a microcantilever (monolayer or dual layer in most cases) that bends according to external stimuli which in turn leads to changes in the surface tension of the sensor. This bending is used with some kind of optical deflection reading to enhance precision and facilitate measurement (Ansari and Cho, 2010).

The structure is often polymeric but with a surface metal deposit (silver, copper, gold or a highly reflective substance) that assists the optical measuring system. Some additional thoughts on the design of these kinds of cantilever sensors are included further on.

13.4 Design Aspects: Combining Theoretical Models and CAD-CAE Tools

13.4.1 Characterisation to Obtain Information

Most microstructured material suppliers have theoretical models, occasionally interactively available online, apart from characterisation sheets that provide an approximation of the behaviour and operational ranges of the sensors and actuators they market.

Whatever the case, it is a good practice to perform one's own additional characterisation tests to validate the supplier's information or analyse how those sensors or actuators behave in less than ideal operating conditions once they have been integrated into a specific device. Figures 13.3 and 13.4 show an example of how to characterise a bimetallic cantilever with the aid of a comparator and a thermocouple to control temperature, as well as the differences in the theoretical response and the information obtained from tests.

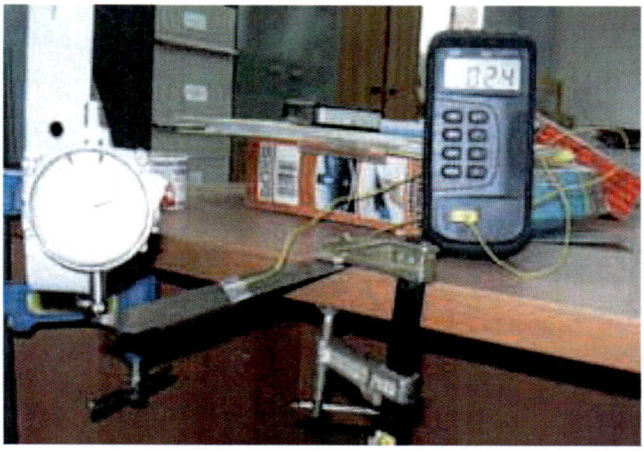

Figure 13.3 Preparing a bimetal test bench. Clamping tools and thermocouple for measuring temperature and a comparator for measuring the displacements of the end.

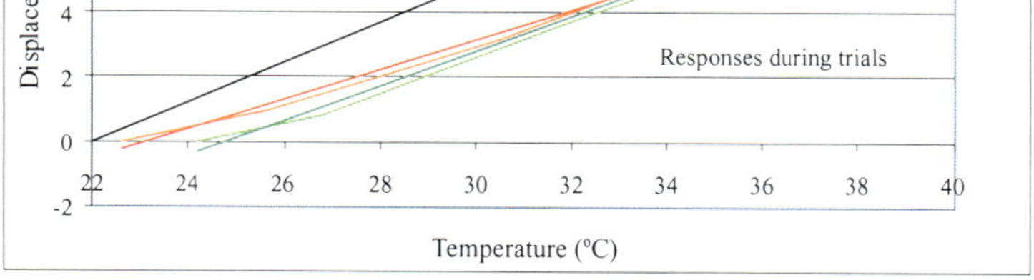

Figure 13.4 Characterisation test results of the bimetallic actuator (unrestricted).

The use of infrared thermography tools to control the process and homogeneous heating of the whole bimetallic surface is also of use. It has already been demonstrated to be a valuable aid for the characterisation of other active materials that show a response to thermal stimuli.

13.4.2 Theoretical Models of Some Microstructured Materials

Different researchers have developed behaviour models of bimetallic materials that can aid the design of devices based on these types of microstructured materials by taking account of the boundary conditions, the thermal loads applied and the forces to be overcome by the actuator. Thus, Timoshenko's general theory of multilayer actuators for the design of thermostats comes into play (Timoshenko, 1925) and other more recent works concerning the development of thermoactive microcantilevers (Chu *et al.*, 1993; Matovic, 2006; Ansari and Cho, 2010).

Below we include a brief theoretical approximation using general equations from the cited models, as well as some equations proposed by the suppliers of these kinds of actuators (Hood & Co. – Arcelor Group, Kanthal AB and others). By taking these analytical equations for dual-layer materials it is simple to implement programs that can compute the results for other multilayer active materials and even for FGMs. However, as the complexity of the system increases, the analytical models gradually become devoid of usefulness. In this situation, it may be of interest to turn to numerical resolution methods (as detailed in the following section).

Taking a differential component of a bimetallic actuator subjected to a temperature ($\Delta T = T - T_0$), where α_1 and α_2 are the coefficients of thermal expansion of the two materials, E_1 and E_2 being the modules of elasticity, I_1 and I_2 the moments of inertia of the section of each film, t_1 and t_2 (with $h = t_1 + t_2$) being the thicknesses of each film and b_1 and b_2 the width of each film, a bending of the film will be produced that will show a curvature of ρ as a function of the following ratios. Let us suppose that $\alpha_2 > \alpha_1$, and that a moment M_1 and a force P_1 (traction) will act on the section of metal 1 (concave) and a moment M_2 and a force P_2 (compression) will act on the section of metal 2 (convex).

For there to be mechanical and thermal equilibrium, the following expressions must be met, which, by reordering the terms will let the radius of curvature of the bimetallic film be found:

$P_1 = P_2 = P \qquad P\,h/2 = M_1 + M_2 \qquad M_1 = E_1\ I_1/\rho$

$M_2 = E_2\ I_2/\rho$

$P\cdot (t_1 + t_2)/2 = E_1\cdot I_1/\rho + E_2\cdot I_2/\rho$

$\alpha_1 \cdot\Delta T + P_1/(E_1\ t_1\ b_1) + t_1/(2\ \rho) = \alpha_2\ \Delta T - P_1/(E_1\ t_1\ b_1) - t_2/(2\ \rho)$

Taking the expression for the radius of curvature, the deflection at the end can be simply found according to the geometry of the deformation or by direct integration (Timoshenko, 1925).

Apart form the deflection d resulting from the changes in temperature (important in detection tasks), the force generated by a bimetallic cantilever (micro)actuator at its end is also of interest (especially for activation tasks). Although the force is usually generated throughout the entire length L of the cantilever, we can consider the specific case of actuation at the end, which provides an equivalent force F_{eq}, according to cantilever theory:

$F_{eq} = 3\ E\ I\cdot d/L^3$

We also believe it is of interest to proceed to a brief explanation of two other simple models for calculating bimetallic actuators (under torque and bending) that help in the task of selecting specific components from a manufacturer, in this instance Kanthal AB (Kanthal Bimetal Handbook, 2008). The results are similar to using the models described above, although they include concepts such as specific deflection associated with specific types of bimetals and dual-layer materials, which simplify calculating an approximation to these problems. This approach is more like that laid down in standard DIN 1715 regarding bimetallic actuators.

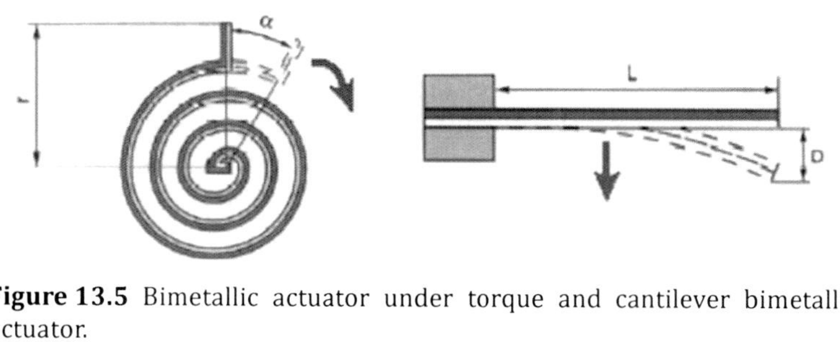

Figure 13.5 Bimetallic actuator under torque and cantilever bimetallic actuator.

(A) ***Bimetallic spring under torque***

Figure 13.5 represents a bimetallic spring under torque that is proposed as an alternative for activation for a range of active devices.

where

α is the rotation of the bimetallic strip (°);

a, specific deflection for the bimetal under torque (K^{-1});

b, bimetal width (mm);

t, bimetal thickness (mm);

L, length (mm);

T_2, maximum temperature of cycle (K);

T_1, minimum temperature of cycle (K);

ΔT, $T_2 - T_1$ (K);

E, Modulus of elasticity (MPa);

P, activation force (N); and

r, radius (mm).

According to these parameters the "unrestricted thermal rotation" of a bimetallic spring under torque is given by the following expression:

$$\alpha = \frac{360 \cdot a \cdot L}{\pi \cdot t} \Delta T$$

(B) *Bimetallic cantilever*

Figure 13.5 depicts also a bimetallic film proposed as an alternative for the activation of a wide range of devices. It may be necessary to use additional rotational linear movement transformation mechanisms (connecting rod-crank or similar type), for use in some applications.

where

D is the deflection (mm), and

a, the specific deflection for bimetallic cantilever (K^{-1}).

The other parameters are represented by the same symbols and units as in the previous case. According to the parameters, the "unconstrained thermal deflection" of a cantilever bimetallic film is governed by the following expression:

$$D = \frac{a \cdot L^2}{t} \Delta T$$

In the event of their being constrained, most manufacturers (Hood & Co. – Arcelor Group, Kanthal AB and others) provide characterisation curves that include the attainable deformations according to the force that the bimetal must overcome, as the theoretical models in these cases become complicated to a point that they are hardly functional. Once again, it is not out of place to remember the benefits to be had from conducting one's own characterisation tests for the active materials that are component parts of the device, as well as for the final application, since quite often these materials' linear range of behaviour is less than 10°C of variation in temperature.

13.4.3 Design Optimization Using CAD-CAE Tools

The typical linear geometries for sensors and cantilever actuators or the spiral geometries also supplied by many manufacturers do not allow an optimised response when solving a diagnostic, surgical or therapeutic problem. In order to address different specific situations, it is highly advisable to use customised geometries.

In these cases, by using an analytical approach, preliminary design estimates can be made that provide guidance on the most suitable combinations (metal–metal, metal–polymer) and on the approximate thicknesses (order of magnitude).

However, for more effective comparisons and for validating the final geometry and the materials selected, it is important to make use of CAD-CAE (computer-aided design and calculation) tools. The thermomechanical calculation modules integrated into many of these software packages allow analysing the rises in temperature required for a particular deformation, the stresses appearing in the structure during activation or the heating power required. The benefits of these kinds of tools are obviously more clearly appreciated when the geometries involved are too complex for an analytical approach to be effectively used.

Moreover, transitory state simulations allow analysing the response speed of this kind of actuator, as can be seen in Figs. 13.6 and 13.7, as well as making comparisons between the different possible combinations of geometries and materials for the dual-layer (or multilayer) actuator and choosing the most appropriate heating system.

Depicted in Fig. 13.6 is the design and finite-element model of a claw-shaped dual-layer microstructure designed for minimally invasive surgical operations. It also includes the solution for displacement obtained when activation is triggered through thermal effect.

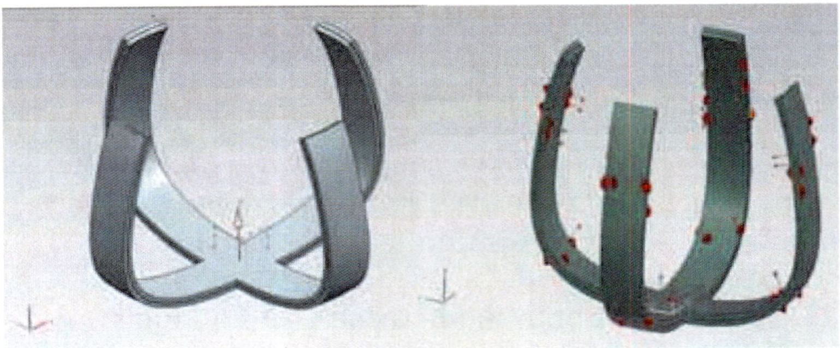

Figure 13.6 FEM design and model of a claw-type dual-layer microstructure.

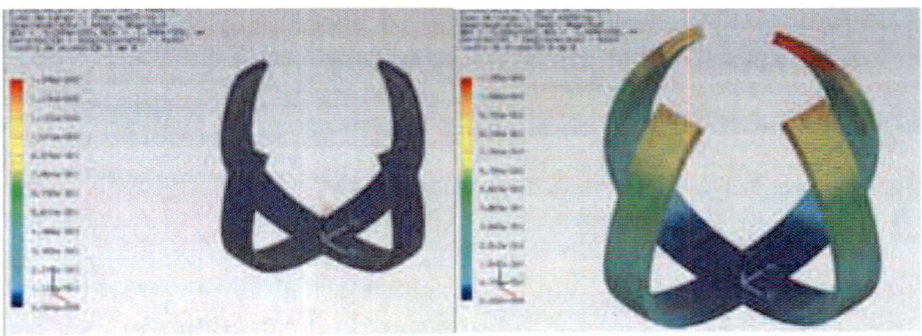

Figure 13.7 Solution for displacements before and after triggering activation through thermal effect.

Figures 13.8 and 13.9 show another possible example where the pincer comprises three passive sections (that do not change their geometry), joined to one another by two bimetallic or thermoactive prismatic joints to which they are welded and which take charge of the activation through a more localised heating.

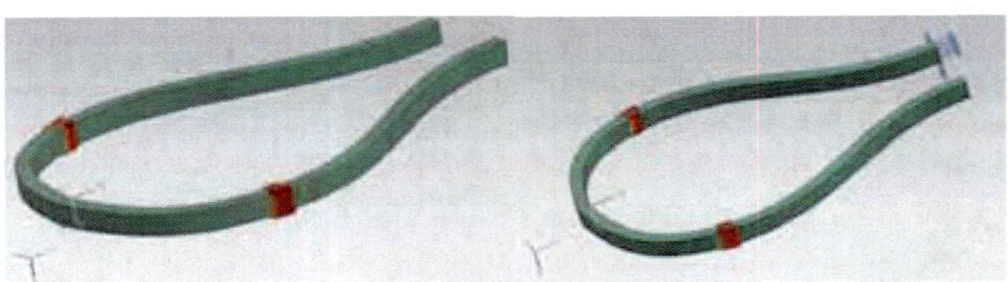

Figure 13.8 FEM of a pincer-type microstructure with two active prism-shaped elements with a trapezoidal base (Meshing, load conditions and boundary conditions).

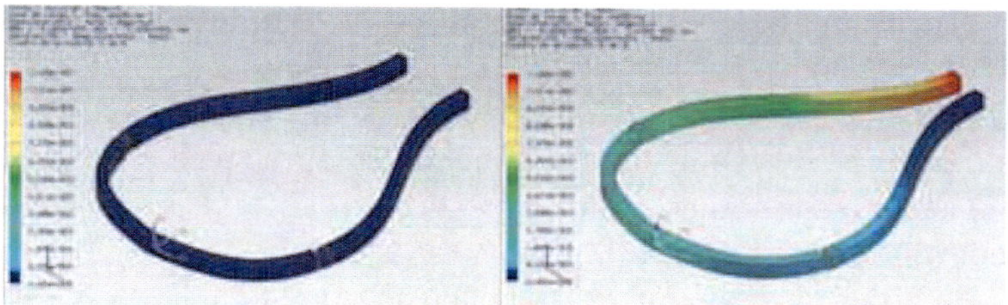

Figure 13.9 Solution for displacement before, during and after triggering thermal activation.

As an additional possibility we should again mention that these computer-aided design tools can be combined with manufacturing or rapid prototyping technologies so that physical parts can be directly produced from the CAD geometry of the parts.

They usually use layer manufacturing or high speed machining processes that have marked advantages especially when the geometries are complex and are difficult to make using a lathe or more conventional milling or shaving tools. Therefore, when the geometry has been designed the two layers of the actuator can be separately made and then welded to obtain the required device.

Another alternative option to dual-layer structures consists in using layer-by-layer sintering processes (e.g., selective laser sintering) using a tank containing powders with radially varying properties, thereby enabling functional gradient structures to be obtained that will also provide thermomechanical responses like those already described.

In these cases, using CAE programs to evaluate device activation becomes complicated, although the functional gradient material (with varying properties throughout its thickness) can always be divided into superposed layers with intermediate properties.

13.4.4 Designing Biostructured Biomimetic Surfaces

As an aid to obtaining substrates for tissue engineering and for developing implantable active devices that have optimised contact with the organs and tissue of the receptor organism, surfaces with fractal geometry can be designed to simulate the geometrical irregularities to be found on biological surfaces. These kinds of surfaces have already proven to be of use in other geographic engineering-linked applications, as they help simulate the textures to be found in woods, rivers and mountains for geographic simulators and information systems (GIS) (Falconer, 2003).

Their application to Bio-GIS or GIS applied to living organisms can be beneficial particularly in combination with CAD design and rapid manufacturing tools with which tissue engineering scaffolds can be directly obtained that can be directly produced or textured implants (among other examples). A foretaste of this is shown in the following brief examples.

In order to obtain micro- and nanostructured flat surfaces with a controllable texture that can be adapted to the receptor organ or tissue, we suggest using Brownian fractional fractal surfaces with a generic equation like that shown below (height z depending on the position given by the components x and y of the horizontal plane):

$$z(x,y) = z_0 + \sum_{k=1}^{\infty} C_k \cdot \lambda^{-\alpha k} \cdot \sin(\lambda^k [x \cdot \cos(B_k) + y \cdot \sin(B_k) + A_k])$$

In order to obtain micro- and nanostructured surfaces that will adapt to a micrometric pre-pattern, equations like the following can be used:

$$z(x,y) = z_0 + 10 \cdot \left|\sin(\pi x/10) \cdot \sin(\pi y/10)\right|$$

$$+ \sum_{k=1}^{\infty} C_k \cdot \lambda^{-\alpha k} \cdot \sin(\lambda^k [x \cdot \cos(B_k) + y \cdot \sin(B_k) + A_k]) / 100$$

where C_k are functions that are randomly independent of each other, with mean 0 and variance 1; A_k and B_k are functions that are randomly independent of each other with uniform distribution in the interval $[0,2\pi]$; where λ and α are constants to control the roughness and which meet the requirements: $\lambda > 1$ and $0 < \alpha < 1$. The values 10 and 100 as numerators and denominators in this example adjust the dimensions of the initial micrometric wave and the superposed nanometric texture, simulating a lotus leaf-based superhydrophobic surface (see Fig. 13.10).

This biomimetic approximation to the design of surfaces for implants and other medical devices can provide a better implant-organism interaction, make complex procedures such as osseointegration easier, optimise the geometry of surface electrodes for active devices and enhance the various tribological phenomena related to friction, lubrication, corrosion and wear of the devices involved.

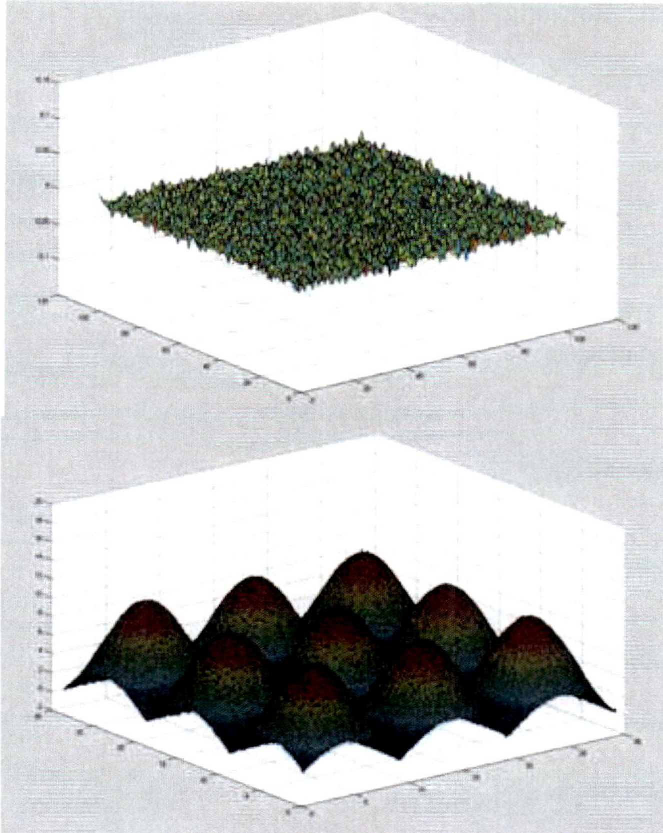

Figure 13.10 Fractal geometry-based biostructured biomimetic surfaces. Top image: Proposal for a substrate for tissue engineering and cell growth. Bottom image: Lotus leaf-based superhydrophobic surface biomimetic model.

13.5 Manufacturing Technologies

This section describes some of the manufacturing and processing technologies most commonly used for preparing microstructured materials, and detailing their possible applications. These range from traditional bonding techniques like welding to modern thin layer deposition technologies using gas deposition processes (physical or chemical) and other solution deposition processes.

13.5.1 Bonding Processes

As described when dealing with the main types of microstructured and functional gradient materials, the main bonding processes between macroscopic layers are welding and the use of adhesives and diffusion bonding technologies depending on the kind of material to be bonded or the characteristics required of the bonding.

Sintering is also a conventional process that takes materials in powder form to achieve gradual variations in composition throughout the structure to produce materials that are especially complex on a microscopic level. The emergence of rapid manufacturing technologies (selective laser sintering or SLS) in the last decade of the 20th century, capable of "layer-by-layer" sintering following a pre-set pattern to automatically achieve complex three-dimensional structures from the part geometry stored in a CAD file has made sintering more popular as a bonding process.

Listed below are several deposition processes where different film or powder material is not the starting point, but which let layers be shaped by the chemical or physical superposition of deposits on a substrate, as well as letting the substrate be structured by different attacks.

13.5.2 Chemical Vapour Deposition (CVD) Technology

A standard chemical vapour deposition process brings about deposition through the deposition on a substrate of a composite generated from a gaseous reaction. Other volatile by-products are usually produced in this reaction and are removed from the reaction chamber. On other occasions the chemical reaction of the gases introduced into the chamber with the substrate material is encouraged so that the product of reaction can be then condensed on that surface (Smith, 1995; Albella, 2003, 2006).

By using these processes, thin layer deposits of micrometric thicknesses (and even nanometric) can be obtained that possess a range of microcrystalline, polycrystalline, amorphous and epitaxial structures. A range of materials are usually deposited in this way, such as silicon, fibres, nanofibres and carbon nanotubes, silicon dioxide, tungsten carbide and various oxides and nitrates with a high surface hardness. However, the consistency and adherence of the thin layer depends to a large extent on the compatibility of the substrate and the surface deposit.

To encourage this compatibility, multilayer structures are often used in which the transition from substrate to the required final coating includes several intermediate layers for a better transition with fewer residual stresses that can cause the appearance of cracks in many thin coatings (Bunshah, 1994; Glocker, 2002).

Operating pressures for standard CVD equipment range from atmospheric (APCVD) to high vacuum (UHVCVD) and on occasions aerosols and plasmas are used to favour the chemical reaction or focus it on the substrate zone for a more effective process. All this increases the complexity of the systems whose installation and maintenance costs are usually high.

Although the CVD and PVD systems mentioned below are expensive, there are different suppliers who offer the chance to subcontract their services for depositing different materials on to metallic, ceramic or polymer substrates. This can be very convenient in research projects on a new implant or special material for medical applications, provided it is required to compare the mechanical, chemical and biological behaviour of possible surface coatings before choosing the most suitable substrate-deposit combination for the end application.

A good web page for locating different services and information on technological supply and demand in the surface coating sector is "The Society of Vacuum Coaters" (www.svc.org) web site. There is also detailed information on teaching resources, seminars, and specific conferences and congresses where specialised information on these tools can be found. It has free resources on vacuum generation techniques, surface and thin film characterisation and matters related to the preparation of substrate, deposition using different technologies and the major surface coating and multilayer structure applications.

13.5.3 Physical Vapour Deposition (PVD) Technologies

In physical vapour deposition processes, the vapour to be deposited and condensed on the substrate to be coated is not the result of a chemical reaction, but is generated as a result of the different physical processes conducted on a solid sample of material to be deposited, without involving the formation of new species. Standard processes that might be mentioned are vapour deposition by evaporation, vapour deposition by electron bombardment, deposition by sputtering the vapour from plasma discharge, the deposition of vapour from a pulsed arc or the vapour deposition produced by laser ablation (Smith, 1995; Albella, 2006). Materials such as metal alloys, pure elements and composites like tungsten carbide, chrome nitrate or titanium nitrate are usually deposited by these PVD processes (Bunshah, 1994; Glocker and Shah, 2002).

In general, PVD processes lead to deposits of higher purity since they start out from solid samples as a source of the material to be deposited and because there is no contamination from other reacting species as is often the case in CVD techniques. Deposits can also usually be done at a lower temperature using PVD rather than CVD, which is important for polymer or biological substrates.

However, effects resulting from the directionality of PVD processes usually result in somewhat less homogeneous depositions than by using CVD processes.

The different processes and most suitable materials have been dealt with in a high level of detail in the references mentioned and fall outside the scope of this handbook. Using them depends on the pressures and temperatures admitted by the substrate during processing, as well as the end quality and coating thickness required, among others. However, being able to consult expert suppliers that can be subcontracted to do the coating of a specific device is always very convenient for research teams that require a coating to enhance properties but who do not have access to the facilities and equipment necessary.

Most materials deposited using PVD or CVD are oriented towards obtaining very hard wear-resistant surfaces, on strong substrates that show good performance in the face of vibration and impact. It is also often sought to minimise the friction coefficient to obtain machine parts with a longer useful life. However, these technologies can also be applied to produce active materials with optimised detection or activation capabilities.

For example, a surface deposit may contribute certain conductive properties to a shape-memory polymer substrate and achieve a thermo-electromechanical coupling to enable the device to be activated by applying a voltage across the coating ends, which is heated by Joule effect until the surrounding polymer is activated.

Small thickness and small size actuators for minimally invasive surgery can also be obtained by using substrate and coating materials with widely varying thermal expansion coefficients.

13.5.4 Chemical Attack Technologies Combined with Photolithography

Photolithography has been used for several decades in the electronics industry for transferring the micrometrically detailed pattern of a mask to a film with the aid of a photosensitive resin and a high intensity ultraviolet light. The base material or substrate is coated with a thin metallic layer usually deposited by CVD or PVD technologies. The substrate is then coated with a layer of photosensitive resin and is then exposed to UV light through a mask, which cures the resin with the required pattern. The next step consists in using a developer to eliminate the uncured resin in the zone, thereby leaving zones with exposed metal and zones where the metal is protected by the resin. A selective chemical attack can be therefore carried out with acid to remove the metal in the exposed zone. Finally, the layer of resin hardened with other agents is removed leaving the initial substrate with a metal deposit with a specific pattern and with details that reach an accuracy of around 5 to 15 μm (depending on the photoresin used and the precision of the mask).

The masks for selective exposition are usually glass plates or some other transparent material on which the image that needs to be transferred is drawn with chrome or opaque metals. However, a direct method has been developed by the University of South Florida called "Smart Filter", which allows photolithography without a mask. Instead of the pattern being printed on a glass mask, it is projected directly from a computer screen using a controllable selective filter. The system has been marketed since 2001 under the name of "SF-100" from "Intelligent Micro Patterning", a spin-off created for that purpose.

One marked application of microstructured active material development is the possibility of obtaining specific electrodes or ones with complex surface patterns so they can be more easily integrated into integrated circuit boards. A film of electroactive material can be used, for example, on which the electrode metal is deposited by CVD or PVD. Photolithography is then used to make the electrode with the required pattern. The now metallised active material film is coated with a polyimide photosensitive resin layer using a centrifuge or spinner. It is exposed to high intensity UV light through a mask which transfers the pattern from the mask to the photosensitive resin and activates the photopolymerisation or curing reaction. A developer is then used to eliminate the resin from the uncured zone, thus leaving zones with exposed metal and zones with metal protected by the resin. A selective acid attack can be carried out to eliminate the metal from the exposed zone, but the attack times and acid concentration need to be carefully adjusted to prevent any irreversible damage to the polymer base layer.

Another less risky option for the integrity of the substrate is to deposit the photosensitive layer on the substrate itself and structure it using photolithography. Electrolyte deposition or CVD and PVD technologies can then be used to coat the space left by the uncured resin that was eliminated after developing. Finally, the structure of the photosensitive material that had been protected by the mask can be removed using the right solvents.

13.5.5 Deposition Technologies in Solution

Some of these technologies were already been described in Chapter 12, when explaining hydrogel processing to obtain multilayer actuators based on these materials. A brief reminder is included here that can be expanded by consulting some of the references enumerated at the end of the chapter (Albella, 2006; Díaz Lantada, 2005–2006).

Sol-gel

These sol-gel processes are characterised by their transition from a sol phase to a gel phase, usually by various hydrolysis reactions, and are used to produce vitreous and ceramic materials. The sol is made up of solid particles (usually around 0.1 to 1 μmin diameter) dispersed in a liquid, while the gel comprises a solid network of macromolecules immersed in a solvent (Brinker and Scherer, 1990; Hench, 1998; Albella, 2006). One of the advantages of sol-gel processes for depositing thin layers is the wide range of attainable thicknesses (from tens of nm to several mm), the excellent adhesion between substrate and coating, low operating temperatures and the economical process. From a research point of view the outstanding feature is that the end properties can be widely varied by making simple parameter changes such as the initial concentration, precursor size and the working temperature and sol viscosity.

Spin coating

This is used to deposit dissolved polymer film (using solvents like chloroform or trichloroethylene) or even liquid state monomer layers in order to then activate the polymerisation reaction using heat or UV light. It can also be used to complement deposition in the sol phase of sol-gel processes as different substrates can be used. If the process is repeatedly performed homogeneous multilayers of different materials can be obtained.

The process consists in supplying a liquid resin or dissolved polymer drop-by-drop on to the substrate that will be centrifuged.

The centrifuge or spinner is then switched on and the material spreads over the substrate to form the film and is then left to dry. It is sometimes subjected to heating at different temperatures to evaporate the volatile elements and cure the film (soft bake and hard bake processes).

The greater the viscosity of the liquid or resin supplied to the spinner, the greater the thicknesses attained. High rotation speeds lead to thinner layers. The process can be used to obtain varied samples with very different properties in very short times, which for research is a major added value.

Dip coating

The process consists in immersing a film vertically into a tank containing the polymer to be deposited in solution form, as liquid state monomers or in sol phase with dispersed particles. The film is then extracted at constant speed to achieve constant thickness (Newtonian fluid) and is left to dry.

At the end, thermal processing can be applied to finally cure the polymer. Greater viscosities and higher extraction speeds (due to the short time the fluid has to become arranged and compact) give rise to thicker layers.

It is used to deposit dissolved polymer film or liquid state monomer layers to then activate the polymerisation reaction through heat or UV light, as is the case with spin-coating. The immersion or dip-coating process can also be used for sol-phase deposition in a sol-gel process and various metal, ceramic or polymer substrates can be used.

Electrolytic/electrochemical deposition

The basic principle of electrolytic or electrochemical deposition processes for obtaining coatings consists in converting the metal of the anode into metallic ions that are distributed in the solution. These ions are deposited on the cathode (device, part or substrate to be coated) forming a metal layer on its surface. The different coating properties as well as the most suitable fields of application depend on the type of crystalline structure of the metal deposited.

The electrolytic coating of the parts is produced almost entirely through immersion in a bath. For this purpose the parts are immersed in the tanks of electrolyte, current is applied as a cathode and they are then coated and dried. When the parts are removed from the bath some of the electrolyte becomes attached to the surface of the parts. This surface film is then eliminated by a washing process so that it will not interfere in any subsequent operations and will have the required finish.

Deposition using Langmuir-Blodgett technology

This is a very exact deposition technology (performed by the superposition of monolayers) using different organic coatings, such as fatty acids, phopholipids and polymers with long lateral hydrophobic chains. Nanostrucures can be produced with molecular alignment and controllable roughness and thickness and are widely used for producing biosensors. Their high precision means that the materials obtained can either be microstructured or nanostructured.

It can also be used for surface micro-engraving that can be combined with other CVD or PVD technologies to produce electrodes with special geometries. New research proposes using them to produce multilayers with ferroelectric polymers for non-volatile RAM memories and mass storage devices. By means of this technology extremely thin layers of ferroelectric polymer have been deposited, PVDF as well as various copolymers, attaining thicknesses of 10 Å with properties similar to those of thicker multilayers but showing additional phase changes.

Ionic self-assembled monolayering techniques

Developed by Decher and Hong in 1991 for polyelectrolytes and then extended to the production of multilayer structures with many electroactive polymers, fullerenes and other materials. Layers can be deposited on a substrate by consecutively alternating the adsorption of catatonic and ionic species. It is a relatively cheap and simple technology for controlling the molecular structure of materials and influencing their macroscopic properties. It has recently been used to obtain multilayer structures by bonding very different materials like polyelectrolytes, metal colloids, biological molecules, conductive polymers and light emitting polymers.

The process begins by taking a clean substrate with a negative surface charge. This material is submerged in a solution with polymer molecules dissolved in it that have functional groups bonded to a polymer chain with a net positive charge. These molecules are attracted to the surface of the substrate, which is left coated with a layer that is neutral as a whole but with a positive charge on its upper surface. When this cationic layer has been deposited, the external charge then incites the deposit of another anionic layer, and in this way a multilayer structure can be produced.

By adding appropriate functional groups to the substrate or using surface patterns, deposition can be encouraged in certain zones. By adjusting immersion times, solute concentration and dissolution temperature, 3D structures can be obtained by depositing material layers of controlled thickness that generally have more stable properties than those obtained by Langmuir-Blodgett technology (Madou, 2002). It can then be subjected to chemical attack to eliminate zones of unwanted deposits.

This technology together with the production of multilayer deposits with electroactive polymers has succeeded in optimising the performance of light emitting diodes (LEDs), as well as enhancing the stability of luminescent organic pigments compared to films obtained by spin-coating (Bar-Cohen, 2004). Medical applications combined with active material substrates are also promising as they are of use in work to functionalise substrates for biosensors and for improving the biocompatibility of active implantable devices (Saliterman, 2006).

13.5.6 Rapid manufacturing technologies

Vacuum casting

By taking prototypes manufactured using rapid prototyping technologies or layer manufacturing technologies silicon moulds can be made for rapid shape copying to reproduce the geometry of the original model with precision using polymer materials with different kinds of micro- and nanocharges or micro- and nanoforces. These moulds can be used to make short runs of 10 to 50 units, usually to make concept samples and verify functions before proceeding to manufacture prototypes with the definitive process.

Vacuum casting makes it easier to fill the mould, improves the final precision and helps to eliminate the bubbles that form during the curing process of many of the dual component polymers usually used for this type of casting. During the mixing process, before casting, the micro- or nanocharges can also be added (like those in Fig. 13.11) using mechanical and ultrasonic agitators to improve the dispersion of the particles and achieve more homogeneous properties.

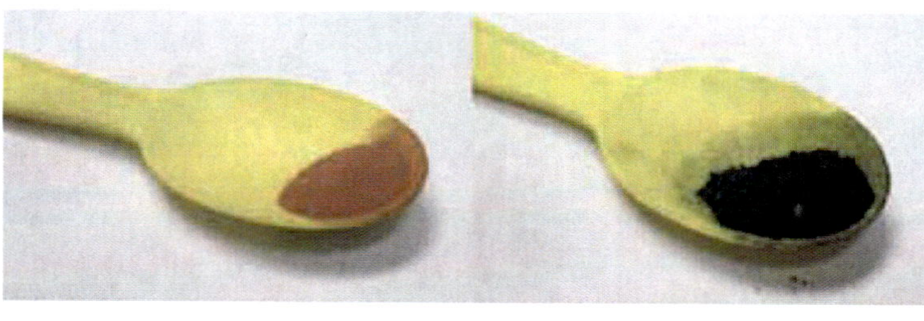

Figure 13.11 Photo of copper and graphite microcharges.

By way of example, Figs. 13.12 and 13.13 show a comparison between active rings produced by using shape-memory polyurethane (white) and shape-memory polyurethane and graphite powder (12% by weight), to optimise the thermal conductivity and other mechanical properties of the original polymer.

Figure 13.12 shows the two recently cast prototypes, while Fig. 13.13 includes an image of the training process (by heat traction and subsequent cooling of the ring with a graphite charge) as well as its subsequent recovery to its original geometry by heating. It is included next to the polyurethane ring with no charge so that the geometry after the activation process and its recovery can be compared to its original geometry.

Additional information on using charges at the core of shape-memory polymers can be found in Chapter 5.

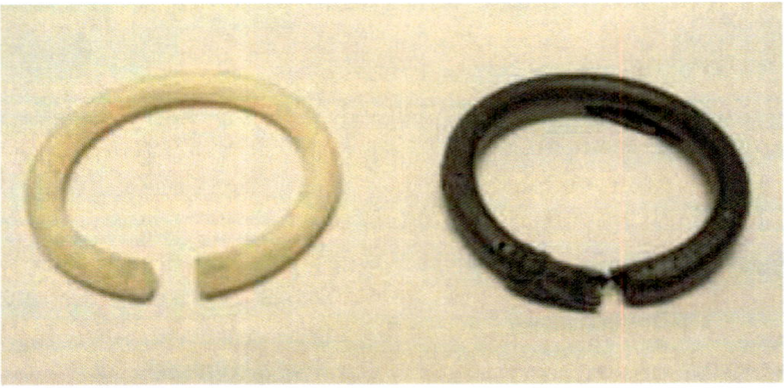

Figure 13.12 Polymer rings with shape-memory properties (original geometry). Left: Polyurethane ring. Right: Polyurethane ring with 12% of graphite powder by weight.

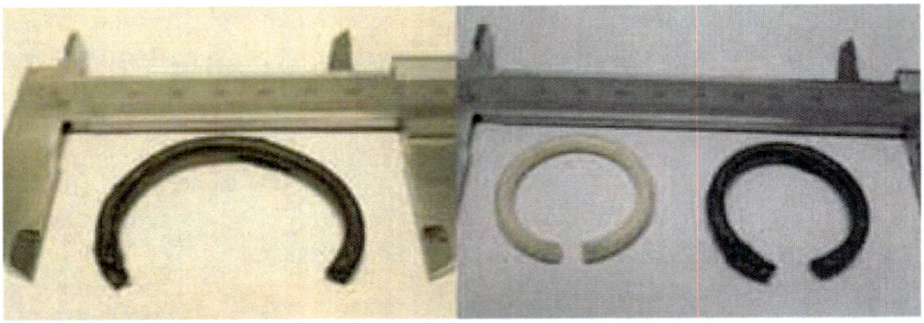

Figure 13.13 Example of temporary geometry after training and of the resulting final geometry after the activation processes and recovery followed by the ring with charge, compared to the original.

13.5.7 Surface Treatment Technologies

Laser ablation

Laser ablation consists in eliminating the surface material of a substrate, usually solid, using a laser beam to produce evaporation, sublimation or to convert the zone exposed to the beam to plasma. The process is performed by laser pulses (that last from ms to fs), which means the elimination of material is so precisely focused that the rest of the substrate remains practically unaltered. It is therefore an extremely suitable technology for changing the surface of materials that cannot be subjected to high temperature processes (generally polymers and organic matter).

This process has also been used to produce carbon nanotubes and as a support for PVD processes in which a laser acts on the substance to be deposited and the plasma generated is projected on to the substrate to be coated (Phips, 2006).

Ion implantation

The process consists in coating a substrate with the ions of another material to change the physical properties of the substrate. This has numerous applications in the electronics industry for manufacturing semi-conductive devices. To do this an ion source is required and an accelerator to project the ions into a chamber where the substrate to be implanted has been placed (Rimini, 1995).

With regard to active materials for medical devices, ion implantation is usually used to make the surface of different polymers become locally conductive. This avoids deposition of the electrodes that cover the whole surface as this is usually accompanied by an unwanted stiffening effect which limits the capacity for deformation and the activation capabilities of microstructured polymer actuators. This technology is an alternative to photolithography when micromanufacturing electrodes with complex patterns or geometric shapes.

13.6 Main Conclusions

This chapter has dealt with different active materials whose activation and detection capabilities with a view to developing diagnostic or therapeutic devices are strengthened by their microscale structure. These materials usually have a dual-layer structure or one whose properties gradually change. This makes them into materials that respond in a very special way to electrical, thermal, mechanical or magnetic stimuli and which can amplify some responses to produce more effective sensors or actuators than others previously analysed.

We have looked at the basic applications for these kinds of microstructured active materials to be mainly found in the medical industry and in the development of electro-mechanical microsystems, which encompasses all kinds of robots, micromachines, microactuators and microsensors, whose accuracy and speed benefit from acting on a microscale.

As an aid to the development of devices or structures that integrate these kinds of materials, some theoretical approximations that are basic to the design and calculation of sensors and actuators have been included. These theoretical models are suitable for simple geometries, but as the complexity of the system under development grows (and its geometry), analytical models gradually become less useful and it is advisable to turn to numerical solving methods. The usefulness of computer-aided CAD-CAE design and calculation tools has been demonstrated.

The thermomechanical calculation modules included in many of these software packages allow analysing the rises in temperature required for a specific deformation, the stresses appearing in the structure during activation, the heating power needed or the attainable response speed, as we have shown in detail for the various case studies.

In addition, we have included some fractal surface models with irregular geometries, as a biomimetic approximation to the design of surfaces for implants and other medical devices that may provide a better implant-organism interaction to make complex tasks such as osseointegration easier, optimise the surface geometry of electrodes for active devices and enhance various tribological phenomena linked to friction, lubrication, corrosion and the wear of the parts involved.

The main manufacturing and most commonly used technologies for preparing microstructured materials have also been explained in detail. Their potential applications have been described, passing from traditional bonding techniques like welding, to modern thin layer deposition technologies using gas deposition processes (physical or chemical) and other solution deposition, rapid manufacturing or surface treatment processes.

Some of these technologies can also be used to obtain nanostructured geometries and materials. Therefore, the topics dealt with here are also closely linked to what will be set out in Chapter 14.

Further information on materials, technologies, processes, research centres and suppliers linked to these kinds of applications can be found by consulting the references enumerated below, as well as the annexes included at the end of the handbook.

References

Albella, J.M. "Preparación y caracterización de recubrimientos y láminas delgadas". Programa de Doctorado en Ciencias Físicas de la Universidad Autónoma de Madrid – Instituto de Ciencia de los Materiales de Madrid (CSIC), Material Docente. Madrid, 2006.

Albella, J.M.; Gómez-Aleixandre, C.; Ojeda, F.; Martí, F.J. "Síntesis de materiales cerámicos mediante técnicas químicas en fase de vapor (CVD)". Boletín de la Sociedad Española de Cerámica y Vídrio, 42(1), 27–31, 2003.

Ansari, M.Z.; Cho, C. "A study on bimetallic effects in microcantilever biosensors". Proceedings of the 3rd International Conference on Biomedical Electronics and Devices, Biodevices 2010, Valencia, Spain, 2010.

Bar-Cohen, Y. "Electroactive polymer (EAP) actuators as artificial muscles: Reality, potential and challenges". SPIE Press, Second Edition. Washington, 2004.

Begley, M.R. "The impact of materials selection and geometry on multi-functional bilayer micro-sensors and actuators". Journal of Microelectromechanical Microengineering, 15, 2379–2388, 2005.

Bove, T.; Wolny, W.; Ringgaard, E.; Pedersen, A. "New piezoceramic PZT–PNN material for medical diagnostics applications". Journal of the European Ceramic Society, 21(10-11), 1469–1472, 2001.

Brinker, C.J.; Scherer, G.W. "Sol-Gel Science: The Physics and Chemistry of Sol-Gel Processing". Academic Press, 1990.

Bunshah, R.F. "Handbook of Deposition Technologies for Films and Coatings: Science, Technology and Applications". 2nd Edition. Noyes Publications, Materials science and process technology series. Park Ridge, N.J., 1994.

Chu, W.H.; Mehregany, M.; Mullen, R.L. "Analysis of tip deflection and force of a bimetallic cantilever microactuator". Journal of Microelectromechanical Microengineering, 3, 4–7, 1993.

Decher, G.; Hong, J.D. "Buildup of ultrathin multilayer films by a self-assembly process. II: Consecutive adsorption of anionic and cationic bipolar amphiphiles and polyelectrolytes on charged surfaces". International Journal of Physical Chemistry, 95(11), 1430–1434, 1991.

Decher, G.; Hong, J.D.; Schmitt, J. "Buildup of ultrathin multilayer films by a self-assembly process. III: Consecutively alternating adsorption of anionic and cationic polyelectrolytes on charged surfaces". Thin Solid Films, International conference on Langmuir-Blodgett films, 1992.

Díaz, A.F.; Rubinson, J.F.; Mark, H.B. "Electrochemistry and electrode applications of electroactive/conductive polymers". Advances in Polymer Science, 84, 113–139, 1988.

Díaz Lantada, A. "Procesos de transformación para polímeros electroactivos". Master Thesis, Universidad Politécnica de Madrid, 2005–2006.

Falconer, K. "Fractal Geometry". John Wiley & Sons Ltd. West Sussex, 2003.

Gad-el-Hak, M. "The MEMS Handbook". CRC Press. New York, 2003.

Glocker, D.A.; Shah, S.I. "Handbook of Thin Film Process Technology". Institute of Physics Pub. Bristol, UK, 2002.

Hafez, M. "Polymer based actuators as artificial muscles". FSRM Training in Microsystems Course. Teaching Resources. Zurich, 2006.

Hench, L.L. "Sol-Gel Silica: Properties, Processing and Technology Transfer". William Andrew, 1998.

Kanthal, AB. "Kanthal Thermostatic Bimetal Handbook". Hallstahammar, Sweden, 2008.

Madou, M. "Fundamentals of Microfabrication: The Science of Miniaturization". CRC Press, 62–63, 2002.

Manzo, J.E.; García, E. "The smart joint: Model and optimization of a shape memory alloy / shape memory polymer composite actuator". ASME Conference on Smart Materials, Adaptative Structures and Intelligent Systems. Maryland, 2008.

Matovic, J. "A simplified method for analysis of MEMS bimaterial cantilever elements". Proceedings of the 25th International Conference on Microelectronics (MIEL 2006), Belgrade, 2006.

Ngernchucklin, P.; Safari, A. "Bilayer piezoelectric/electrostrictive dome unimorph". IEEE Transactions on Ultrasonics, Ferroelectrics and Frequency Control, 56(12), 2744–2749, 2009.

Ojeda Diaz, C. "Estudio de la influencia de estabilidad primaria en el diseño de vástagos de prótesis de cadera personalizadas". PhD Thesis. Universidad Politécnica de Madrid, 2009.

Ojeda Díaz, C.; Osuna López, J.; Lafont Morgado, P.; Díaz Lantada, A. "Estudio de la estabilidad primaria, influencia en el diseño de vástagos de prótesis femorales personalizadas: Aplicación a paciente específico". 3° Congresso Nacional de Biomecânica. Sociedade Portuguesa de Biomecânica. 11–12 February 2009 in Braganza.

Phips, C.R. "Laser ablation and its applications". Springer Series in Optical Sciences, 2006.

Puchades, I.; Fuller, L.F. "Design and evaluation of a MEMS bimetallic thermal actuator for viscosity measurements". University/Government/ Industry Micro/Nano Symposium, 2008. UGIM 2008.

Rimini, E. "Ion implantation: Basics to device fabrication". Kluwer Academic Publishers. Massachusetts, 1995.

Saliterman, S. "Self-assembled monolayers (SAMs)". Fundamentals of BioMEMS and Medical Microdevices, SPIE Press, 94–96, 2006.

Sansiñena, J.M.; Olazábal, V. "Conductive polymers". In Bar-Cohen's Electroactive polymer (EAP) actuators as artificial muscles: Reality, potential and challenges, 2004.

Schwartz, M. "New materials, processes and methods technology". CRC Press, Taylor and Francis Group. Florida, 2006.

Shirzadi, A.A.; Wallach, E.R. "A new method to diffusion bond superalloys". Science and Technology of Welding and Joining, 9(1), 37–40, 2004.

Shirzadi, A.A.; Assadi, H.; Wallach, E.R. "Interface evolution and bond strength when diffusion bonding materials with stable oxide films". Journal of Surface and Interface Analysis, 31(7), 609–618, 2001.

Smith, D. "Thin-Film Deposition: Principles and Practice". McGraw-Hill, 1995.

Timoshenko, S. "Analysis of bi-metal thermostats". J.O.S.A. & R.S.I., 233–255, September, 1925.

Zhu, X.; Xu, J.; Meng, Z.; *et al.* "Microdisplacement characteristics and microstructures of functionally graded piezoelectric ceramic actuator". Materials & Design, 21(6), 561–566, 2000.

Chapter 14

Nanostructured Active Materials in Biodevices

Andrés Díaz Lantada
Mechanical Engineering Department, E.T.S.I. Industriales, Universidad Politécnica de Madrid, c/ José Gutiérrez Abascal 2, 28006 Madrid, Spain
adiaz@etsii.upm.es

14.1 Introduction

Richard P. Feynman, winner of the Nobel Prize in Physics, is widely recognised as the father of nanoscience, since his talk, "there is plenty of room at the bottom" (1959) moved scientists into doing active research, on a nanometric scale, into the "curious" or somewhat unconventional properties and phenomena of material. Nanotechnology may be defined as the science that studies the control of matter on an atomic and molecular scale. This means that structures of less than 100 nm, in at least one of their dimensions, have to be used, which also means developing devices of that size.

Inorganic, organic and biological nanostructured materials have been around in Nature ever since the beginning of the evolutionary chain on Earth. This can be seen if the crystallised minerals forming the rocks, the component parts of micro-organisms or the particles in suspension in smoke or fog are examined in detail (Schwartz, 2006). However, real progress in this discipline and the control of material on a nanoscale began to emerge at the beginning of the

Handbook of Active Materials for Medical Devices: Advances and Applications
Edited by Andrés Díaz Lantada

www.panstanford.com

1970s, and was closely linked to the developments in electronics and computing, which were continuously seeking circuits with ever tinier connections and sizes so that more information could be stored in a smaller volume.

During the first decades of development, nanotechnology basically focused on the use of semi-conductor materials, particularly silicon, due to the ease and precision that could be attained when processing it with acid attacks, thanks to its peculiar crystallography. From the 1980s, however, attention began to focus on other materials, especially polymers. The intention was to obtain nanosystems that were cheaper to mass produce and that would be suited to other applications, particularly in health sciences, because of their good behaviour when in contact with human tissue.

On these very tiny scales, the quantum effects between particles begin to take on considerable importance, and the typical physical, chemical and biological properties of the materials undergo a surprising alteration as their size gets smaller. This means that nanosystems and nanostructures can be obtained with very high mechanical strength, which makes amazingly fast chemical reactions possible, with extraordinary optical and chromic effects, among many other properties, and remarkable responses to external stimuli that can be managed (or controlled) by simple changes to size, shape or the relative geometric layout of the grain forming these materials.

Generally speaking, any material containing fibres, layers, particles or granules of a size less than 100 nm may be considered as a nanostructured material. If, moreover, the material is oriented to exploit some of the remarkable variations in the properties mentioned, depending on the different external stimuli, we can speak of the concept of "nanostructured active material".

Some of the manufacturing and processing technologies like CVD and PVD techniques, sintering and powder metallurgy in the preceding chapter also have multiple applications for the development of nanostructured materials, by limiting the thickness of the layers deposited to a few tens of nanometres by using shorter exposure times.

This chapter details the different families of active materials whose behaviour depends directly on their structure on a nanometric level, which endows them with special innovative properties for developing medical devices that are more effective for performing diagnostic or therapeutic tasks. Due to operational limitations, we will deal with some of the families of nanostructured, active materials that are giving rise to most interest, particularly in the area of health sciences. The main current and potential medical applications of each family dealt with are also analysed together with the limitations and trends of current research.

It is hoped that the inclusion of various excellent texts and handbooks specifically devoted to nanotechnology and nanomaterials will be of use to any researchers wishing to examine these topics in greater detail than we have been able to do.

14.2 Carbon Nanotubes

14.2.1 Introduction to These Materials

Nanotubes are allotropic forms of carbon with a cylindrical structure and with a length that is millions of times greater than their diameter. They were officially discovered in 1991 by Ijima and his collaborators (Ijima, 1991, 1993), although, there had been some evidence of their existence since the 1950s (Monthioux and Kuznetsov, 2006). In principle, a carbon nanotube (CNT) is made up of a single layer of graphite rolled into a tube shape with fullerene ends. Depending on the synthesis and processing, either single-walled nanotubes (SWCNTs or SWNTs) can be obtained or concentric multiwalled nanotubes (MWCNTs or MWNTs).

Although producing multiwalled nanotubes usually entails simpler processes, they usually possess a higher number of defects that limit their mechanical properties and change their electrical properties (from conductors to semi-conductors, which, however, makes them more suitable for some other applications). In whichever case, SWNTs are still more expensive (200–300 €/kg) than MWNTs (10–30 €/kg) and if high purity is required these prices can rise by up to 10-fold, although these prices are expected to fall considerably in the coming years due to advances in the synthesis and processing procedures.

The enormous interest being shown in these materials is closely linked to the remarkable properties deriving from their structure, which enable them to be used in a wide range of fields. Their tensile strength (with values of up to 150 GPa) is at least 10 times higher than for conventional carbon fibre, and, in addition, they are very light (densities from 0.7 g/cm^3 to around 1.9 g/cm^3), which is encouraging research, with a view to their use as reinforcement fibres for all kinds of polymer matrix composites.

Depending on their structure they can exhibit metallic behaviour, electrical conductivity or semi-metallic behaviour which means they can be used to replace semi-conductors. They are also excellent heat conductors with a conductivity as high as that of diamonds. All this makes them first class candidates for the development of passive structures with enhanced properties, as well as for numerous multifunctional systems that make full use of their capabilities as sensors or actuators, which will be examined further on.

Moreover, the marked influence of their structure on these properties opens up the way to "a la carte" approaches, as is the case with the polymer industry, so that their properties can be designed and tailor-made to the specific application being developed.

More detailed information on synthesis, processing and properties can be found in the references included at the end of the chapter (Schwartz, 2006; Spinks *et al.*, in Bar-Cohen, 2004), as well as by consulting the suppliers' characteristics sheets cited in the annexes, since the different synthesis processes used by each manufacturer lead to SWNTs and MWNTs that can show differences of up to 50% in the values assigned. The characteristic sheets almost always refer to pure material, which means that if they are to be used for reinforcement, thorough additional characterisation testing may be required.

Suppliers usually provide the material in powder form (see Fig. 14.1) or as a solution, depending on the end use and the processing to be followed. In its solution form it usually incorporates some kind of functional group to aid percolation when used as reinforcement nanofibres to change conventional mechanical, thermal or electrical properties.

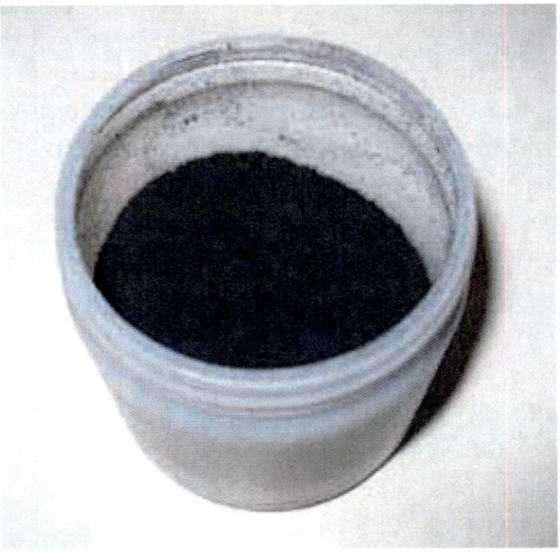

Figure 14.1 Carbon nanotubes (multi-walled) for use as reinforcement fibre

We will now include information on some potential applications for these materials in the medical sector, with emphasis on the main scientific-technological progress regarding nanotubes in recent years, and include some reflections on current research trends.

14.2.2 Proposals for Application to Medical Devices

Apart from the proven use of carbon nanotubes in multiple applications, one very marked use is as fibre in the development of compound materials with optimised properties.

They are also used in electronic devices for their conductive and semi-conductive properties, or for their military potential, and are opening up the way to new diagnostic and therapeutic possibilities in the medical industry, like those enumerated below.

Applications as sensors

Major leaps forward in exploiting the capabilities of nanotubes as biosensors are emerging as a result of producing DNA-nanotube hybrids. Connecting nanotubes to a pathogen's DNA sequence enables the presence of those pathogens in the body to be electrically recorded through contact and be accurately located (Harutyunyan *et al.*, 2002; Schwartz, 2006).

Applications as actuators

Carbon nanotubes have been put forward as drug carriers, either in their interior or adhered to their surface, for very localised actions (due to their tiny size which means they can even pass through cell membranes) aimed at eliminating cancer cells, for example (Harutyunyan *et al.*, 2002). The bond between nanotubes drug-carriers and magnetic nanoparticles has been proposed as another possible solution for guiding these nanostructures inside the body so they will reach their target.

In recent years many nanotube-based nanometric-sized actuators have been developed, either in the form of a film with the ability to bend or through the bonding of antagonistic linear components that bend (Baughman, 1999; Hunt, 2001; Spinks *et al.*, in Bar-Cohen, 2004; Schwartz, 2006). Among the uses proposed, we can cite their possible use as atomic force microscope ends and for the development of nanomanipulators or nanotweezers that can act at a cell and sub-cell level to manipulate viruses, molecules etc.. These structures, principally intended for activation tasks, have also demonstrated capabilities as sensors when their properties are changed under mechanical stimulus.

14.2.3 Main Progress Achieved

Synthesis and transformation processes

There are a large number of ways to synthesise carbon nanotubes, such as by generating an electric arc between pure carbon cathodes and carbon anodes with metal components, through the combustion of cyclical hydrocarbons, laser vaporisation using carbon samples or CVD deposition techniques. Each of these methods can be used to obtain SWNTs or MWNTs with different structures and properties. For research teams focusing on product development work (and medical devices) that integrate the benefits of these materials, either as structural elements or transducers, it is usually sufficient to purchase the nanotubes from manufacturers that are solely devoted to this task, with synthesis remaining beyond the scope of the project.

With regard to the processing required to obtain nanotube-reinforced polymer, several aspects must be borne in mind that will be of help in obtaining homogeneous and repetitive results. One of the usual problems is that the nanotubes normally supplied "as powder" adhere to one another to form micro-particles. If the nanotubes are directly added to the core of the polymer to be then cured to produce the composite, these microparticles fail to break up properly, leading to the loss of the enormous benefits of the nanotubes as reinforcement particles.

By encouraging a correct dispersion, the properties of a polymer can be varied with only a small percentage of nanotubes (0.1%–1 %). To ensure this, before the mixing process, it is usually sufficient to use crusher mills to break these micrometric aggregates, as well as ultrasonic agitators once the material has been added to the core of the polymer (sometimes for several hours) to produce percolation and obtain polymer composites with optimised properties.

Marked properties

To supplement the introduction to carbon-nanotube properties on the preceding pages, we will now include a comparative table (Table 14.1) showing some of the remarkable mechanical properties of these materials found from the characterisation testing conducted by various groups (see references).

Table 14.1 Some of the Different Typical Properties of Carbon Nanotubes and other Materials

Note. Some data from the references included at the end of the chapter and manufacturers' data (annexes).

	Tensile strength (GPa)	Young modulus (GPa)	Poisson coefficient	Stretch to break (%)
SWCNT	10–100	500–2000	0.16	5–20
MWCNT	10–150	200–900	0.27	5–15
Carbon nanotube-reinforced polymer	20–40	6–600	0.3–0.33	3–6
Carbon fibre-reinforced polymer	2–7	15–50	0.35	1.7–3.5
Glass fibre-reinforced polymer	0.5–4	5–40	0.35	2.2–3.5
Kevlar – Epoxy (50% vol.)	2–3.5	70–150	0.35	2–3
Spider's web	2	12–34	0.3	26
Conventional stainless-steel	0.6–3	210	0.28–0.33	8–12

The data in the table may be of use as an approximation when conducting feasibility studies. However, for more detailed designs it is important to contact the suppliers or perform your own characterisation tests, as the direction and proportion of reinforcement fibre used has a major influence on the end properties.

14.2.4 Main Lines of Research

Property characterisation

Much of the information available up to now is the result of simulations based on quality outcome models (although in some cases, the theoretical predictions differ enormously from the actual data), due to the difficulty of characterising isolated nanotubes. However, in spite of the goodness of these models, it is always a good idea to compare the theoretical predictions with tests performed using real samples, particularly when the conditions under which they are used vary widely, as this normally leads to slight model misfits under boundary conditions.

Moreover, the large number of formulations for polymers that are candidates for having their properties enhanced by using nanotubes as reinforcement, combined with the different kinds of properties of nanotubes, leads to an enormous number of combinations. Thus, characterisation tasks takes on major importance if material data bases are to be compiled that will provide designers with the information they really need.

For example, already existing data bases, such as Campus Plastics, that contain information on the mechanical, electrical, thermal, optical and chemical properties of a wide range of polymers and reinforced polymers, could be completed with the information related to nanotubes as reinforcement material. To this end, collaboration among researchers is particularly vital.

Search for new applications

Since the integration of nanotubes as dispersed elements in polymer matrices, and even ceramic matrices, is giving rise to innovative materials with special properties, it is important to monitor progress in the sectors that are seeking new applications for them. Taking steps to protect the intellectual property, in parallel to the development of new materials (patents, utility models and industrial designs), is highly advisable.

Nanotubes of other materials

The special properties resulting from the structure of carbon nanotubes has encouraged the synthesis of inorganic nanotubes in materials like copper, gold, silicon, titanium, dioxide and others.

The high surface/volume ratio of these materials usually gives an enormous boost to the speed of reaction in the presence of certain components or composites, for which reason, sensors fabricated with nanotubes are normally far more sensitive than other more conventional sensors. Therefore, they are beginning to be used to detect hydrogen, as the integral parts of lab-on-a-chip devices and in various kinds of installations to alert the presence of gases (dangerous leaks, terrorist attacks, pollution, automotive emissions etc).

Safety in nanotechnology

It is important to look very closely at some issues related to the effects on health and the environment of using nanotubes, both in the laboratory and on an industrial scale. Some research has begun to show results in this respect (Zhu, 2008). Although the results of cytotoxicity are not conclusive, it is important to act with caution. While possible harmful effects are still being investigated, it is essential to continue to use protective gloves, face-masks and goggles, in addition to extractor hoods, during processing and follow the additional safety recommendations contained in the characteristic sheets supplied by the manufacturers.

14.3 Quantum Tunnelling Composites

14.3.1 Introduction to These Materials

Quantum tunnelling composites or QTCs are polymer matrix composites (elastomeric) with metal particle filling and were discovered by the scientist David Lussey in 1997, when he was trying to develop an electrically conductive adhesive. The surprising properties of this new material led to the founding of Peratech Ltd., a company dedicated to research work, the search for applications, and technology transfer regarding these materials.

The working principle of QTCs differs from that of other conductive polymers obtained through percolation (using metal particles, carbon nanotubes, smoke-black and other fillings). These latter attempt to bring into contact the metal-filled particles to obtain electrical conductivity or, at least, considerably reduce the electrical resistance of the polymer matrix (Blythe and Bloor, 2005; Takele *et al.*, 2008). However, QTCs usually obtained by integrating Ni particles of around 100 to 500 nm into an elastomeric matrix, act differently. In a state of rest these metal particles are not in contact and the polymer acts as an insulator, but when the material is deformed in an appropriate way, the particles come together (without actually touching) and the material becomes an excellent conductor (electrical resistance is reduced by several orders of magnitude).

An explanation for this behaviour was contributed by researchers from Durham University (Bloor *et al.*, 2005, 2006; Hands *et al.*, 2001). Since the Ni particles embedded in the polymer matrix have an irregular surface (spiky)—when the material is pressed the particles come together and the electrons can "leap" from the irregularities of some particles to the irregularities of others without any need for contact—due to the "quantum tunnel" effect (overcoming the non-conductive portion of the polymer between particles).

The more the material is deformed, the more marked the reduction in electrical resistance, for which reason the use of elastomeric matrices is particularly effective, although for applications required to support higher pressures, thermoplastic or thermostable materials can be used.

One of the major advantages of these materials is that since they are insulators when in a state of rest, the conditioning electronics fitted to these devices does not consume any energy unless pressure is applied. This helps minimise the size of the power supply required, which opens up a wide range of applications, particularly usage related to the development of implantable medical devices (Mootanah and Bader, 2006) and aeronautic devices (Shadow Robot Company, Peratech Ltd), where end size is a determining factor.

They are also very cheap and easy to obtain, being distributed by various companies at very affordable prices (less than 1 € per sensor), which means that the end applications will not exceed the cost of other solutions available on the market. In fact, apart from Peratech Ltd., various companies have emerged, such as QIO Systems Inc., Elek Tek and Elek Sen to exploit the capabilities of these materials in different sectors of the electronics industry (Connolly, 2004; Boohan, 2005) or the textile industry (Van Lagenhove and Hertleer, 2004)).

14.3.2 Proposals for Application in Medical Devices

Table 14.2 lists the main applications proposed for these materials in the medical sector. It also makes reference to the researchers, companies, universities or research centres responsible for patents, tests and other publicity, marketing or consultancy service tasks, linked to these applications. Some of these proposals have already been tested and are in their commercialisation stage, such as touch switches incorporated into fabric, and into various electronic devices or robot hands, although most of these ideas have not gone beyond the patent stage.

Table 14.2 Some Proposals for Applications for QTC-Based Medical Devices

Sector of application	Specific application	References	Companies/ Bodies
Medical industry	Measuring and controlling blood pressure and heartbeat	Bloor and Lussey, 2005, 2008 Burkitt, 2008US2008289886	Peratech
Medical industry	Measuring pressure distribution in footwear when walking		Peratech
Medical industry	Monitoring sleep apnoea and respiratory conditions		Peratech
Medical industry	Measuring pressures in prosthetic devices	Shadow Robot Company	
Medical industry	Measuring intrabucal pressures for diagnosing TMA problems	Díaz Lantada, 2009	Universidad Politécnica de Madrid
Medical industry	Sensors for diverse physiological checks	Mootanah and Bader, 2006	Anglia Ruskin University

In general, the applications listed in Table 14.2 usually use these materials as "all-or-nothing" switches for their simplicity of design and implementation, while for promoting other uses that need quantifying (and thereby promote their expansion in industry), it is very important to characterise and model these materials in depth.

Other researchers have proposed models based on quantum phenomena that are complex to explain, such as the emission of electrons by the Fowler-Nordheim effect or the Schottky barriers at the polymer-metal interface (Bloor *et al.*, 2005), highly precise in describing the tunnel effect, but which have not included in sufficient detail other thermo-mechanical aspects that affect the physical properties of the material in question and its capabilities as a transducer.

Described below are some tests that were conducted to examine the response of these materials in greater detail, taking account of mechanical, thermal and time aspects.

14.3.3 Characterisation for a Thorough Knowledge of Behaviour

For the detailed studies in this work, tiny 3.6 mm × 3.6 mm × 1 mm QTC pills were taken as the starting point, supplied by the "MUTR Teaching Resources" company (www.mutr.co.uk), in the United Kingdom, associated with Middlesex University (www.mdx.ac.uk). This company also supplies these materials in film and cable form for different applications, but here, we have used them in their pill form which is more suited to analysing combined mechanical, thermal and electrical phenomena.

The sensors used for testing were directly obtained by placing the QTC pills between 75 μm thick Cu film and encapsulating them with adhesive tape, as Fig. 14.2 illustrates, in the same way as proposed by other researchers (Boohan, 2005).

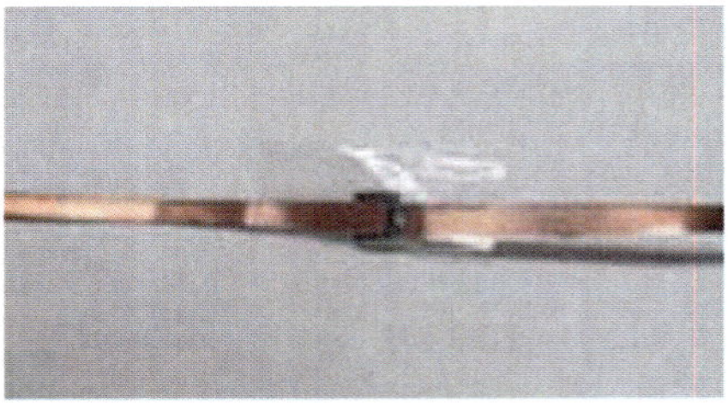

Figure 14.2 QTC pill-based pressure sensor between Cu electrodes.

Encapsulation was done gently without pre-loading the material, since a pre-load would lead to a somewhat compressed initial situation and entail a lower electrical resistance (possibly several orders of magnitude). In this event, the sensor would show a smaller range of property variation, and therefore, of measurement, which would limit its range of application.

To measure the electrical resistance between sensor faces, a "Mastech MY-68" digital multimeter was used with a measuring range of 0.1 Ω to 50 MΩ. As a component for being able to perform tests at different temperatures, a "Fisher Scientific" hotplate was used in combination with a "CME 305" digital thermometer for controlling the test conditions at any instant.

Figures 14.3, 14.4, 14.5 and 14.6 contain the results of these tests, showing the evolution of the electrical resistance of the QTC sensors in accordance with the pressure and time of application for tests conducted at temperatures of 30, 40, 50 and 60°C, respectively.

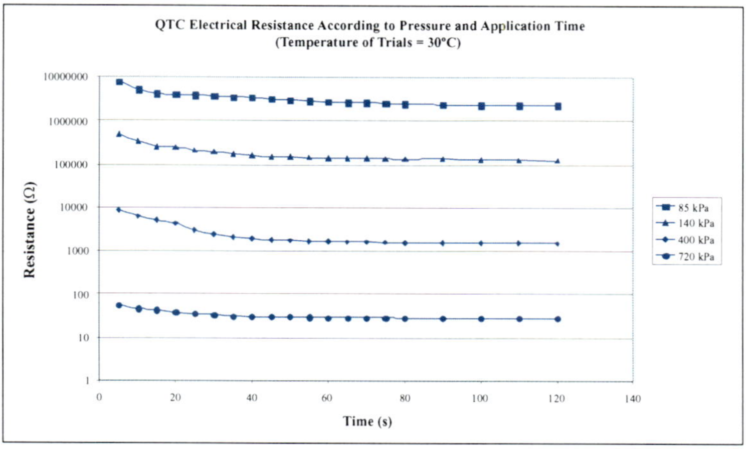

Figure 14.3 Electrical resistance in accordance with pressure and time of application (test at 30°C).

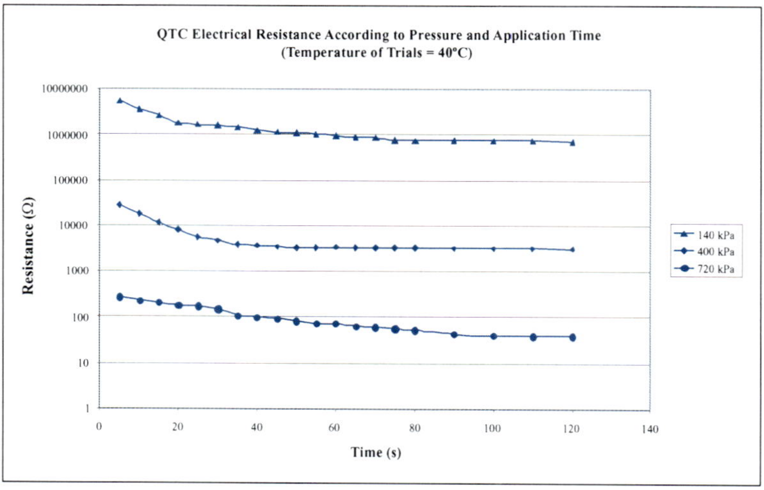

Figure 14.4 Electrical resistance in accordance with pressure and time of application (test at 40°C).

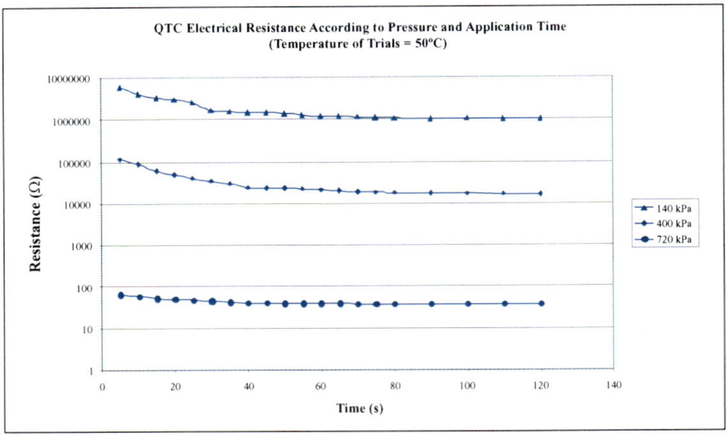

Figure 14.5 Electrical resistance in accordance with pressure and time of application (test at 50°C).

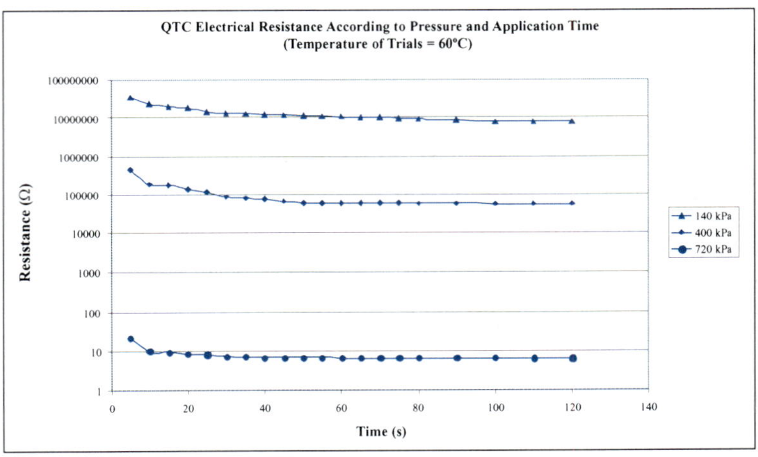

Figure 14.6 Electrical resistance in accordance with pressure and time of application (test at 60°C).

Moreover, Fig. 14.7 also reveals a drop in electrical resistance with pressure in a more than exponential manner, going from practically insulating values for pressures of around 100 MPa to the typical values of above 700 MPa for good conductors. Behaviour in relation to this variable is similar to that described in other references (Hands, 2001, 2003; Boohan, 2005; Bloor *et al.*, 2005).

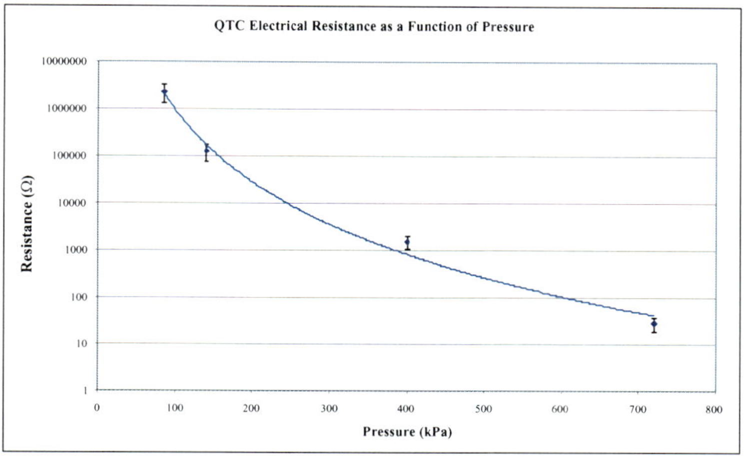

Figure 14.7 Electrical resistance in accordance with pressure (at ambient temperature = 30°C).

The results of these tests have also allowed a deeper analysis of certain phenomena described concerning the in-service response of QTCs, as is the case with the "thermostatic positive temperature coefficient" or "PTC effect" (Hands *et al.*, 2001; Boohan, 2005) and the acceptance limits of this behaviour.

According to this phenomenon, the electrical resistance of the material shows a linear growth with temperature, a phenomenon detected previously in other polymer-carbon-black/metal particle conductive composites (Boiteux *et al.*, 1999; Li and Cheng, 2000), which can also have applications for measuring temperature.

In fact, a summary of the results in Fig. 14.8 reveals a remarkable non-linear behaviour due to thermo-mechanical effects, which is noticeably accentuated for high pressures. This behaviour does not coincide with what is found in other references (Hands, 2001, 2003; Boohan, 2005; Bloor *et al.*, 2005), probably due to having characterised the material this time by varying the temperatures in a wider range. Therefore, the effect of the "thermostatic positive temperature coefficient," or "PTC effect", can be inverted simply by working at around 25°C above standard conditions. This can limit the ranges of application of these materials as pressure sensors (or even temperature). In whichever case, this change of tendency must be borne in mind for design work when defining the specifications for sensors based on these materials, particularly with a view to developing highly responsible devices, as is the case with medical devices.

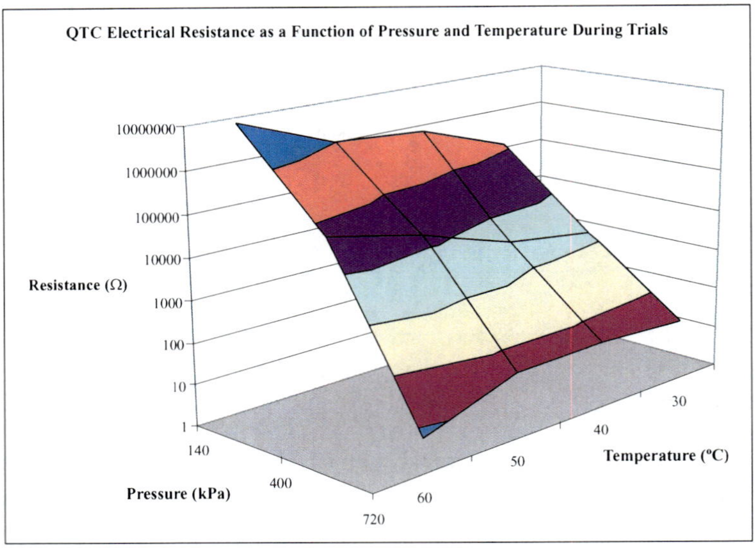

Figure 14.8 Electrical resistance in accordance with the pressure applied and test temperature. Additional details can be found in Díaz Lantada, 2010a, 2010b.

14.3.4 Main Lines of Research

The main lines of research into these polymer-metal composites seek to obtain behaviour models for simulating their response in order to lead to applications able to quantify pressure and even temperature. It is also sought to optimise synthesis processes by seeking more homogeneous dispersions of the metal particles in the core of the polymer, so as to produce sensors that are repetitive and suited to precise, safe end devices.

To achieve this, it may be useful to use artificial neural networks as support tool since they are usually applicable for modelling systems that are dependent on multiple parameters where non-linearities are very marked. To illustrate these possibilities, we offer a detailed example of QTC modelling with the aid of artificial neural networks in Chapter 15.

14.4 Nanocharges as a Way of Adding Functionalities

14.4.1 The Advantages of Nanocharges as a Way of Adding Functionalities

Some advantages of integrating nanocharges into the core of the material, which becomes an "active or intelligent material", were already described while dealing with electro-magneto rheological fluids and elastomers in Sections 10.2 and 10.3.

In these cases, we have seen how nanoparticles help to change the electromagnetic properties of the materials used as matrix, integrating new functionalities to bring about responses through electro-mechanical magneto-mechanical coupling, which enables them to be used as sensors and actuators.

Also, in Sections 11.4.1 and 11.4.3, we analysed the changes to the optical properties that can be brought about by glass that incorporates nanoparticles whose orientation can be changed under electrical stimulus.

These nanoparticles are often used as reinforcement, which is the case with many applications using carbon nanotubes, as they help to enhance the mechanical properties of the base material.

It should be pointed out that very small amounts of nanocharges (often less than 1% by weight) dispersed in a conventional material matrix are now able to produce these couplings, without any noticeable worsening of the other beneficial properties (usually mechanical, such as flexibility, high durability and others) of the original material.

14.4.2 Nanocharges for Shape Memory Polymers

Recent studies on the activation process of shape-memory polymers have focused on a more homogeneous distribution of heating elements (micro and nanoparticles, carbon nanotubes and other approaches) for obtaining magneto/electro active shape-memory polymers and the related improvement in activation and end-size reduction (Leng *et al.*, 2007, 2008, 2009; Liu, 2009; Lv *et al.*, 2009; Vialle *et al.*, 2009; Weigel *et al.*, 2009).

Those improvements can be used in combination with other proposals based on the use of conductive heating threads for improving activation ability (Díaz Lantada, 2010). Such particles and fibres can also be used as reinforcements for improving the mechanical properties and response of these interesting materials within more complex intelligent structures (Lan, 2009).

In this way, materials can be produced with electro-thermo-mechanical coupling that can provide solutions to diagnostic or therapeutic needs, due to their marked multifunctionality that lets different stimuli be related to different responses.

The results described in the references underline the benefits of using nanocharges compared to the micro-charges used in the previous chapter (see the last three Figures of the chapter), since the influence of nanoparticles on the appearance of problems during manipulation, casting and curing in the moulds, is much less, as is the fragility of the end devices.

One of the main limitations (and therefore the subject of major research work) continues to be the biocompatibility of the end devices and the methodology followed to evaluate such biocompatibility. Many comparative *in vitro* studies have been made using multiple combinations of polymers with shape memory and nanocharges. However, on occasions, extrapolating these conclusions to the final *in vivo* performance is asking too much.

14.5 Nanosensors, Nanoactuators and Nanomachines: New Horizons Based on Biological Components

For the last few decades attention has been focused on the combined use of inorganic nanostructures and biological nanostructures to promote the development of biosensors and bioactuators that exhibit an optimised response to different stimuli or parts of the body. These have an enormous potential for the medical industry.

These sensors or actuators usually comprise a measurement or activation chain with the following components:

- **Bioreceptor or bioactuator.** Usually enzymes, proteins, DNA, RNA or microorganisms either able to recognise materials and detect the presence of any harmful element (viruses, bacteria, antigens etc.) on a molecular level, or act on them. It is usually the organic part of the nanobiosensor or nanobioactuator, as well as being the smallest part.
- **Transducer.** Organic or inorganic material that receives the signal from the bioreceptor and usually transforms it into

electric current, in the case of a nanobiosensor, or either transforms an electrical impulse from the control unit into a stimulus that triggers the activation of the biological component. Many of the materials explained in this handbook can perform this function in this kind of device.

- **Control unit.** Its mission is to receive the electrical signal from the transducer and analyse it or either generate an electrical signal able to activate the transducer.

The most frequently used principles of detection or activation are based on piezoelectric, electro-chemical, thermo-chemical and optical phenomena. The most outstanding applications are linked to diagnostic and clinical work, detecting harmful elements in the environment and quality control in the food industry. In each of these sectors, precision and speed are key factors that are boosted in these kinds of devices due to the large surface/volume ratio of their components, which increases the speed of reaction and interaction (Huefner, 2006).

Some interesting works have shown how to obtain dual or multilayer sensors based on "self-assembled nano-thin films", simple to produce, stable and robust. The last layer can incorporate selective molecules that react with a specific substance for chemical analysis tasks (Ribeiro *et al.*, 2009). On other occasions, carbon nanotube electrodes have been used that have a surface deposit of different types of enzymes to detect specific biochemical reactions (Razumiene *et al.*, 2009). This kind of nanostructured functionalisation of the electrodes in a device lets more specific and sensing approaches be adopted for a very rapid detection of very specific pathologies or phenomena.

With regard to bio-nanoactuators, the different mechanical responses of single-cell organisms to different stimuli are being used, such as motor elements in nanoactuators and nanomachines. The conceptual degree of complexity of these machines is small and their consumption practically zero. However, if bionanoactuators showing an adequate response to a specific purpose are to be designed, it is still important to continue researching into the modelling, simulation and characterisation of the electromagnetic, electromechanical and vibroacoustic phenomena among others (Lyshevski, 2003).

Once all these current difficulties have been overcome, it is hoped that the use of swarms of nanomachines, managed by single-cell, interrelated organisms will lead to solving many medical, biological and environmental problems, and even help human beings to solve any kind of complex problem (micro and nanorobots with a biological brain) (Warwick, 2008).

14.6 Main Conclusions

This chapter has focused on the different families of active materials whose behaviour depends directly on their structure on a nanometric level, which endows them with innovative and special properties for the development of medical devices that will perform diagnostic or therapeutic work much more effectively.

We have limited ourselves to some of the families of nanostructured active materials that are giving rise to most interest particularly in the field of health sciences. We have analysed the main current and potential applications of each family dealt with, together with the limitations and trends of current research. Some of the materials already dealt with in this handbook (like electro/magneto rheological fluids or some types of optoactive materials) also base their activation capabilities on their structure on a nanometric level. Therefore, this chapter links up with other previous ones, but focusing on certain more innovative families and on some more specific aspects.

So, we have attempted to give different introductions to materials like carbon nanotubes, quantum tunnelling composites and the potential contribution of different nanocharges, with a view to the development of innovative biosensors and actuators.

New horizons open up concerning the ability to combine these kinds of nanostructured synthetic materials and other kinds of active materials already dealt with, together with biological nanostructures that can perform activation detection tasks directly on components that form the basis of life.

Among the main research trends regarding the development of nanostructured materials on a nanoscale, we can mention the effort being put into finding manufacturing technologies (subtractive or additive) that are sufficiently exact to go beyond the capabilities of chemical lithography technologies for Microsystems or the use of nanocharges randomly dispersed in the core of a conventional material. Therefore, atomic force microscope ends are being more and more frequently used to generate surface nanotextures to endow a material with different functionalities or for local substrate oxidation (Campbell, 1999).

The CVD and PVD technologies already detailed in the previous chapter are evidently useful in this respect, as they allow depositing layers with thicknesses that fall within the nanometric range, which can be subsequently worked on with some kind of physical attack to make nanostructures. It has been successfully demonstrated that nanostructures can be produced by following these ideas by using electron beam and X-ray lithography techniques (Mc Cord and Rook, 1997; Cerrina, 1997).

We suppose that new steps forward and improvements to the precision of manufacturing and rapid prototyping technologies based on the concepts of "layer manufacturing" and "solid free-form fabrication" will let nanometric precision be achieved in the near future and lead to the fabrication of nanostructures with much more complex geometries and very special functionalities that even use biological materials. If this is combined with a more detailed observation and understanding of how Nature is able to synthesise macromolecules to generate biological structures, then maybe, in the future, we will be able to carry out similar processes in a controlled manner. The chance to improve the welfare of human beings if the present limitations are overcome makes it well worthwhile to continue researching in this direction.

References

Bar-Cohen, Y. "Electroactive polymer (EAP) actuators as artificial muscles: Reality, potential and challenges". SPIE Press, Second Edition. Washington, 2004.

Baughman, R.H., Cui, C.X., Zakhidov A.A.; *et al.* "Carbon nanotube actuators". Science, 284, 1340, 1999.

Bloor, D.; Donnelly, K.; Hands, P.; *et al.* "A metal-polymer composite with unusual properties". Journal of Physics D: Applied Physics, 38, 2851–2860, 2005.

Bloor, D.; Graham, A.; Williams, E.J. "Metal–polymer composite with nanostructured filler particles and amplified physical properties". Applied Physics Letters, 88, 102103, 2006.

Blythe, A.R.; Bloor, D. "Electrical properties of polymers". Cambridge University Press. 2nd Edition, Cambridge, 2005.

Boiteux G.; Fournier J.; Issotier D.; *et al.*"Conductive thermoset composites: PTC effect". Synthetic Metals, 102(1), 1234–1235, 1999.

Boohan, R. "QTC a remarkable new material to control electricity". Gatsby Technical Education Projects. Science Enhancement Program. London,

2005. Burkitt, J. "Position detection". Patent Document US2008289886, 2008.

Campbell, P.M.; Snow, E.S.; Mc Carr, P.J. "AFM-based fabrication of Si nanostructures". Physica B: Condensed Matter, 227(1–4), 315–317, 1999.

Cerrina, F. "X-ray Lithography". SPIE Handbook on Lithography, 1997.

Connolly, C. "Switches and pressure sensors benefit from novel composite material". Sensor Review, 24(3), 261–264, 2004.

Díaz Lantada, A.; Lafont Morgado, P.; Muñoz Sanz, J.L. Muñoz García, J.; Munoz-Guijosa, J.M.; Echávarri Otero, J..- "Intelligent expandable structures based on the improved activation of shape memory polymers". Biodevices 2010 – Third International Conference on Biomedical Electronics and Devices. IEEE Engineering in Medicine and Biology Society. January 20–23, in Valencia, 2010.

Díaz Lantada, A.; Lafont Morgado, P.; Echávarri Otero, J.; Munoz-Guijosa, J.M.; Munoz-Sanz, J.L. "Neural network approach to modelling the behaviour of quantum tunnelling composites as multifunctional sensors". Smart Materials and Structures, 19(12), 125007, 2010.

Díaz Lantada, A.; Lafont Morgado, P.; Echávarri Otero, J.; Munoz-Guijosa, J.M.; Munoz-Sanz, J.L. "Quantum tunnelling composites: Characterisation and modelling to promote their applications as sensors". Sensors & Actuators A: Physical, 164(1–2), 46–57, 2010.

Gad-el-Hak, M. "The MEMS Handbook". CRC Press. New York, 2003.

Díaz Lantada, A. "Methodology for the structured development of biodevices based on intelligent polymers". PhD Thesis, Universidad Politécnica de Madrid, 2009.

Hands, P. "Vapour sensing applications and electrical conduction mechanisms in a novel metal-polymer composite". PhD Thesis. Department of Physics, Durham University, 2003.

Hands, P.; Bloor, D.; Donnelly, K.; *et al.* "Quantum tunnelling conductive metal-polymer composites". Poster – SET for Britain. House of Commons, London, 19th March 2001.

Harutyunyan, A.R.; Pradhan, B.K.; Sumanasekera, G.U.; *et al.* "Carbon nanotubes for medical applications". European Cells and Materials, 3(2), 84–87, 2002.

Huefner, S. "Nanobiosensors". (http://www.chem.usu.edu), 2006.

Hunt, B.; Noca, F.; Hoenk, M. "Carbon nanotube bimorph actuators and force sensors". NASA Tech Briefs, p. 33, September 2001.

Iijima, S. "Helical microtubules of graphitic carbon". Nature, 354, 56–58, 1991.

Ijima, S.; Ichihashi, T. "Single-shell carbon nanotubes of 1-nm diameter". Nature, 363, 603–605, 1993.

Ko, F.K.; Kawabata, S.; Inoue, M.; *et al.* "Engineering properties of spider silk". (http://web.mit.edu).

Lee, H.; Mall, S.; He, P.; *et al.* "Characterization of carbon nanotube/nanofiber-reinforced polymer composites using an instrumented indentation technique". Composites Part B: Engineering, 38(1), 58–65, 2007.

Leng, J.S.; Huang, W.M.; Lan, X.; *et al.* "Significantly reducing electrical resistivity by forming conductive Ni chains in a polyurethane shape-memory polymer/carbon black composite". Applied Physics Letters. 92, 206101, 2008.

Leng, J.S.; Lan, X.; Liu, Y.; Du, S.Y. "Electroactive thermoset shape memory polymer nanocomposite filled with nanocarbon powders". Smart Materials & Structures, 19, 074003, 2009.

Leng, J.S.; Lv, H.; Liu, Y.; Du, S. "Electro-active shape memory polymer filled with nanocarbon particles and short carbon fibers". Applied Physics Letters, 91, 144105, 2007.

Leng, J.S.; Lv, H.; Du, S.; Liu, Y. "Synergic effect of carbon black and short carbon fiber on shape memory polymer actuation by electricity". Journal of Applied Physics, 105, 129903, 2009.

Leng, J.S.; Lv, H.; Liu, Y.; Du, S. "Shape-memory polymer in response to solution". Advanced Engineering Materials, 10 (6), 592–595, July, 2008.

Leng, J.S.; Lv, H.; Liu, Y.; Du, S. "Qualitative separation of the effect of solubility parameter on the recovery behavior of shape-memory polymer". Smart Materials & Structures, 18, 085003, 2009.

Li, B.; Cheng, G. "The mechanism of PTC effect in polyethylene/carbon black composite". 6th International Conference on Properties and Applications of Dielectric Materials, 2000.

Liu, Y.; Lv, H.; Lan, X.; Leng, L.S. "Review of electro-activate shape-memory polymer composite". Composites Science and Technology, 69. 2064–2068, 2009.

Lyshevski, L.E. "Nanoactuators: Novel synchronous reluctance nanomachines". IEEE Nano2003, 2, 295–298, 2003.

Mc Cord M. A.; Rooks, M.J. "Electron Beam Lithography," in Handbook of Microlithography, Micromachining, and Microfabrication, Vol. 1,

Ch. 2, ed. by P. Rai-Choudhury, 139–249, SPIE Optical Engineering, Bellingham, WA, 1997.

Monthioux, M.; Kuznetsov, V.L. "Who should be given the credit for the discovery of carbon nanotubes?". Carbon, 44, 1621–1625, 2006.

Mootanah, R.; Bader, D.L. "Pressure sensors". Wiley Encyclopedia of Biomedical Engineering. John Wiley & Sons, 2006.

Razumiene, J.; Gureviciene, V.; Barkauskas, J.; *et al.* "Novel combined template for amperometric biosensors with changeable selectivity". Second International Conference on Biomedical Electronics and Devices, Special Session on Active Materials for Medical Devices (AMMD), Biodevices 2009, Porto, Portugal, 2009.

Ribeiro, C.; Gomes, P.J.; Ribeiro, P.A.; Raposo, M. "Polymeric film sensors based on PAH-PAZO ionic self-assembled multi-nanolayers". Second International Conference on Biomedical Electronics and Devices, Special Session on Active Materials for Medical Devices (AMMD), Biodevices 2009, Porto, Portugal, 2009.

Schwartz, M. "New materials, processes and methods technology". CRC Press, Taylor and Francis Group. Florida, 2006.

Selmi, A.; Friebel, C.; Doghri, I.; Hassis, H. "Prediction of the elastic properties of single walled carbon nanotube reinforced polymers: A comparative study of several micromechanical models". Composites Science and Technology, 67(10), 2071–2084, 2007.

Shadow Robot Company. "Tactile sensors as compact as a human fingertip". Press release (www.shadowrobot.com), 8th May 2007.

Spinks, G.M.; Wallace, G.G.; Baughman, R.H.; Dai, L. "Carbon nanotube actuators: Synthesis, properties and performance". In Bar-Cohen's "Electroactive polymer (EAP) actuators as artificial muscles: Reality, potential and challenges", 2004.

Takele, H.; Jebril, S.; Strunskus, T.; *et al.* "Tuning of electrical and structural properties of metal-polymer nanocomposite films prepared by co-evaporation technique". Applied Physics A: Materials Science and Processing, 92, 345–350, 2008.

TMC News. "Peratech: The upcoming technology of RFID for contactless access control, passports and credit cards is too easy to compromise warns Peratech; Peratech's ultrathin QTC switch technology prevents financial and identity theft". 5th September 2008.

Van Lagenhove, L.; Hertleer, C. "Smart clothing: A new live". International Journal of Clothing Science and Technology, 16(1/2), 63–72, 2004.

Vialle, G.; Di Prima, M.; Hocking, E.; *et al.* "Remote activation of nanomagnetite reinforced shape memory polymer foam". Smart Materials & Structures, 18, 115014, 2009.

Warwick, K. "Outthinking and enhancing biological brains". Biodevices 2008 – First International Conference on Biomedical Electronics and Devices. IEEE Engineering in Medicine and Biology Society. Madeira, January, 2008.

Weigel, Th.; Mohr, R.; Lendlein, A. "Investigation of parameters to achieve temperatures required to initiate the shape-memory effect of magnetic nanocomposites by inductive heating". Smart Materials & Structures, 18, 025011, 2009.

Zhu, Y.; Li, W.X. "Cytoxicity of carbon nanotubes". Science in China Series B: Chemistry, 51(11), 1021–1029, 2008.

Chapter 15

Novel Techniques, Methods and Processes for Active Materials in Medical Devices

Pilar Lafont Morgado and Andrés Díaz Lantada
Mechanical Engineering Department, E.T.S.I. Industriales,
Universidad Politécnica de Madrid, c/ José Gutiérrez Abascal 2,
28006 Madrid, Spain
plafont@etsii.upm.es, adiaz@etsii.upm.es

15.1 Introduction

The preceding chapters have focused on an explanation of the different families of active materials, whose use as sensors in medical devices or actuators can enormously enhance the diagnostic or therapeutic capabilities of more standard solutions.

After the three general introductory chapters, the first topics on materials have looked in very close, specific detail at the families with the largest range of medical applications to date (alloys and shape-memory polymers, electroactive polymers and ceramics). Many particularly innovative materials with a great potential for the future medical industry have been left for the topics at the end, although materials possessing properties in common have been grouped together to make study easier.

Up to now, specific aspects have been explained regarding the modelling, simulation, characterisation and processing of these main

Handbook of Active Materials for Medical Devices: Advances and Applications
Edited by Andrés Díaz Lantada

www.panstanford.com

families of intelligent materials. We have also shown how to design, manufacture and test medical devices that integrate these materials. The techniques, methods and processes dealt with have sometimes been very specific and only applicable to a specific family of active materials.

This chapter details different techniques, methods and processes that are the most multidisciplinary, and therefore applicable to many families of intelligent materials. Using these new tools can be of great benefit throughout the development of active material-based medical devices for sensors or actuators, and most particularly, for the stages of modelling and simulation, device design, prototype manufacture and *in vivo* and *in vitro* testing.

In this way, we hope to include a short review of the different tools that are coming to the fore (as a result of more powerful computers for calculations, the recent advances in materials science and the advent of new manufacturing technologies). Used in combination, these tools can provide a support for the entire development process of a new active medical device from the moment of conception right up to its first use.

These technologies complement the proposal for methodology included in the next chapter. So, having started out from the first introductory chapters on the development processes of products and standard medical devices, and taking the knowledge acquired of the main active materials as a basis, we have now arrived at a methodology that is more focused on medical devices whose activation for diagnostic or therapeutic purposes is based on intelligent materials as transducers.

15.2 New Trends in Modelling and Simulation

15.2.1 Artificial Neural Networks as a Modelling and Simulation Tool

The conventional approach to modelling, simulating and controlling dynamic systems, based on the development (and subsequent resolution) of theoretical analytical models, can be complemented by a proper use of the tools that fall within the framework of "artificial intelligence". Essentially, "artificial intelligence" uses a computer to attempt to reproduce what a human would do when tackling and solving a problem. Its advantages are now beginning to be appreciated, thanks to the enormous calculating capability acquired by computers in the last two decades.

The heading, "artificial intelligence", covers a set of techniques developed in the computer engineering sector, which is referred to globally as "soft computing" techniques. They are aimed at solving problems that are especially difficult due to the effects of non-linearities, which lead to excessively complex theoretical models. They are also of use for simulating new phenomena whose physical-chemical principles are still not known in detail or cannot be modelled mathematically.

Among these "soft computing" techniques we cannot fail to mention artificial neural networks, genetic algorithms and "fuzzy logic" techniques. Their foundations and applications are detailed in some excellent texts (Aminzadeh and Jamshidi, 1994; Yager and Zadeh, 1994; Jang *et al.*, 1997).

This section describes the use of artificial neural networks in more detail, due to their more direct application to the modelling of active materials. However, it may still be of interest to examine the use of other materials in order to provide continuity of the research described in this handbook.

Artificial neural networks, or ANN, are designed to emulate the behaviour of biological or natural neural networks. Each artificial neuron or node in the network has connections to other neurons from which it receives or transmits information. Each connection is assigned a specific weighting and each neuron has an activation threshold and a characteristic input/output function. One basic feature of neural networks is their ability to "learn" when subjected to a training process based on existing data (inputs and results) to arrive at a set of weights and thresholds suited to the neural network reproducing the required behaviour.

Once it has been trained, the ANN works as an input/output system with the ability to manage multiple inputs and outputs, which makes it especially suitable for simulating complex systems. They have remarkable applications in a wide range of areas like philosophy, psychology, economics, engineering and science, in general (Schalkoff, 1997; Haykin, 1999).

Some materials that are especially suited to modelling and simulation using artificial neural networks are the so-called multifunctional materials, either active or "intelligent". They are able to respond in a controlled way to different external physical or chemical stimuli, changing some of their properties.

As already analysed, the properties of these active materials help a wide range of functions to be integrated into a system, which, in combination with the major advances in micro and nano-fabrication technologies, has promoted the expansion of micro-electromechanical systems (MEMS) during the last two decades.

These systems are based on integrated functions and a reduction of size in order to attain optimised responses of materials and processes in terms of time and cost. Modelling these microsystems usually requires a thorough knowledge of various domains (mechanical, electrical, thermal, fluidic, magnetic etc.) and since their response usually exhibits major non-linear effects, analytical models can become too complicated to be of any practical use.

In order to solve these problems some researchers have begun to use neural networks to obtain models that allow approaching the in-service performance of these microsystems. A specific example was the application of ANN to modelling (so that it can then be controlled in real time) a micro-heat exchanger in which the thermal, fluid, electrical and mechanical couplings were a barrier to producing an accurate analytical model (Díaz, 1999, 2001; Gad-el-Hak, 2003).

Other researchers have also shown the usefulness of using neural networks to analyse information from sensors monitoring the behaviour of complex systems. Such networks have also been used to find anomalies when making a real-time prediction of the system being monitored, and detect problems by making comparisons with the measurements recorded by the sensors (Gulati, 2000; Rakowski, 2006).

They have also proven to be of use for processing the information from sensors (or sensor networks) that are sensitive to different stimuli and recognising the kind of stimulus that has generated a specific signal, as we have described earlier on for mobile robots with audio-tactile micro-sensors (Manoonpong, 2004) and for therapeutic robots with multiple pressure sensors, electrical field and temperature (Stiehl, 2005).

A clear example, chosen in this work, to show the benefits of using this type of approach to modelling multifunctional materials is quantum tunnelling composites. Their recent discovery, added to the complexity of producing a theoretical model to combine the quantum effects and the thermo-viscoelastic properties of the material, makes neural networks an excellent choice for achieving an especially good fit.

15.2.2 Application to Modelling Quantum Tunnelling Composites

Chapter 13 has dealt with different characterisation tests for quantum tunnelling composites, analysing the influence of such factors as applied pressure, application time and environmental temperature. As a result of these tests we now have 240 pieces of data (results of the electrical resistance of the material according to applied pressure, application time and environmental temperature) that can be used to train different artificial neural networks. Once they are trained, these neural models reproduce the system's behaviour within the range of variation of the properties studied.

In order to prepare, train and adjust the tests, and validate and simulate different neural models, we used the Mablab R2009b "nftool", an interactive tool from Neural Network Toolbox™ to adjust the functions. Seventy-percent of the 240 test samples (168 pieces of data) were used to train the various neural networks, 15% (36 pieces of data) as validation during the training process and the remaining 15% (36 pieces of data) to test the training received.

Training was done using the Levenberg–Marquardt back-propagation method. Having trained the neural networks, the response of each one was simulated by entering all the pressure, temperature and time conditions of the tests as inputs so as to be then able to compare the outputs of the networks with the electrical resistance values measured in the tests.

In the models, the input layer has three inputs, pressure, temperature and time, while the results layer provides a single value or output corresponding to the electrical resistance between the sides of the QTC sensor. As a transfer function, we chose the sigmoid function for the hidden layer as well as for the results, while it was the structure generated by Matlab that was entrusted with normalising the inputs in the range [0, 1], to optimise the calculation results with the "mapminmax" tool, as this usually results in faster learning and training (Gad-el-Hak, 2003). Figure 15.1 shows the schematic layout of a neural model with ten neurons for simulating these materials.

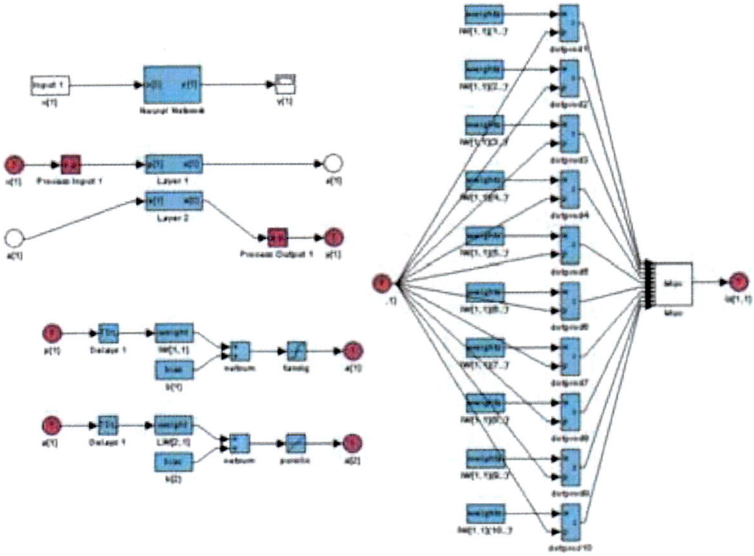

Figure 15.1 Simulink layout of a neural model used for modelling QTCs.

Figure 15.2 shows the goodness of the simple linear regression; on the one hand, of the data from a simulation based on an analytical model and test results, and on the other hand, of the data from a simulation based on a neural model and test results. The fit using the neural model is clearly more accurate due to the marked non-linearities of the system which lead to very complex analytical models. A logarithm scale was used to represent the values for electrical resistance as a function of pressure, due to its wide range of variation (several orders of magnitude).

Neural network-based models can also be used as part of a Matlab or Simulink model program to evaluate material behaviour in greater detail, even going a little beyond the test range. As an example, Fig. 15.3 shows a more complete representation. To produce the chart, the neural model was integrated into a Matlab program which was used to vary the applied pressure from 100 to 800 kPa (with 50 kPa increments), material temperature from 30 to 60°C (with 5°C increments) and the time taken was set at 120 s (for a quasi-permanent state evaluation).

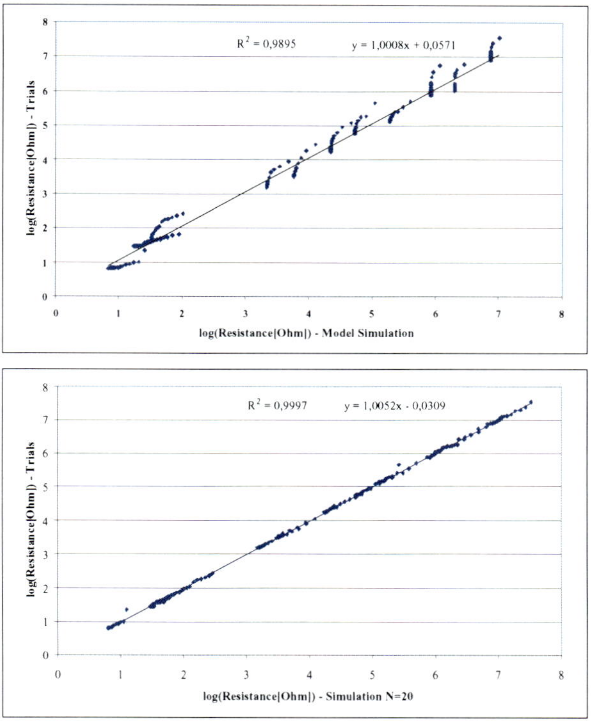

Figure 15.2 Simple linear regression between the analytical and test data-based model (upper image) and between the neural and test data-based model (lower image).

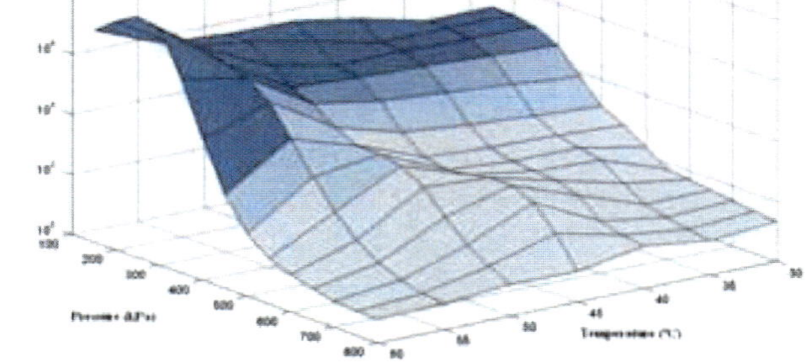

Figure 15.3 Electrical resistance as a function of pressure and temperature a in steady state. Simulation using the 20 neuron network. Additional details can be found in Díaz Lantada, 2010.

The fit shown was adequate in general terms, particularly for design work intended to evaluate the capability of this material as a sensor for the specified pressure range and for estimating the thermal effects of the environment on measurement. On some occasions, during the first few seconds of data collection, a slight misfit can be appreciated. We attribute this to the rapid variation in electrical resistance and the difficulty encountered by the measurement system to respond to variation rates above 1 MΩ/s. However, in a state of rest, the sensor exhibits such a high resistance that it is outside the measurement range of the device used. This adds further difficulties to measuring the first 5 seconds of each test, especially when the resistance values exceed 20 MΩ.

Nonetheless, these misfits are considerably reduced after 10 seconds of charge being applied, with the differences between steady state tests and simulations being very little, particularly for the 10 and 20 neuron models, although networks with an even smaller number of neurons can supply data of sufficient quality for a large number of studies and applications.

It should be pointed out that a more detailed knowledge of the properties of these materials combined with the use of high-capacity measuring and data recording equipment will allow gradual improvements in fitting the integration of other effects. These effects may well be of significance when expanding the ranges of variation of the variables of influence.

Moreover, using signal conditioning electronics in conjunction with measuring circuits designed ad hoc may help optimise the accuracy of measurement and fit the measurement range to the required application.

Some recently proposed solutions can be consulted in this regard (Shadow Robots' tactile sensors) or the alternatives that are typically used for conventional piezoelectric sensors (Elwenspoek and Wiegerink, 2001; Tekscan: Pressure mapping and force measurement).

However, the main objective of this study is to validate the use of artificial neural networks as a tool for simulating the behaviour of quantum tunnelling composites, and set out a standard methodology for simulating active materials by means of these tools.

Instead of resorting to analytical equations that include quantum effects and other thermomechanical factors such as the influence of the viscoelasticity of the polymer matrix on sensor response, the influence of pressure and temperature on the elasticity modulus and dynamic viscosity of the material, or certain thermal dilation-related effects, we opted to use neural networks because of the outstanding non-linearity of the aforementioned effects.

These non-linearities involve carrying out numerous characterisation tests on both the material and the devices into which it is integrated, as well as using different fitting constants, which makes it very difficult to attain accurate analytical models. However, simulations based on neural networks that have been properly trained with the data resulting from the characterisation, allow high precision fits, even with a small number of neurons and without any unnecessary increase in calculation time needed to be used.

It should be underlined that the neural network-based approach does not claim to replace complex analytical models, which are extremely useful for understanding the coupling between thermal, electrical and mechanical properties in these materials and the their subsequent response under ideal conditions. Our proposal is to use these neural models to complement the theoretical-analytical models when evaluating the behaviour of these sensors in wide ranges of applications where the effects of non-linearities are particularly marked and lead to analytical models that are too complex to be of practical use.

Thus, neural models can be highly suited to a more rapid simulation and comparison of prototypes manufactured from different active materials. This is because they do not require multiple property characterisation tests to be performed on the different materials used as sensors or actuators. All that needs to be characterised is the response of these prototypes to conditions of pressure and temperature in order to obtain sufficient data to ensure the neural networks are adequately trained.

Moreover, by using Matlab's Neural Network Toolbox™ after building and training a neural network, .m and .mdl files can be directly generated and integrated as sub-systems into more complex Matlab and Simulink models. This makes it simpler to design devices that use these materials as sensors and compare them with the existing alternatives when selecting a specific transducer.

We also think it would be interesting to consider using models with various neuron layers for optimising the precision-calculation time ratio, in addition to having a more detailed look at the influence on the results of the various fits of the training method as well as of the percentages of data used for training, validation and verification.

15.3 Novel Design Technologies

15.3.1 New Horizons for Customised Prosthesis Design

The leaps forward of the last decades in the different systems of medical image acquisition (principally computerised tomography, Doppler echography and magnetic resonance) have considerably increased the diagnostic capability of these systems as well as the reliability of the diagnoses based on these data and the ensuing decisions made regarding the therapy to be applied.

Computerised axial tomography (CAT) resulted from the research of two teams. One team led by Dr. Alan McLeod Cormack (who disclosed the theoretical formulation in 1962, 1963 and 1964) and the other by the engineer Godfrey Newbold Hounsfield (who built the first prototype in 1971), for which they received the Nobel Prize for Medicine in 1979.

The conventional CAT provides axial planes of the body by way of sections of a quality that is often higher than anatomical slices. This is achieved by using the simultaneous rotation of the tube producing the ray beam and the corona detectors. A computer calculates the dose absorbed at the different points of the slice during the rotational motion of the whole system, which displays an image on a screen.

Since the first TAC images in 1976, different generations have appeared in the search for ever faster processing speeds and better image quality while attempting to obtain reconstructions on other different axial planes that are of an acceptable quality, with a larger number of detectors and shorter study times.

Thanks to the important advances in hardware during these years a new computerised tomography (CT) has been developed, helical CT (HCT), which uses the continuous rotation of the detector and the X-ray source in combination with the continuous movement of the examination table. With this method of examination, 100% of the time is put to use. Moreover, with this system, data capture is not slice-by-slice as in axial CT, but results in the entire volume being captured so that slices can be reconstructed in all three dimensions of space.

One of the limitations of present-day CTs (64 detectors) is the radiation associated with cardiological examinations which require simultaneous gating with the patient's electrocardiogram. The latest generation models (256 detectors) have greatly improved the time resolution compared to the 64 detector models, and axial acquisition models ("step and shoot") are now being tested that allow reducing the dose of radiation received by the patient, but at the cost of limiting acquisition to one single cardiac cycle.

Combining this new hardware with the progress in software for processing the images taken enables more efficient diagnoses to be made from the more realistic and exact reconstructions achieved with 3D textures and images. An HCT 64 detector model was used for this work due to its having the precision required for subsequent customised design.

In fact, medical circles are now benefiting from the ability to exchange information from different medical image acquisition systems between centres and researchers. This is due to the "DICOM" (digital imaging and communication in medicine) standard having been set up and its now generalised use as a working format for a range of three-dimensional image reconstruction software, particularly since the introduction of version DICOM 3.0 in 1993.

"Mimics" (Materialise NV) programs have also appeared which not only perform three-dimensional reconstruction from medical images but also carry out simple operations on the reconstructions and convert them to other formats that can be accessed by "CAD-CAM" computer-aided design and manufacture programs. These CAD-CAM programs (Solid Edge, Catia, NX-5, I-DEAS, Rhino, Solid Works and others) form a wide range of computer tools that are at the service of engineers, architects and design professionals.

The power of these software packages together with their ability to manage information from medical images as a basis for design, means that at present, customised prostheses can be designed in a matter of hours, while comparing alternative designs is also made easier (Hieu *et al.*, 2002).

However, the use of customised prostheses or implants has been historically sporadic, practically always the fruit of research projects. This is basically due to problems of cost and timescale which have always prevented these customised prostheses or implants from competing with standard mass-produced designs.

Nonetheless, in recent years a set of technologies known as "rapid prototyping" have made major inroads into industry. This has led to reduced time scales and costs by manufacturing parts directly from the information on their geometry stored in the files of programs like CAD-CAM or Mimics and to the advent of new capabilities for a customised response in the design of implants and prostheses, with a social impact that is likely to be highly positive (Schwarz, 2005; Kucklick, 2006).

15.3.2 Application Case: Personalised Design Adapted to Hard Tissue

The case study set out in this sub-section as an example details the process for producing a customised hip prosthesis design from the information from a nuclear magnetic resonance. The aim was to produce a non-cemented prosthesis where the metal part is pressure-mounted inside the femur and must therefore be made to fit the space.

The design was made in the Machine Engineering Division of Universidad Politécnica de Madrid Polytechnic University with the aid of the available CAD-CAE-CAM technologies (www.dim.etsii.upm.es). More detailed information may be found in the references (Osuna, 2008; Ojeda, 2009).

The usual procedure for carrying out a customised examination with a view to using a prosthetic device usually begins either by taking a computerised tomography (CT) or a nuclear magnetic resonance (MRI/NMRI) of the patient needing the prosthesis.

Then, with the aid of .dicom or .dcm (Digital Communications in Medicine) format, the information from the CT or MRI can be transferred to a program such as "Mimics" so that it can be displayed in 3D, as Fig. 15.4 shows.

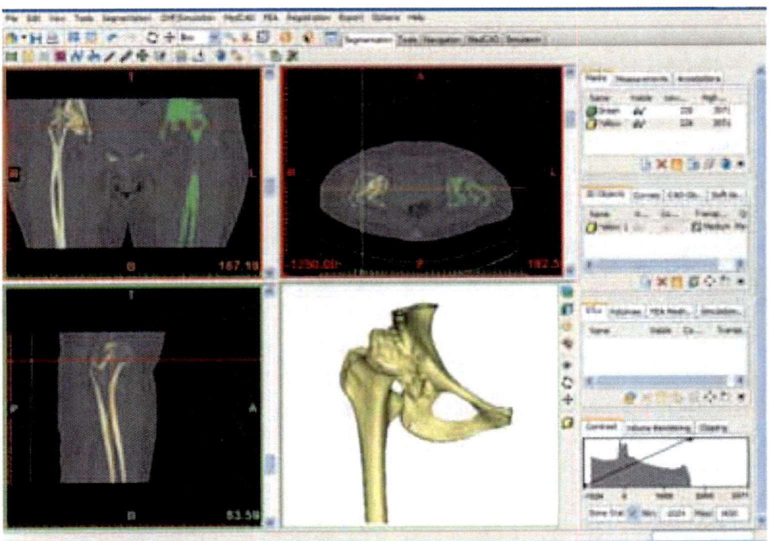

Figure 15.4 3D digitisation of the hip prior to an arthroplasty (Mimics, Materialise NV).

These programs usually include modules that allow selecting part of the patient's bone geometry and storing it in .stl or .igs formats that can be read by other CAD programs after processing the images "slice by slice".

Having selected the relevant part of the patient's femur (in this example, the internal cavity to which the metal part of a customised prosthesis must be adapted), this three-dimensional geometry can be transferred to a format that is valid for a design program and this femoral zone can be used as the basis for a customised prosthesis design, as can be seen in the Fig. 15.5 (Ojeda *et al.*, 2009).

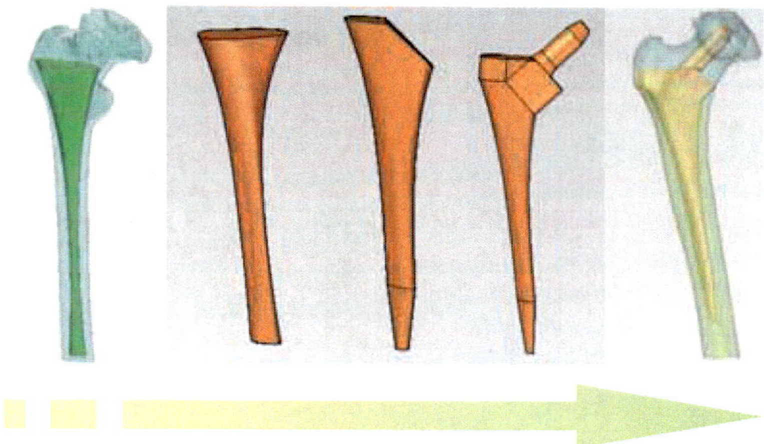

Figure 15.5 Customised femur design process using a three-dimensional reconstruction of the patient's femur based on the information from a magnetic resonance.

Taking the designs produced by CAD programs, this geometry can be converted into files that are recognised by CAE programs, that is, computer–aided calculation to which the finite-element method can be applied as a simulation tool for verifying that the design is adequate for the in-service loads to be borne by the final implant.

Until just a few years ago, this conversion was not always direct and the use of .igs or .stl formats led to some loss of information. However, the most widely used CAD design programs are becoming more and more flexible in saving files and using different formats that are compatible with other CAD and CAE programs with FEM capabilities (Catia, NX-6, Solid Works, Rhino, Ansys, Nastran etc.). In fact, some programs like "Mimics" with the ability to reconstruct the information from medical images in 3D, cannot only transfer files to other design programs (and rapid prototyping machines) through their use of .stl format, but are also beginning to include specific outputs for finite-element calculation and simulation programs.

Figure 15.6 shows an example of how the femoral part of a hip prosthesis behaves where the ball receives the load from the acetabulum (2000 N is the value usually chosen for critical situations), and where the metal part is pressure-mounted inside the femur. The simulations were performed using the NX-6 program (Siemens PLM Software Solutions), taking an initial CAD design produced by Solid Edge v.20. The model and the movement solution (enlarged scale) are shown in the figure.

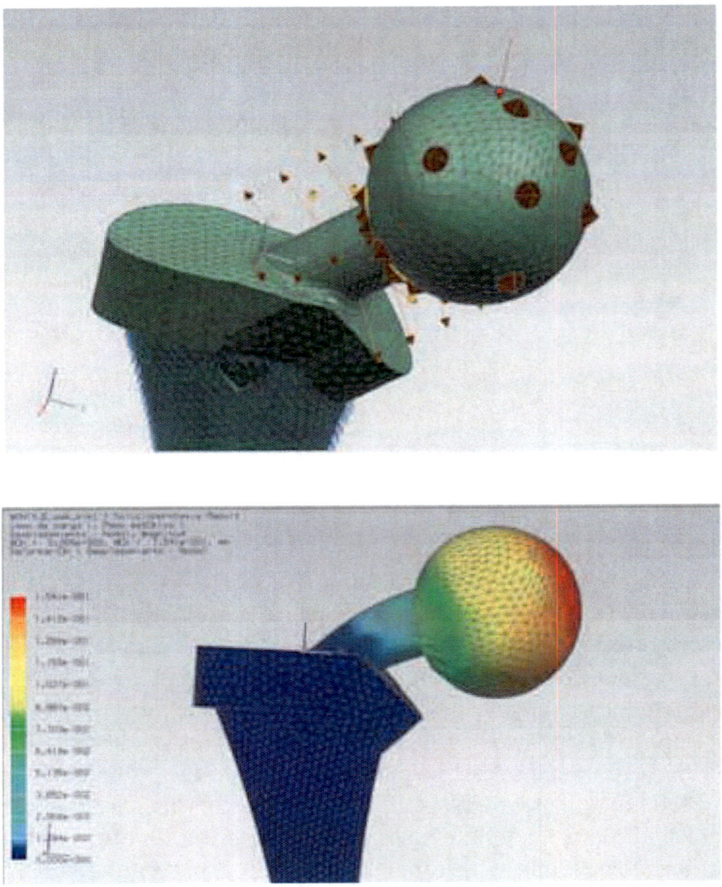

Figure 15.6 FEM model and the simulation result of a customised femur implant under load.

These FEM simulations can be also used to evaluate the effect on tissue, both rigid and soft. To do this, not only the implant but also the whole set comprising the geometry of the implant and surrounding tissue needs to be exported to the calculation program. By using different contact models, the in-service behaviour of the implant and its effects on the surrounding tissue can be reproduced. This is essential for evaluating any harm that may be caused to the receptor organism by the implant.

Recent research has focused on using simulation to evaluate the effects of implants on body tissue, both during surgical operations and the immediate postoperative period, in the case of conventional implants (Ojeda, 2009), as well as during the process of activating and modifying the geometry of active implants (Díaz Lantada, 2009). We have already mentioned the results of this work in Chapter 5, although the process has become directly generalised to other families following the same methodology as that described.

However, the importance of using samples and prototypes for validating the results of computer-aided simulation should not be forgotten. Making some prior estimations "by rule of thumb" with simple performance models is also helpful for ruling out calculation errors and keeping an eye open for unexpected deviations. On the other hand, when using FEM programs, it is always good practice to go by the widely used International System of Units, when entering model data and properties, in order to avoid operational errors. This is especially important when developing devices with a high responsibility, like those used in the Medical Industry.

15.3.3 Application Case: Personalised Design Adapted to Soft Tissue

The major advances in customised prosthesis design have traditionally been linked to bone structures, since bone tissue density is easily identifiable, making it easier to produce the associated design more easily than for soft structures and tissue. Bone tissue appears as a very distinct white on the Hounsfield Scale. This is an advantage when processing information from medical imaging tools, with programs like "Mimics".

However, in soft organs the difference in density between tissues is very small and does not let the different structures be identified separately, which is an enormous barrier to customised design work. This is the case with cardiac prostheses and in particular, for the mitral annuloplasty rings shown here as an example of application (Díaz Lantada, 2009).

In these cases, some reference point needs to be found in the medical images that will help the three-dimensional reconstruction of the target zone of the organ or soft tissue. In the example shown, cardiac CT images were used to identify in each "slice" the points of insertion of the valve leaflets in the patient's mitral ring (see Fig. 15.7). These points were inserted through CAD program coordinates in order to get an idea of the three-dimensional morphology of the patient's mitral ring to which the prosthetic annuloplasty ring is to be adapted; this can be seen in the figure. The design was made in the Machine Engineering Division of Universidad Politécnica de Madrid, with the aid of the available CAD-CAE-CAM technologies (www.dim.etsii.upm.es).

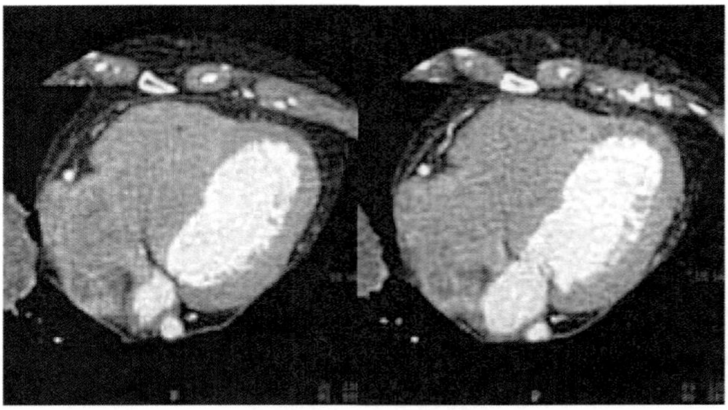

Figure 15.7 Cardiac CT images: two cross-sections are shown as an example (from a total of 30 images used to reconstruct the valve ring).

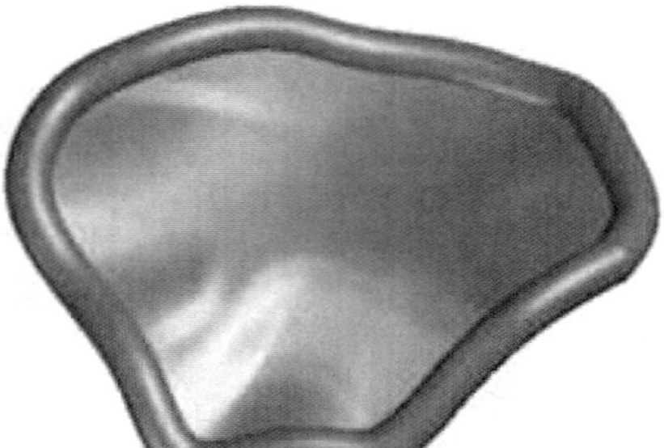

Figure 15.8 Design of a customised annuloplasty ring for the treatment of mitral valve insufficiency. It was obtained from CT information (Annals of Biomedical Engineering, 2010).

Further information on the complete design process of prostheses adapted to soft tissue and the customised design methodology proposed may be found in the references section.

But whatever the case, the information from medical imaging technologies combined with rapid prototyping technologies, mainly layer manufacturing technologies (as already mentioned in the handbook), are not only enormously useful in planning surgical work (Binder, 2005; Gilon *et al.*, 2002; Mottl-Link *et al.*, 2008; Kim *et al.*, 2008), but also have considerable advantages when rapid customised implants are required.

From these first solid models manufactured by LMT, other rapid prototyping technologies denominated as "second stage" can be used to produce rapid shape-copying moulds. These moulds can be obtained from numerous materials such as silicones, ceramics, ceramics with a metal load and others, and allow casting stronger materials inside them than the original models. They enable prototypes to be produced that meet the in-service specifications.

Among the many materials that can be cast in rapid moulds for producing end parts are a large number of polymers (especially a wide range of polyurethanes), metals and alloys. The ability to produce prototypes in both stiff and flexible materials means that the different requirements of cardiologists and surgeons can be met, as well as there being more likelihood of being able to offer patient-customised adaptations. Customised prototypes can also be obtained in shape-memory materials by casting polymers or alloys possessing these properties that will admit the postoperative geometric changes, as has recently been proposed (Lafont *et al.*, 2000, 2006, 2008; Díaz Lantada, 2008, 2009).

There are also major implications for teaching, since models of different organs can be cheaply produced to conduct practical surgical sessions on these models, also using implant prototypes with different geometries and mechanical properties.

As an alternative to the combined layer manufacturing technologies described above, high speed numerical control machine tools can be used. According to the information received from a 3D CAD file, they enable prototypes to be produced, usually in metal materials that can be processed by tooling to eliminate material from a starting block.

When the prototypes have been produced in the final materials, various surface deposits can be used by means of physical or chemical vapour deposition technology (particularly the new DLC "diamond-like carbon") coatings, as well as textile coatings to ensure the biocompatibility of the device and facilitate its implanting (Salgueiredo *et al.*, 2008).

In all cases, to optimise the safety of customised devices and ensure they can be used, they are required to comply with the guidelines of the "European Directive on Medical Devices – 93/42/EEC". It is also advisable to follow the recommendations of ISO Standard 13485 on medical device quality, as well as specific regulations on material characterisation tests (ISO and ASTM Standards).

Future improvements to medical image acquisition systems regarding the exchange of information between these systems and rapid prototyping machines will promote the use of customised medical devices in the coming years. The prototypes will be also produced with greater precision and speed.

15.4 New Manufacturing Technologies: Combining Synthetic and Biological Materials

15.4.1 Medical Applications of "Rapid Prototyping and Manufacturing" Technologies

Previous chapters have dealt with the advantages of using rapid manufacturing and prototyping technologies to complement the product development process as a way to reduce time scales and costs, particularly when active materials are involved whose response to different stimuli is still being studied.

They also have a major use in different areas of the Biomedical Industry. With further research, they may well complement the specific applications for these technologies described in the handbook and give rise to new application proposals for intelligent materials.

For the time being, the main applications for rapid prototyping technologies in relation to medical device development can be grouped into the following categories:

- **Biological models for clinical diagnosis.** On occasions, it is appropriate to reproduce a diseased organ by combining the information from medical imaging and rapid prototyping technologies to make a better diagnosis (Mottl-Link *et al.*, 2008).

- **Models for training, planning and surgical aid.** As a teaching aid or for conducting pre-surgery tests, the use of models produced by rapid prototyping is becoming more and more widespread, especially for maxillofacial surgery and dentistry. Sometimes support or guide tools are also produced that can be adapted to the surface of a specific organ to help make incisions and perform operations (Momi *et al.*, 2005; Naranjo *et al.*, 2010).
- **Biological models as an aid to *in vitro* tests.** Some complex physiological and anatomical examinations can be more simply conducted by using synthetic biological models of certain body structures, particularly those connected with hemodynamic studies (Freitas *et al.*, 2010).
- **Direct manufacture of implantable devices.** The feasibility of customising implantable devices that combine medical imaging technology and RP tools has led to research being conducted into the direct manufacture of a very wide range of implants to complement mass-produces ones. This is particularly true for dentistry due to the lower risk of these operations (Kai *et al.*, 2000; Ovsianikov *et al.*, 2007).
- **Direct manufacture of active implantable devices.** Some works have shown the feasibility of directly producing active implantable devices using RP technologies. However, the commercialisation of these products is still pending certain steps forward in device biocompatibility and the activation/detection capabilities of the active materials used (Díaz Lantada, 2009).
- **Direct manufacture of support material for tissue engineering.** As will be explained further on, these technologies are especially suitable for obtaining biodegradable supports on which to cultivate tissues for use in transplants and operations (Mironov *et al.*, 2006, 2009; Bartolo, 2009; Gómez Ribelles *et al.*, 2010).
- **Validating active material behaviour.** The original activation principles of different active material families make prototypes extremely useful for comparing sensors or actuators that are the possible candidates for a specific active medical device (Díaz Lantada, 2010).

However, attention is being more and more focused on the new techniques that it is hoped will come along in the next three decades for the production of complex geometry three-dimensional prototypes using biological materials, which will even be able to generate artificial tissues and organs, as we shall now describe.

15.4.2 Tissue and Organ Prototyping using Synthetic and Biological Materials

We have seen that in the context of medical device development and the biomedical industry, one of the major areas of application for these rapid prototyping technologies is tissue engineering. Since the 1980s, outstanding researchers like Eugene Bell and Robert S. Langer, both professors at the MIT, began looking at how to produce scaffolds with materials and geometries that were suitable for cell culture and tissue growth and could be used in surgical operations (Langer *et al.*, 1993).

The gradual progress in the field of biodegradable polymers together with the advances in more flexible rapid manufacturing technologies, means that at present, complex geometry scaffolds can be obtained to which living cells with growth factors adhere, and which multiply until they cover the scaffold. Having reached this stage, the set (scaffold + coating) is implanted into the damaged parts of the body. After being implanted, the cells adapt to their environment and reproduce the functions of the surrounding tissue, while the scaffold is gradually reabsorbed (Hollister, 2005; Gómez Ribelles *et al.*, 2010). All this has led to changes in the approach to solving many surgical problems.

It is hoped to continue work on this progress with a view to obtaining three-dimensional biological structures that will one day lead to the additive fabrication of human organs. The firm Enviosiontec GmbH has already developed the Bioplotter®, with which small three-dimensional structures are being obtained by the "layer-by-layer" deposit of cells together with the biocompatible material, and the initial use of the concept of a "bioprinter" looks promising.

A larger number of printing technologies based on appropriately modified conventional RP technologies are being sought, which, it is hoped will lead to more affordable machines.

This progress may open up new horizons to the treatment of many diseases by combining synthetic and biological materials to produce veins, capillaries, arteries, bones and soft organs or at least part of them. By using machines with several heads that can deposit different materials biological tissue could be directly obtained with synthetic implants pre-integrated into them. This would endow the newly generated tissue with mechanical consistency.

However, there is still a long way to go, not only regarding the precision of these "bioprinters" and the biological and biomedical materials they are capable of depositing, but also regarding the manufacture of structures larger than 1 cm^3. It would appear that the development of a capillary network to provide the newly generated three-dimensional cell structures with nutrients is currently one of the major limitations (Mironov *et al.*, 2006; Bartolo, 2008, 2009).

Organising specific work sessions to facilitate information exchange among researchers is a particularly useful idea, usually within a framework of bioengineering congresses where rapid prototyping applications in the medical sector can be discussed, and people can join forces to go forward together.

Worth mentioning are the "World Bioprinting Congresses", the "International Workshop on Bioprinting and Biopatterning" and the "International Conferences on Biomedical Electronics and Devices – Biodevices 2008, 2009, 2010", as part of which, they have developed the "Special Session on Rapid Prototyping for Improving the Development of Biodevices".

15.5 Advances in *In vivo* and *In vitro* Testing

The advances in multidomain simulation tools that use FEM calculation, combined with the progress in computer-aided design and manufacturing technologies for prototype production, have provoked recent changes of approach towards the testing of a newly developed medical device.

We have already mentioned how programs like ANSYS Multiphysics, NX-6, Abaqus, Comsol Multiphysics and others help provide customised design and simulation solutions, including couplings between mechanical, electrical, thermal, fluid and magnetic domains. Furthermore, these packages are incorporating working environments that are specifically focused on micro-electromechanical systems (MEMS) that have a whole range of biomedical applications (Gad-el-Hak, 2003).

A little more than a decade ago, most physiology and anatomy laboratories resorted to using animal models directly, while nowadays simulation tools are being used to measure and simulate how a system responds to different stimuli. This is helping to reduce the number of animals sacrificed for scientific purposes to the absolute minimum necessary. Decisive in this respect is the work of major teams who are using numerical methods to model and simulate the chemical-electrical-mechanical-fluid behaviour of various body organs. This can be seen in various references on cardiac modelling developed with the collaboration of different departments of the University of Karlsruhe (Schenkel *et al.*, 2009).

Becoming more and more common is the construction of test benches using models of different organs and structures (often obtained through a combined use of medical imaging technologies and computer-aided rapid manufacturing tools) to reproduce the geometry and function of a part of the body intended to receive an active implant. These test benches are less costly and more immediate than tests on animal models. Test conditions can also be controlled to conduct thorough studies on the influence of different design parameters. The reproduction of body conditions must be as exact as possible, although it is usually sufficient to maximise certain load effects to test the devices in more unfavourable circumstances in order to achieve safe designs (Reul *et al.*, 1996; Wojnarowski and Mirota, 2006).

To assist this progress in obtaining realistic models for *in vitro* tests, many multinationals devoted to medical device production are developing synthetic tissues (usually polymers for soft organs and ceramics for hard tissues) and biological tissues (using controlled cell growth on appropriate scaffolds), that can be purchased for this research.

Outstanding is the Edwards Lifesciences' "Bovine Pericardial Patch" shown in Fig. 15.9, whose use has led to exceptional results, both *in vitro* and *in vivo*, even when implanted in human patients (Banbury *et al.*, 2002). Developing these materials obviously involves exhaustive biomechanical and biological testing (Vesely and Mako, 1998; Pires, 1992; Cunanan *et al.*, 2001; Obermiller *et al.*, 2004), which allows validating how the properties adapt to the final purpose, either by *in vitro* tests, *in vivo* tests or implantation into a living organism.

Quite logically, there are innovative centres for minimally invasive surgery devoted to research work that have adequate staff and resources (medical imaging teams, operating theatres, animal house, different species etc.), which are valuable when carrying out the pre-approval testing of an implantable device. These centres usually participate in teaching work in collaboration with faculties of biology, medicine or engineering and also provide support for research projects, frequently by doing the *in vivo* testing of a new product.

However, just to give one example, the cost of asking of these centres to test a new implantable device in a swine model can easily reach €50,000 to 250,000 until satisfactory results are achieved, depending on the death toll associated with the device in the initial tests, the preparation and post-surgical monitoring required and the staff and equipment needed for the test.

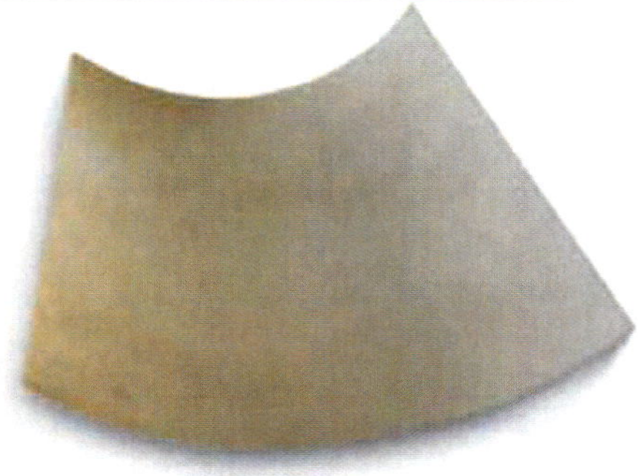

Figure 15.9 Edwards "Bovine Pericardial Patch" (www.edwards.com).

For all these reasons, it should be borne in mind that working with animals is a privilege that should not be taken lightly (Kucklick, 2006). It is always essential to plan every issue involved, right down to the last detail, with the aid of reference data, simulations and prior *in vitro* tests, until unknowns such as the following can be properly answered:

- The parameters of interest for statistical validation and pre-commercial studies
- The number of animals required
- The organ involved
- The species that are most like human beings
- The animal models used in similar cases
- The equipment needed, especially when tools are required that are not usually used in operating theatres
- The advance preparation required for the animals (cleaning and looking after, drugs, the induction of pathologies etc.)
- Post-surgical needs
- The overall cost of the tests, both in time and money

It is always a very good practice to discuss all issues thoroughly with the members of the team involved in the development, and to take on external consultants specialising in *in vivo* testing if the end results are to be optimised. Some additional advice can be consulted in the last Chapter 16, which aims to summarise the concepts set out in this handbook.

15.6 Main Conclusions

The challenge of using new materials as an aid to solving problems of technology is both exciting and formidable. New materials, such as intelligent or multifunctional materials bring with them risks and uncertainty, as they might not work in the expected manner, which for medical applications is particularly critical.

For this reason, the preceding chapters have focused on detailing methods, techniques and processes that are suited to the principle families of active materials, regarding characterisation, modelling and processing, together with some notions on the design, manufacture and testing of the medical devices based on these materials.

Although the new materials require investment in research and experimentation to gain sufficient knowledge of their in-service response, the new horizons they have to offer make all the effort worthwhile, as we have seen from the applications and case studies described for the different types of intelligent materials. As an aid to the research and experimental work required to understand these materials in sufficient detail, various multidisciplinary tools have been described in this chapter that are beginning to prove themselves useful for studies focused on numerous families of active materials.

Related to the field of modelling and simulating the response of these transducers to external stimuli, we have shown the efficacy of properly trained artificial neural network-based approaches using precise information from characterisation tests.

Regarding "state-of-the-art" design tools, we have shown the benefits of using the information from medical imaging technologies combined with computer-aided design tools, to obtain customised implantable device designs (passive or active) for better and less invasive treatment. The process can be directly applied to implants adapted to bone tissue, due to the excellent definition of the medical images. Although some additional precautions need to be taken, the process is beginning to show promising results for implants adapted to organs and soft tissues.

Linked to design technologies are manufacturing technologies which are also experiencing very significant advances that can now be put to good use to produce rapid prototypes to be used for testing throughout the development process. It is expected that in the near future, these technologies will be used to make combinations of synthetic and biological materials to develop more effective active biodevices.

Finally, some forms of activation for device testing have been dealt with that are becoming more and more based on the combined use of simulation tools and exhaustive *in vitro* testing before setting out on costly *in vivo* testing, which is also necessary but in the right measure. For conducting the *in vitro* testing of active devices, it is of enormous help to obtain three-dimensional biological models of the organs involved by using "layer manufacturing technologies" followed by second phase rapid prototyping technologies to produce replicas using synthetic biological tissue to simulate the properties of body tissue.

Further and more specific information on the issues dealt with can be found by consulting the references included in the following section. Consulting Chapter 16 after this chapter, is also of interest as a summary of the knowledge acquired throughout the handbook, with a view to developing active material-based medical devices.

References

Aminzadeh, F.; Jamshidi, M. "Soft computing: Fuzzy logic, neural networks and distributed artificial intelligence". Prentice Hall. Englewood Clifs, NJ, 1994.

Banbury, M.K.; Cosgrove, D.M.III; Thomas, J.D.; *et al.* "Hemodynamic stability during 17 years of the Carpentier-Edwards aortic pericardial bioprosthesis". Annals of Thoracic Surgery, 73, 1460-1465, 2002.

Bartolo, P.J.S.; Almeida, H.; Laoui, T. "Rapid prototyping and manufacturing for tissue engineering scaffolds". Tissue Engineering, 36(1), 1–9, 2009.

Bartolo, P.J.S.; Bidanda, B. "Biomaterials and prototyping applications in medicine". Springer Verlag, 2008.

Binder, T.; Moertl, D.; Mundigler, G.; *et al.* "Stereolithographic biomodeling to create tangible hard copies of cardiac structures from echocardiographic data: *In vitro* and *in vivo* validation". Journal of the American College of Cardiology, 35, 230–237, 2005.

Cormack, A.M. "Representation of a function by its line integrals with some radiological applications". Journal of Applied Physics, 35, 2908–2913, 1964.

Cunanan, C.M.; Cabiling, C.M.; Dinh, T.T.; *et al.* "Tissue characterization and calcification potential of commercial bioprosthetic heart valves". Annals of Thoracic Surgery, 71, 417–421, 2001.

Díaz Lantada, A. "Metodología para el desarrollo de dispositivos médicos basados en el empleo de polímeros activos como sensores y actuadores". PhD Thesis. Mechanical Engineering Department, Universidad Politécnica de Madrid, 2009.

Díaz Lantada, A.; Lafont, P.; *et al.* Treatment of Mitral Valve Insufficiency by Shape-Memory Polymer Based Active Annuloplasty. Biodevices 2008 – International Conference on Biomedical Electronics and Devices. INSTICC Press, 1, 17–22, 2008.

Díaz Lantada, A.; Lafont Morgado, P.; Echávarri Otero, J.; *et al.* "Neural network approach to modelling the behaviour of quantum tunnelling composites as multifunctional sensors". *Smart Materials* and Structures, 19(12), 125007, 2010".

Díaz Lantada, A.; Lafont, P.; Muñoz-García, J.; *et al.* "Stress-strain simulations for optimising the design of shape-memory polymer based annuloplasty rings". "World Congress on Medical Physics and Biomedical Engineering 2009". 7–12 September 2009 in Munich.

Díaz Lantada, A.; Lafont Morgado, P.; *et al.* "Intelligent expandable structures based on the improved activation of shape memory polymers". Biodevices 2010 – International Conference on Biomedical Electronics and Devices: Special Session on Rapid Prototyping for Improving the Development of Biodevices. IEEE Engineering in Medicine and Biology Society. 20–23 January 2010 in Valencia.

DICOM Standard – Digital Imaging and Communications in Medicine, Strategic Document available from: http://medical.nema.org

Elwenspoek, M.; Wiegerink, R. "Mechanical Microsensors". Springer Verlag, 2001.

Freitas, V.; Queijo, L.; Lima, R. "Rapid prototyping of 3D models to hemodynamic studies". Biodevices 2010 – International Conference on Biomedical Electronics and Devices: Special Session on Rapid Prototyping for Improving the Development of Biodevices. IEEE Engineering in Medicine and Biology Society. 20–23 January 2010 in Valencia.

Gad-el-Hak, M. (Chief Editor) "The MEMS Handbook". CRC Press, New York, 2003.

Gilon, D.; Cape, E.G.; Handschumacher, M.D.; *et al.* "Effect of three-dimensional valve shape on the hemodynamics of aortic stenosis: Three-dimensional echocardiographic stereolithography and patient studies. Journal of the American College of Cardiology, 40(8), 1479–1486, 2002.

Gómez Ribelles, J.L.; Monleón Pradas, M.; García Gómez, R.; *et al.* "The role of three-dimensional scaffolds in the regeneration of joint cartilage". Biodevices 2010 – International Conference on Biomedical Electronics and Devices: Special Session on Rapid Prototyping for Improving the Development of Biodevices. IEEE Engineering in Medicine and Biology Society. 20–23 January 2010 in Valencia.

Gulati, S.; Zak, M. "Neural-network approach to analysis of sensor data". NASA Tech Briefs, November 2000.

Harrysson O.; Hosni, Y.A.; Nayfeh, J.F.; *et al.* "Custom-designed orthopaedic implants evaluated using FEM analysis of patient computed tomography data". BMC Musculoskeletal Disorders, 8(91), 2007. Haykin, S. "Neural networks: A comprehensive foundation". Prentice Hall 2nd Edition, Englewood Cliffs, NJ, 1999.

Hieu, L.C.; Schiller, C.; Rasche, C.; *et al.* Design and manufacturing of personalized implants and standardized templates for cranioplasty applications". Industrial Technology, 2(11–14). 1025–1030. IEEE ICIT '02, 2002.

Hollister, S.J. "Porous scaffold design for tissue engineering". Nature Materials, 4, 518–524, July, 2005.

Hounsfield, G.N. "Computerized transverse axial scanning (tomography): Part 1. Description of system". British Journal of Radiology. 46, 1016–1022, 1973.

Jang, J.S.R.; Sun, C.T.; Mizutani, E. "Neuro-fuzzy and soft computing: A computational approach to learning and machine intelligence". Prentice Hall. Englewood Clifs, NJ, 1997.

Jarrousse, O.; Fritz, T.; Doessel, O. "Implicit time integration in a volumetric mass-spring system for modeling myocardial elastomechanics". World Congress on Biophysics and Biomedical Engineering. 7–12 September 2009 in Munich.

Kai, C.C.; Meng, C.S.; Ching, L.S.; *et al.* "Facial prosthetic model fabrication using rapid prototyping tools". Integrated Manufacturing Systems, 11(1), 42–53, 2000.

Keller, D.; Kalayciyan, R.; Doessel, O.; Seemann, G. "Fast creation of endocardial stimulation profiles for the realistic simulation of body surface ECGs".

World Congress on Biophysics and Biomedical Engineering. 7–12 September 2009 in Munich.

Kim, M.; Klein, A.J.; Carroll, J.D.; *et al.* "Rapid prototyping: A new tool in understanding and treating structural heart disease. Circulation, 117, 2388–2394, 2008.

Kucklick, T.R. "The Medical Device R&D Handbook". CRC Press, Taylor & Francis Group, 2006.

Lafont, P.; Lorenzo, H. "Rapid tooling: Moldes rápidos a partir de estereolitografía". Revista de Plásticos Modernos 79(524), 150–156, 2000.

Lafont, P.; Díaz Lantada, A.; *et al.* Documento de Patente P200603149: "Sistema activo de anuloplastia para tratamiento de la insuficiencia mitral y otras patologías cardiovasculares". Oficina Española de Patentes y Marcas; 2006.

Lafont, P.; Díaz Lantada, A.; *et al.* Patent Document WO/2008/071817: "Active annuloplasty system for the progressive treatment of valvular insufficiencies and other cardiovascular pathologies". World Intellectual Property Organization – International Bureau; 2008.

Langer, R.S.; Vacanti, J.P. "Tissue Engineering". Science, 260, 920–926, 1993.

Lentz, N.; Kikillus, N.; Bolz, A. "A screening method to detect atrial fibrillation with symbolic dynamics". World Congress on Biophysics and Biomedical Engineering. 7–12 September 2009 in Munich.

Leta, R.; *et al.* "Coronariografía no invasiva mediante tomografía computarizada con 16 detectores: estudio comparativo con la angiografía coronaria invasiva". Revista Española de Cardiología, 57(3), 217–224, 2004.

Louis, A.K. "Medical imaging: state of the art and future development". Inverse Problems. 8, 709–738, 1992.

Manoonpong, P.; Pasemann, F.; Fischer, J. "Neural processing of auditory-tactile sensor data to perform reactive behaviour of walking machines". Proceedings of the IEEE International Conference on Mechatronics and Robotics (MechRob' 04), 2004.

Medical Imaging and Technology Alliance, Information available from: http://www.medicalimaging.org

Mironov, V.; Reis, N.; Derby, B. "Review: Bioprinting – A beginning". Tissue Engineering, 12(4), 631–634, 2006.

Mironov, V.; Trusk, T.; Kasyanov, V.; *et al.* "Biofabrication: A 21st century manufacturing paradigm". Biofabrication, 1, 1–16, 2009.

Momi, E. De.; Pavan, E.; Motyl, B.; *et al.* "Hip joint anatomy virtual and stereolithographic reconstruction for preoperative planning of total hip replacement". Computer Assisted Radiology and Surgery, 1281, 708–712, 2005.

Mottl-Link, S.; *et al.* "Physical models aiding in complex congenital heart surgery". The Society of Thoracic Surgeons. Annals of Thoracic Surgery 86, 273–277, 2008.

Naranjo, V.; Lloréns, R.; Alcañiz, M.; *et al.* "MIRACLE: A CAD/CAM system for the manufacture of dental surgical splints". Biodevices 2010 - International Conference on Biomedical Electronics and Devices: Special Session on Rapid Prototyping for Improving the Development of Biodevices. IEEE Engineering in Medicine and Biology Society. 20–23 January 2010 in Valencia.

Narula, J. "State of the art of medical imaging: From molecule to function in heart failure. Circulation Journal, 69(1), 25, 2005.

NEMA - The Association of Electrical and Medical Imaging Equipment Manufacturers, Information available from: http://www.nema.org

Obermiller, J.F.; Hodde, J.P.; McAlexander, C.S.; *et al.* "A comparison of suture retention strengths of three biomaterials". Medical Science Monitoring, 10(1), 1–5, 2004.

Ohnesorge, B.M.; *et al.* "Multi-slice CT in cardiac imaging". Springer-Verlag (p. 15–59). New York, 2002.

Ojeda Diaz, C. "Estudio de la influencia de estabilidad primaria en el diseño de vástagos de prótesis de cadera personalizadas". PhD Thesis. Universidad Politécnica de Madrid, 2009.

Ojeda Díaz, C.; Osuna López, J.; Lafont Morgado, P.; Díaz Lantada, A. "Estudio de la estabilidad primaria, influencia en el diseño de vástagos de prótesis femorales personalizadas: Aplicación a paciente específico". 3° Congresso Nacional de Biomecânica. Sociedade Portuguesa de Biomecânica. 11–12 February 2009 in Braganza.

Osuna, J.E. "Combinación de tecnologías para la optimización del desarrollo de prótesis". Master Thesis. Universidad Politécnica de Madrid, 2008.

Ovsianikov, A.; Chichkov, B.; Adunka, O.; *et al.* "Rapid prototyping of ossicular replacement prostheses". Applied Surface Science, 253(15), 6603-6607, 2007.

Pires, A.C.; Saporito, W.F.; Cardoso, S.H.; Ramaciotti, O. "Bovine pericardium used as a cardiovascular patch". The Heart Surgery Forum. 2(1), 60–69, 1992.

Rakowski, W.A.; Zimowski, S. "Polyesterimide composites as a sensor material for sliding bearings". Composites Part B: Engineering, 37, 81–88, 2006.

Reul, H.; Eichler, M.; Potthast, K.; Schmitz, C.; Rau, G. "*In vitro* testing of heart valve wear outside of the manufacturers laboratory--requirements and controversias". Journal of Heart Valve Disease, 5, 97–103, 1996.

Reumann, M.; Morris, C.; Keller, D.; *et al.* "Towards run time visualization in cardiac modeling". World Congress on Biophysics and Biomedical Engineering. 7–12 September 2009 in Munich.

Salgueiredo, E.; *et al.* "Biocompatibility evaluation of DLC-coated Si3N4 substrates for biomedical applications. Diamond and Related Materials, 17(4-5), 878–881, 2008.

Schenkel, T.; Krittian, S.; Spiegel, K.; *et al.* "The Karlsruhe Heart Model KaHMo: A modular framework for numerical simulation of cardiac hemodynamics". World Congress on Biophysics and Biomedical Engineering. 7–12 September 2009 in Munich.

Schalkoff, R.J. "Artificial neural networks". McGraw Hill, New York, 1997.

Schwarz, M. "New Materials Processes, and Methods Technology". CRC Press. Taylor & Francis Group, 2005.

Seemann, G.; Rombach, C.; Keller, D.; Doessel, O. "Effect of the drug cisapride on human ventricular cardiomyocytes: A simulation study". World Congress on Biophysics and Biomedical Engineering. 7–12 September 2009 in Munich.

Stiehl, W.D.; Liebermann, D.; Breazeal, C.; Basel, L.; Lalla, L.; Wolf, M. "Design of a therapeutic robot companion for relational, affective touch". Proceedings of the 2005 IEEE International Workshop on Robots and Human Interactive Communication, 408–415,2005.

Vesely, I.; Mako, W.J. "Comparison of the compressive buckling of porcine aortic valve cusps and bovine pericardium". Journal of Heart Valve Disease, 7, 34–39, 1998.

Wojnarowski, J.; Mirota, K. "Generalized criterion for in vitro testing of artificial heart valves". Journal of Biomechanics, 39, 619–619, 2006.

Yager, R.R.; Zadeh, L.A. "Fuzzy sets, neural networks and soft computing". Van Nostrand-Reinhold. New York, 1994.

Chapter 16

A Proposal for Structured Methodology

Andrés Díaz Lantada
Mechanical Engineering Department, E.T.S.I. Industriales,
Universidad Politécnica de Madrid, c/ José Gutiérrez Abascal 2,
28006 Madrid, Spain
adiaz@etsii.upm.es

16.1 Introduction

This chapter contains a detailed description of a proposal for a structured methodology for developing active material-based medical devices, such as sensors or actuators. The intention is to promote the industrial expansion of these materials and put their special characteristics to full use in the development of devices with remarkable diagnostic or therapeutic capabilities. For this purpose, the use of systematic processes can be highly beneficial for optimising all the associated developments.

This proposal is not only a result of the examination made at the beginning of the handbook of the use of systematic methodologies for product development and of the current state of technology related to the use of active materials in medical devices, but is also a result of the knowledge acquired during the specific developments covered in previous chapters.

Solutions are put forward for the different problems encountered that affect the development of any medical device together with an analysis of how the use of active materials has influenced the different stages of the systematic design methodologies already set out.

Handbook of Active Materials for Medical Devices: Advances and Applications
Edited by Andrés Díaz Lantada

www.panstanford.com

16.2 The Need for Multidisciplinary Teams

16.2.1 The Need for Multidisciplinary Teams: Associated Benefits

A typical medical device development team is usually made up of doctors, pharmacologists, engineers, computer experts, physicists, chemists, and biologists as well as economists and law graduates, to provide financial and legal advice, respectively. Some of the main benefits of having multidisciplinary teams are

- Creativity is encouraged
- More varied responses to problems
- The division of labour makes finding the right solutions easier
- It is easier to assign responsibilities
- It is more difficult to take key design aspects for granted
- The end solution is checked from different points of view

The development process undoubtedly benefits from such a wealth of approaches; however, having experts in specific areas can also give rise to problems of communication (misunderstandings, imprecision, lack of information false assumptions) and of organisation that can lead to specific work schedules and budgets not being adhered to and even personal conflicts that affect the project. Explained below are diverse instruments that may serve to avoid these kinds of problems.

16.2.2 Communications Problems

A lack of understanding, frequently arising from a wrong use of language has resulted in economic, political, social, religious and many other types of conflict throughout history. This has caused many scholars to undertake a systematic, in-depth examination of the roots of these conflicts as a way of seeking solutions in order to avoid future problems.

Analytical philosophers, starting in particular with Bertrand Russell and Ludwig Wittgenstein, focused attention throughout the 20th century on the importance of language and how it is used, and placed these topics at the core of philosophy. Both coincide in stating that the duty of philosophy is to clarify language, by which many of the traditional problems of this discipline of knowledge can be eradicated, since most problems are due to a wrong use of language, which means they are lacking in any sense.

As occurs in other fields, communication problems (often the result of not using a common terminology or language) also give rise to problems in product development projects in any industry. Medical device development-related work teams, in particular, are usually made up of experts in many different fields that can generally be classified as "specialists in technological sciences" and "specialists in medical sciences" among whom communication is not always precise and effective.

On the other hand, the small number of training programmes existing in Europe until only recently on bioengineering topics (in its widest sense) is making it difficult to find people who can liaise between medical science specialists and technological science specialists as part of medical device development teams. This means that establishing a fluid dialogue between these teams is no easy matter.

16.2.3 Proposals for Improvement

The use of a common language

Preparing an initial document to suitably define the medical condition under study has been proved to be very useful for the developments put forward in previous chapters as a tool for facilitating communication from the very start of the development process.

This handbook should deal with the various aspects related to the condition in question as a way of facilitating the search for new diagnostic or therapeutic solutions that can benefit from the new possibilities to be had from using active materials, by comparing the advantages and disadvantages of the different families. We propose a common framework for these initial documents which should include the following issues:

- General aspects of the condition
  - Definition and physiopathology
  - Main types or manifestations
  - Aetiology
  - Diagnosis (also differential diagnosis when appropriate)

  - Prognosis
  - Treatment
- Available diagnostic or therapeutic products
  - Passive commercial devices
  - Active commercial devices
  - Non-commercial devices and designs
  - Other devices under development (competitor analysis)
  - Devices used in other related conditions
- Main national and international researchers
  - Hospitals
  - Research centres
  - Universities
- Main related publications
  - Books
  - Scientific papers
  - Papers presented at congress
  - Related web pages
- **Patents**
  - National patents
  - International patents
  - Patents pending
- Diagnostic proposals or alternative therapies
  - Diagnostic proposals
  - Therapeutic proposals
  - List of requirements
  - Possible use of active materials
  - Benefits associated with the use of active materials
- Annexes: Proposal for the terminology to be used
  - Dictionary of basic terms
  - Abbreviated notations
  - Basic units to be used (it would be interesting to encourage the use of the International Unit System)

Preparing these documents is a considerable learning process in itself and provides an overall vision of the conditions for which diagnostic or therapeutic solutions are being sought. Once prepared, and throughout the entire development process, this document acts as a point of reference for the whole team taking part and helps provide a common terminology between the experts in technology and the experts in health.

Teaching requirements

As commented in Chapter 2, the medical device industry in Europe employs around 350,000 people, which is some proof of the social importance of this sector. However, this high demand is not completely satisfied from an educational point of view, particularly in countries like Spain where the journey along the path to teaching in matters of bioengineering is only just beginning.

If this industry is to evolve properly, a major issue is to have a choice of graduates available from training programmes that provide their students with the knowledge, skills and aptitudes required to effectively carry out (among other things) the supervision, communication and information management tasks associated with medical device development projects.

Since we are dealing with experts in technological sciences and health sciences, it is exactly this type of bioengineering programme graduate that can most help to minimise the problems from an imprecise use of language by taking on the role of "communication facilitator" on the multidisciplinary teams working in this sector.

It is important for these training courses to be officially recognised (with clearly identified job competencies), with a degree and postgraduate degree structure like other branches of engineering, which may encourage students to choose this option.

To only depend on postgraduate programmes intended to supplement graduate training in different branches of engineering, often in too specific aspects, can result in a mistaken strategy, since it limits the job spectrum open to students, as is currently the case with various postgraduate courses in bioengineering.

Cooperation among technology branch and health-branch teachers in the preparation and teaching of these courses is also important. It is in this respect that the participation of departments from different universities is very positive as they can make their laboratories and research centres available to students. In addition, having the support of sector companies and hospitals to serve internships linked to final degree or end-of-course projects is also very positive for achieving the teaching aims of this type of course (Díaz Lantada *et al.*, 2008).

16.3 Preliminary Studies: The Importance of Addressing a Medical Need

As mentioned, when analysing systematic development methodologies and the special considerations for medical devices, it is essential to have a medical need requiring a solution as the main objective. This factor needs bearing in mind from the very beginning of the "defining objectives and planning" stage as well as in the "preliminary studies". If there is no such need it is not logical to start developing a new product to provide a solution to a non-existent problem or one that is being adequately solved by other methods.

The appearance of new technologies or other materials, which is happening now with numerous examples of multifunctional or "intelligent" materials, normally arouses tremendous expectation as to the different fields in which these technologies or materials can be applied. A use obviously needs to be found for this scientific-technical progress, but on occasions a desire to find an immediate use can lead to awkward situations or to the offering of solutions to problems for which there is no demand either by medical specialists or society.

When using active materials as a basis for the development of medical devices with detection capabilities or enhanced activation, one should act prudently. A real goal arising from a real medical need should be pursued and the materials used for this end should be properly characterised and tested despite their novel properties. If this is borne in mind and selection is made according to specific criteria in the "conceptual design" stage, the rest of the development process will be a straighter road with fewer obstacles that leads to a successful solution.

To ensure that new technological supply meets the existing social and medical demand we must once again focus attention on the importance of encouraging these issues to be taught on courses. The creation of new bioengineering syllabuses with the cooperation of doctors and engineers and the active participation of universities and medical centres would be of tremendous help for this purpose, since it is precisely in hospitals and health centres where diagnostic and therapeutic needs are detected. Then, once the technical schools have been informed of these needs, they can set about finding technological solutions through research and development projects into new devices.

Especially in the United States there are noteworthy examples of hospitals that have major engineering departments that actively collaborate not only in health science-related teaching work but also in purely technological aspects. Some examples are the "John Hopkins Hospital", the "Mayo Clinic", "Massachusetts General Hospital" and the "Cleveland Clinic".

Similar moves in this direction, to take advantage of the period of change which European Universities are going through (Madrid Technical University's Biotech initiative and others) could be highly beneficial for promoting major advances in this issue.

16.4 Conceptual Design

Complementary to the work described in the paper on systematic product development methodologies (Roozenburg and Eeckels, 1995; Pahl and Beitz, 1996; Ulrich, Eppinger, 2007), this subchapter analyses in finer detail the importance of making a correct initial choice of materials that have the right diagnostic and therapeutic characteristics for the active medical devices under development.

When choosing any multipurpose material and comparing the different candidates, the following characteristics must be looked at in detail as they can mark the difference between which materials are suitable for the device to be developed and which are not.

For activation purposes:

- Attainable deformations.
- The stresses that must be faced.
- Response speed.
- Power required.
- Feed voltage.
- Feed current.
- Reversibility.

For detection purposes:

- Useful measurement range.
- Sensitivity.
- Signal/noise ratio.
- Frequency response.
- Time resolution.

- Amplification requirements.
- Packaging requirements.

Whatever the case, the following properties should be taken into account:

- Mechanical strength.
- Thermal resistance.
- Chemical resistance.
- Density.
- Effects on the receiver organism.
- Evolution of properties over time.
- Availability (time period and despatch facilities).
- Cost (repercussion on the price of the end device).
- Additional difficulties.
- Data on its interaction with tissue and sterilisation possibilities.

It is then useful to construct a decision matrix based on these characteristics where the candidate materials are ordered in columns and the relevant properties in rows. In this way, each material can be scored according to different criteria, and after due consideration of the relative importance of the different properties, the ideal material or group of materials can be chosen objectively for a specific medical use. In conventional medical product processes this initial choice of materials is based on the information of similar devices and similar materials to those of existing products are usually chosen. However, if a medical device with novel characteristics is to be developed that incorporates an active material for detection or activation purposes, this prior information is generally not available, which means this stage is fraught with more difficulties.

On the other hand, these active materials have been only recently developed and are not fully characterised and the manufacturers' information is not always complete. So, when choosing possible candidates, it is important right from the conceptual design stage to ensure that there is an availability of suppliers of these materials and that delivery schedules and prices are reasonable.

Furthermore, it should be checked that suppliers are willing to supply basic information about the properties of these materials as well as processing and design instructions that may be useful in the following stages of development. If information on certain essential material properties required for the work is lacking, an appropriate solution is to obtain a sample of the material and carry out a study or pre-characterisation using the raw material to evaluate the crucial properties. Once a list of possible candidate materials has been made it is advisable to contact the main suppliers and ask them if they would be willing to collaborate in the development process. In this way the suppliers that are most willing to help their customers can be selected and more formal collaboration agreements reached, which in turn can lead to better results on completion of the research and a more effective end device.

As an aid to future researchers who may wish to use multi-purpose materials, a list of the main suppliers of active materials is included in the annexes, classified by families, as well as information on manufacturers of the additives that can aid the synthesis process of these materials and result in new active compounds being obtained.

16.5 The Protection of Intellectual Property

The competitive edge of a new product often lies in its reaching the production stage and then being marketed before any of its competitors' products. This is particularly the case when conventional products conceptually similar to others already on the market are developed, but which have some slight differences in design, shape, ergonomics, colour, and appearance that could boost sales due to subjective factors.

It is not unusual for the success of a conventional product to depend on such peculiarities as appearance, brand image, the stamp of exclusivity, the feeling of belonging to a group, the advertising used and other emotional criteria that are difficult to predict. In these cases protecting intellectual property is not especially relevant since there is not sufficient novelty or inventive genius for the product to be patented. Occasionally the new form of product can be entered in a special register for such under the heading of "industrial design", which gives the title holder the exclusive right to make, manufacture, produce, sell, utilise and exploit the object registered, including the possibility of preventing the importation of any products copying the protected design. The "brand" and "brand names" register can eventually take on a significant commercial value for new products as well as for future developments in the event of the manufacturer having sufficiently outstanding growth.

However, products that are the result of notable technological progress (and the new fields opened up by that progress) usually have more objective competitive edges based on conceptual or functional originality that involves a radical change of focus in the sectors where they will be used. These notable original ideas of outstanding inventive genius usually specified as products or procedures (manufacturing procedures, for example), can benefit from being registered as a "patent". A patent gives the holder the exclusive right to prevent others from making a commercial use of the patented invention, thereby reducing the uncertainty, risk and competition from imitators by providing a means of protection for the intellectual property but with major additional benefits, which are listed below:

- For companies that invest large amounts of time and money in research and development work, protecting any inventions with a patent usually means costs are recovered and greater returns are had on the investment.
- Additional income can be obtained by granting a licence on the patent or its surrender, usually to other more powerful sector companies that wish to counter any threat to their privileged position.
- Certain companies that are interested in technologies that are the property of others can use the patents of which they are holders to negotiate agreements to transfer crossed licences.
- Transferring patents to others under licence can open up access to new markets that would be otherwise inaccessible. If this is done, the invention must also be protected in the corresponding foreign markets.
- Being in possession of a patent considerably increases the chances of obtaining financing at a reasonable rate of interest. This, in turn, increases the chances of placing the patented product on the market.
- Being in possession of a patent considerably increases the chances of taking successful legal action against those who copy or imitate the protected invention.
- Being in possession of patents gives a positive corporate image. Some companies mention or enumerate their patents

in their advertising as a way of projecting an innovative image to the public.

- In academic circles it is an additional tool for assessing the quality of research of universities and research groups, often with positive financial repercussions on these institutions.

It should be underlined that the scope of this handbook, which is focused on the use of active materials in the development of medical devices with new detection or activation capabilities for novel diagnostic or therapeutic work, is open to major intellectual property–related activities. Since many active material formulations are the fruit of recent research in search of applications and given the intrinsic difficulties of any medical device development process, any medical devices that integrate active materials such as sensors or actuators usually have features that are subject to protection by patent. These developments can therefore benefit from the advantages set out above.

It is precisely at the end of the conceptual design stage after completion of the preliminary-studies (which include existing product and patent analysis, as already stated) and after choosing the working principle and the active material most suited to the diagnostic and therapeutic work, when it is the right moment to apply for a patent for the product. At least this is what we have learned from our experience in developing the products presented in earlier chapters.

If the patent is not applied for until later stages of development (like basic engineering, detailed engineering or *in vitro* or *in vivo* tests) it is very likely that other research teams working on a similar topic will patent a similar invention that will strip our development of its novelty and inventive genius and may block any future projections after having invested large sums of time and money.

Neither is it advisable to make any type of public announcement giving any information about the active medical device under development until a patent has been applied for, as once it has been made public the fundamentals of such a device cannot be patented.

For this reason, it is important to prepare and apply for the patent in the early stages of development, since after doing so the work can be made known, the preliminary results published, congresses and conferences attended to seek possible collaborators, and other type of actions taken to publicise the originality of the device being developed. All this also facilitates the search for financing to complete and develop the product launch onto the market under more beneficial circumstances.

Throughout the design process, significant new issues can emerge that may also require various forms of intellectual property protection. Having completed the development of the device and made an objective analysis of its benefits and limitations, different future actions or modifications can be considered, which if sufficiently original and utilitarian from an industrial and medical point of view, may also require a patent.

It is also necessary to underline the scientific importance of patenting any inventions arising from research and development. To exemplify this importance we will mention the following issues that demonstrate the positive outcomes for the scientific community of using patents, which go well beyond the purely financial and strategic purposes of having a patent from an entrepreneurial point of view:

- Patents are an excellent source of updated technological information since different data bases (easily accessible in the Internet and free) place over 60 million documents at the disposal of researchers, both patents granted as well as those applied for. In principle, the information in a patent document must be sufficiently complete and exact for the invention to be reproduced, which from a scientific and teaching point of view is highly valuable.
- Furthermore, searching these data bases by field of application lets the researcher find the products and procedures that are quite often aimed at solving technical problems similar to their own. It also helps find the most recent emerging technologies and locate strategic sectors by analysing the applications for a patent submitted for a particular subject (as was done at the beginning of the handbook for the active materials used in medical devices).
- Applying for a patent is one of the most effective ways of publicising an idea that is to the benefit of Society, as it is presented as a document with an international standardised framework. It includes an abstract, a description of the invention, some explanatory diagrams, at least one way of making the invention and the inventor's claims concerning what they consider to be their own creation. As no prototypes or tests are required, as is the case with other documents, such

as scientific papers or congress communications, but simply to explain an idea on paper, publishing the information is also quicker, which is yet another advantage.

- On many occasions, the information that can be extracted from patents is unique, often the fruit of unfinished research or proposals made to continue along specific lines of research. As an example, we can cite a study from the United States Patent Office which found that around 70% of the technology described in patents documents in the United States between 1967 and 1972 had not been described in any other media. However, whatever the case, drawing up patents documents is a valuable way of generating knowledge as a foundation for future developments.

We have so far explained the benefits of utilising patents in the development processes of medical devices based on the new possibilities opened up by active materials, particularly at the end of the conceptual design stage. In the next section, we shall now go on to examine further aspects to ensure that the basic engineering stage is successfully embarked upon.

16.6 Basic Engineering

This section covers different issues that are specifically linked to the basic engineering stage in active material-based medical device development projects and which can promote the use of this kind of solution. The issues analysed here complement those already listed in the chapter on an introduction to systematic product development methodologies.

16.6.1 Integrating Patent Information

The new medical image capture technologies combined with the progress made in design and manufacturing tools allows new approaches for developing customised active medical devices. Producing a customised device is in itself an entire development project, and if an active material is included, it may benefit from using the methodology about to be put forward. For producing a unique customised device as well as for setting about developing a device for mass manufacture, it is important to correctly manage any patient-associated information throughout the development process as a whole.

When dealing with a customised device this information has a direct implication on the design because the patient's individual circumstances are a determining factor for the choice of therapeutic approach and may lead to different devices being used according to the severity of their condition. For example, for the treatment of mitral insufficiency one of the solutions chosen may be to utilise annuloplasty rings or full valve prostheses. Both devices can be made to measure, but the choice depends directly on the patient's individual circumstances (Díaz Lantada, 2009).

If dealing with a device for mass manufacture, possessing information on a large number of patients which can be used for demographic studies on a particular condition can help reveal the most appropriate diagnostic and therapeutic approaches and provide information on the devices that can be most beneficial because of the active materials being integrated into them.

In fact, the generalised use of computer tools and data bases has been promoted by the national health systems of the most advanced nations. Diagnosing and treating patients thus becomes much easier as does communication between primary care (in health centres) and specialist care (in hospitals), which enhances the overall efficiency of health systems (Saiz Morón, Lantada Ruiz de Castañeda, Díaz Fernández, 2008).

This progress has been given an enormous boost through doctors, engineers and computer scientists collaborating to develop the tools to manage this information, particularly over the last decade. Some of the most recent major advances can be consulted in the 2008 and 2009 "Biostec - Healthinf" conference reports.

16.6.2 Materials Characterisation

As already explained, active materials are a recent novelty, often resulting from synthesis processes carried out in university laboratories or research centres, and do not always reach the commercial stage. For this reason, it is important right from the conceptual design to ensure there are suppliers of the active materials intended to be used and that adequate information is available.

However, sometimes an active material with much better sensing or activation properties compared to its competitors may be marketed by a supplier that does not provide all the information required for the design, either because they have not examined the properties of the material in depth or because they do not want to disclose certain information about their materials.

This often means that additional characterisation tests need to be done at the beginning of the basic design stage to reveal important information on particular properties required to design the associated device correctly. Characterisation tests can be performed systematically following the procedures set out in ISO standards, some of which have already been described in different chapters of the handbook, depending on the family contemplated.

When characterisation tests lead to little satisfactory information on some property that is crucial to the correct functioning of the device, this material must be replaced by another of the possible candidates selected in the previous stage.

16.6.3 The Use of Modelling and Simulation Tools

These tools are especially useful once the main properties of the active materials used have been characterised and we begin to examine the characteristics required by the sensor or actuator in the design stage in more detail, so that the diagnostic or therapeutic mission will be properly carried out.

These technologies allow constructing simulators that can rapidly and accurately analyse the influence of different factors on the device's end performance and optimise the desired response. Thanks to the use of tools like "Matlab – Simulink" (and others like "Maple" and "Mathematica"), the said simulator construction can be done progressively by encouraging a division of work as a basic problem solving tool. In this way, simple simulators can be had to model a very specific phenomenon. These simple simulators can then be combined with one another in a series of sub-systems to obtain a simulator that will let a much more complex system be modelled where the responses can be analysed in accordance with multiple input variables.

Throughout the developments undertaken different examples of the use of these tools that have demonstrated their usefulness have been described. Just one example are the analyses performed using piezoelectric and pyroelectric simulators to test the right choice of the main values associated with the load amplifiers and to check that the diagnostic systems were performing properly.

In every case, it is very important to compare the simulation outcomes with the preliminary estimates calculated "by hand" and check these results in more detail by carrying out actual tests, either using the materials in isolation or using device prototypes with the active material already integrated. These real tests allow the theoretical models to be adjusted so that their use in later device optimisation operations will be more accurate and effective.

16.6.4 The use of "CAD–CAE–CAM" Technologies

A proper use of the different computer-aided design, calculation and manufacturing technologies ("CAD–CAE–CAM" technologies), throughout the basic engineering stage is a great asset at the design stage and for making a right choice of materials, components, geometries and manufacturing processes so that everything will fit the initial specifications of the device being developed. Recent advances have made it possible to exchange information between the design, calculation and manufacturing programs from different software companies, which makes exchanging information with suppliers or other researchers easier.

Furthermore, the results of simulation programs like "Matlab–Simulink", as well as data from spread sheets like "Excel", can be used as load or shape conditions for the calculations made with the help of "CAE" programs usually based on the finite elements method. So, the various parts of the design can be studied with the aid of different software support tools, each with its own advantages and specific fields of application.

Once again, we cannot overstate the importance of checking the simulation results given by these software tools by comparing them with the results obtained from actual tests to help validate the hypotheses made and inspire greater confidence in the use of these tools for similar calculations in the future.

We have not ceased to state this throughout the handbook as a way of studying the various phenomena and present it as an example for future developments. One clear example is the design process of the heating system for active annuloplasty rings and the validation of the finite elements analyses performed, which were compared with the results of the controlled heating tests with the aid of infrared thermography tools.

16.6.5 The Use of Rapid Prototyping and Manufacturing Technologies

In the last 15 years these new technologies have become powerful support tools for product development processes as they help minimise design iterations thereby reducing delivery schedules and costs, as explained earlier and which can also be seen in other research papers (Freitag, Wohlers, 2003, Kucklick, 2006, Lafont, Lorenzo Yustos, Díaz Lantada, 2007, 2008).

In medical device-associated developments it is especially important to make full use of the customised manufacturing that can be achieved with these technologies. By taking the information from high quality medical image capture technologies and using CAD tools like "MIMICS", geometric models can be obtained of the different parts of live organisms from which physical models can then be made. This customisation not only lets customised implant prototypes be had but also helps in planning surgical work with the manufacture of physical models of the patient's internal organs.

The many examples given help show how these technologies can be used as a support for the different development stages of medical devices and, in general, any product development-associated research. The prototypes obtained in this way are of major importance for validating the outcomes of different simulations as well as design decisions by means of actual tests.

We also propose their being used throughout the entire development process and using them first before turning to conventional product-associated methodologies. In so doing, even in the conceptual design stage, physical models can be had for testing and comparing the properties of the active materials chosen by integrating them into very simple prototypes.

16.6.6 *In vitro* Tests: Characterisation of Materials and Applications

Before setting about any *in vivo* test it must be checked that the basic design decisions made for an active medical device are the right ones and that the design works correctly in general terms. To achieve this, in vitro tests using prototypes of the device under development are essential.

The results will enable the design to be validated or provide guidelines as to what changes are required to optimise its functionality.

These in vitro tests do not involve risks to any living being as they are performed with synthetic tissue or samples taken from corpses. Their combined use with the results from simulation tools has become an essential instrument in the development process of these devices, since many in vivo tests are made unnecessary, leading to reductions in costs, delivery schedules and the suffering caused to the animals subjected to such in vivo tests.

However, carrying out these in vitro tests involves additional design problems to be taken into account that will demand further preparation and work from the research team members. If the results of these tests are to be meaningful, the device must be tested under conditions that insofar as possible recreate the actual circumstances under which it will need to function. It is therefore a good idea to build test benches to reproduce the environment of the device under real working conditions to evaluate its response and propose design improvements. Highly useful are automated devices to perform these tests in a semi-automatic manner in order to optimise the time schedules associated with these tests as well as for enhancing their repeatability.

In vitro tests are also associated with a first approach evaluation of the biocompatibility of the applications designed and the influence of the materials used, as will be seen in detail in the following section.

16.6.7 Deliberations on Safety, Standards and Quality

In the chapters on product and medical device development methodology reference was made to the importance of keeping in mind **safety** and **quality** requirements throughout the development process, above all in the basic engineering stage where the fundamental aspects of the device are decided.

The mandatory directives have been explained (according to the type of medical device), as well as the main regulations, and carefully adhering to these throughout the design process will facilitate obtaining devices that fulfil the requirements of the directives that apply.

We have also analysed many different tools and ways to proceed to assure the quality and safety of the products under development and their implications throughout the design process. It is vital that the entire team should collaborate to optimise these two aspects, with specific responsibilities being assigned according to each member's work area.

Further information on the application of different basic safe design principles to specific cases, such as "the safe life principal", "the safe failure principle" or "the redundancy principle", may be found in other references (Pahl and Beitz, 1996). Their adaptation to medical device design is immediate and was taken into account for certain aspects of the designs produced (protective coatings, duplication of sensors, alternative heating systems and others).

A conclusive factor is the experience acquired beforehand from other development projects where it was learned how to make these reflections as well as all the information gathered from previous research and development work.

When choosing materials for conventional medical devices it is highly recommended to use the materials that have shown themselves to be compatible with organisms in previous developments.

However, if active materials are to be used, this information is often unavailable since we are dealing with recently synthesised materials intended to be placed on the market through research projects. In these cases, extra tests need to be made for *in vitro* as well as *in vivo* evaluations of the device's biocompatibility and safety of usage, as will be explained in the following section.

However, it is always important to bear in mind that the resulting devices must fit the quality management requirements that are part of the National Health System global framework. Again, we must emphasise the need for engineers and doctors to collaborate during the different development stages (which also include marketing, distribution and application to patients) and consult the conclusions of other relevant researchers (Ruíz and Simón 1994, 2004; Simón *et al.*, 1995, 2001; Jiménez *et al.*, 2000).

Taking the above procedures as a basis it should be proceeded to look more closely at how to define the product and improve it, which will constitute a merger between the basic engineering and detailed engineering stages.

Thus, the design stage can be approached as a whole with the precise level of detail being progressively obtained. When developing medical devices certain issues prior to production start-up and traditionally included in the detailed engineering stage, again need to be stressed, as the following section will clarify.

16.7 Detailed Engineering: Deliberations Prior to Production

The proposed methodology is particularly oriented towards obtaining medical device prototypes based on the use of new active polymer materials, usually as part of research projects that are reaching the *in vivo* test or pre-production stage. In whichever case, this section includes certain considerations regarding "pre-clinical research", that must be borne in mind and stages that must be passed before putting medical devices into production. Some of these stages may require entire research projects, particularly if newly synthesised active materials are to be integrated that are not fully characterised.

16.7.1 *In vivo* Tests

Medical devices need to be tested in some living organism (*in vivo* tests) before being subjected to clinical trials, in order to obtain demographic data on their diagnostic capabilities, therapeutic effects or the effect of the device on human beings (Kucklick, 2006).

Once the device has been subjected to preliminary tests in order to evaluate its functionalities, it is advisable to analyse how the device performs *in vitro*. This often means acquiring tissue from living beings or corpse samples to test the device and identify the changes required as a prior step to conducting the *in vitro* tests in order to avoid using animal tissue. As an example of the advances in this respect, the developments of "Edwards Lifesciences LLC" may be quoted for obtaining synthetic pericardial patch tissue, as a support for research work and surgical operations.

After conducting the *in vitro* tests and making the necessary design change, it is essential to make a right choice of the place where the *in vivo* tests will be conducted. This decision is crucial to the success of the tests and the project, since choosing a laboratory with inexperienced staff may lead to unacceptable deviations in costs and schedules.

Again we must emphasise the need for multidisciplinary teams for medical device development and the benefits to be had by occasionally seeking advice and assistance outside the research team for any issues that are beyond their capabilities. A generally good option is to pre-select the most renowned preclinical research centres in the field (province, autonomous region participating team-members' countries) basing choice on objective quality criteria, such as experience, staff and available resources.

The major universities in medicine, biology and veterinary science in the country are always among the candidates, as well as important research centres and laboratories, which quite often are associated with the universities. These centres usually combine research work, training and external services whose founding is usually promoted by public investment to aid the purchase of facilities and equipment.

A good strategy for choosing the right centre is to visit the various pre-selected centres and speak to the people in charge, not only to deal with technical matters but also schedules and costs to help make the final decision. Another key issue for the success of *in vivo* tests is the right choice of animal model to be used. Working with live animals to support a medical device development project is a privilege not to be taken lightly. To help choose the most suitable animal model the following procedure may be followed:

- Study the animals used in similar developments
- Analyse the species whose anatomy is most similar to humans (for the organ associated with the device in question)
- Exchange opinions with other researchers in the same area
- Consult the main scientific publications
- List the equipment needed (which will also help choose the centre for the tests)
- Calculate the number of animals required
- Decide if the operations will be terminal or not
- List all the parameters wished to be studied

Only after an exhaustive planning stage and assigning the right responsibilities to all the participating personnel (particularly regarding the centre where the *in vivo* tests will be conducted, as they are not usually part of the initial development team) the *in vivo* work can be begun. The ethical guidelines contained in the "Helsinki Declaration" may assist and guide the participants in this kind of project in their decision-making.

16.7.2 Verifying Biocompatibility

As already explained, the term "biocompatibility" refers to the interaction between a medical device and the tissues of the patient treated with that device. A biocompatibility evaluation is part of the overall quality assurance and safety process for medical devices. It must be taken into account throughout the development process from the initial selection of materials even though it must be evaluated by using the end device, since the body's response depends on many factors.

Some of the factors that usually influence the biocompatibility of a device are as follows:

- The physical-chemical nature of the device materials
- The type of tissue exposed to the device
- The length of contact
- Device geometry
- Sterilisation method
- The patients themselves

The best starting point to understand the biocompatibility requirements of a medical device and decide the process to evaluate it is probably ISO Standard 10993 on the "Biological evaluation of medical devices". A set of guided steps are described for carrying out this evaluation on the biocompatibility of new medical devices, which in itself makes it a proposal for the methodology of this specific stage.

As certain biocompatibility-related data are always required for devices that are in contact with tissue, it is important to refer to the flow chart included in ISO Standard 10993-1, to examine which type of *in vitro* and *in vivo* biocompatibility tests need to be conducted. In general, the number of tests needed to fulfil the requirements can be reduced if some of the following types of data are available:

- **Data from previous evaluations.** If data is available from previous satisfactory tests on similar devices, certain verification tests will need to be made to check if any significant changes have occurred in the materials used, the manufacturing processes, the nature of the contact or the sterilisation methods.

- **Data from the components or materials suppliers.** If data is available from evaluations made by the suppliers, it is always important to obtain copies of these original studies and it is also advisable to carry out some verification tests.
- **Analytical data**. Usually provided by manufacturers from the chemical characterisation tests conducted to verify the low hazard associated with using certain materials and devices in contact with body tissue.
- **Clinical data.** Having clinical data from tests carried out with devices containing similar components or materials may help satisfy certain biological effect-related requirements to be found in the categories included in ISO Standard 10993-1.

In whichever case, a good strategy for choosing the biological tests to be passed by the device in question is to design the ISO materials biocompatibility matrix. This matrix classifies medical devices according to type and duration of contact. It also provides a list of potential biological effects.

For each device category certain biological effects have to be looked at in detail and satisfactorily addressed by taking previous data or conducting new tests to obtain a positive evaluation that will allow production start-up.

Again, it is highly recommended to enlist the aid of organisations that are experts in these kinds of studies and procedures to provide external advice to the development team. Most sector multinationals have departments exclusively devoted to the biological evaluation work need to fulfil requirements and undertake their own biocompatibility studies.

In fact, many medical device development projects carried out in universities or research centres end up producing a prototype of the device, usually for *in vitro* but sometimes *in vivo* tests. When they have been proved to work properly, it is very often attempted to licence this technology to a sector company which will then take charge of the biocompatibility tests and the official approval procedures, as well as its subsequent production start-up and marketing. Proceeding in this way is the quickest and most effective way of facilitating the transfer of research results to society.

It is also possible to set up technology-based businesses that commit themselves to exploiting the outcomes of medical device development-related research. To this end, many universities are promoting specific actions (like Madrid Polytechnic University's "ActúaUPM" initiative, which provides training and financial support for its researchers so they can set up businesses of this kind). In addition, right from the start of the development project, consideration can be given to enlisting the collaboration of a sector company to help the research team with the many issues related to the market launch.

Another recommended step regarding the biological evaluation of the devices being developed consists in discussing the biocompatibility tests proposed directly with the evaluators of the competent bodies who can always provide guidelines on the safest and most direct way to act.

After a medical device has passed all the different tests required of it in accordance with its classification and the applicable Directive (as explained in Chapter 2), the manufacturer or its authorised representative in the European Union may put the CE mark on its product and begin production and marketing.

In whichever case, it is important to point out that the biological requirements for medical devices as well as the relevant standards are constantly changing and correctly updated information must be used. This information can be found on the web page of the "International Organization for Standardization": www.iso.org.

Other markets are subject to alternative standards, which means the information of other bodies may need to be consulted (particularly the "Food and Drug Administration": www.fda.gov, for the US market).

16.8 Comparisons with Conventional Methodologies

The suggested methodology is in essence an adaptation of structured methodologies for systematic product development, but includes important considerations aimed at making the medical device development process easier for devices integrating these active materials.

Throughout the chapter we have itemised the main issues to be borne in mind when developing medical devices based on the use of active materials such as sensors and actuators, which is what differentiates this proposal from other structured methodologies used for systematic product development.

Of all these issues, the following are worth mentioning once again:

- The importance of multidisciplinary teams
- The importance of using tools to facilitate communication
- The importance of managing information properly, particularly patient-related information
- The benefits of taking measures to protect intellectual property
- The special relevance of making a careful choice of materials suppliers
- The need to conduct property characterisation tests as a design basis
- The benefits of using simulation technologies as a design basis
- The benefits of using "CAD-CAE-CAM" tools in combination with rapid prototyping technologies throughout the basic engineering stage
- The need to validate simulation results with actual tests
- The need to carry out *in vitro* tests to validate materials and applications
- The need to carry out *in vivo* tests to validate the diagnostic or therapeutic benefits
- The importance of keeping in mind safety issues and standards throughout the development

The following page includes in Fig. 16.1 a general outline for this proposal that can be compared to the diagram usually used for more conventional products, as shown in the first chapter when dealing with systematic product development methodology.

The changes made are as a result of the research that gave rise to this handbook and the enquires made into the cutting edge developments of other research centres, universities, technology-based companies and university hospitals. Applying this proposed methodology to future research and development projects will enable it to be improved and its range of applications extended.

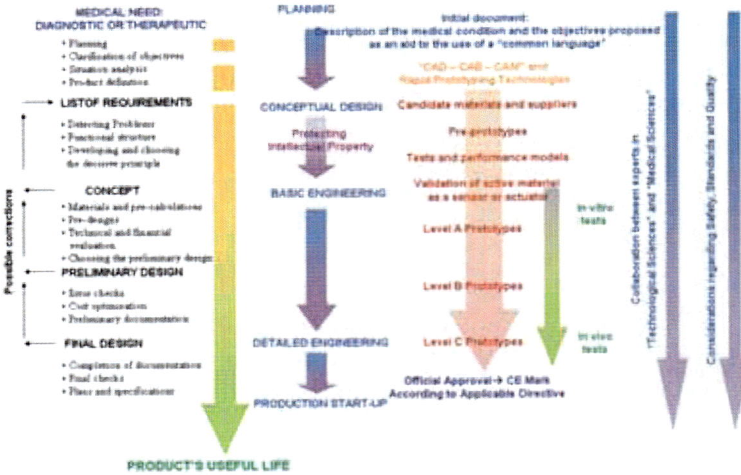

Figure 16.1 Outline of the proposed development methodology.

16.9 The Importance of Collaboration and Information Exchange among Researchers

The following page includes a general outline for this proposal that can be compared to the diagram usually used for more conventional products, as shown in the first chapter when dealing with systematic product development methodology. To promote the industrial expansion of active materials and facilitate their use for the development of new medical devices, it is very important for universities, research centres and major sector companies to collaborate and exchange information in respect of the scientific-technological progress in these materials and their applications.

It is an inherent mission of teachers and researchers to focus attention on these new fields of study and on the importance of examining them together in a coordinated manner and to look on other researchers as companions and never as rivals. Other areas of knowledge have given examples of how joint action leads to rapid scientific progress with no less important socio-economic impacts. Worth quoting as an example is the call for collaboration in matters of micro and nano-manufacturing made by the scientist Richard Feynman in his talk, "There's plenty of room at the bottom" in 1959 at the California Institute for Technology, "Caltech". A little more than two decades after this talk, IBM scientists succeeded in positioning atoms for writing (and reading) words, far exceeding the initial challenges of that call.

In the issue of active materials remarkable efforts of international collaboration have begun to emerge in recent decades. Outstanding events related to the use of electroactive materials may be cited, such as the call to seek answers to the current limitations of these materials made by Yoseph Bar-Cohen from NASA's "Jet Propulsion Laboratory".

Outstanding forums have also been created to exchange information on the advances in materials science, such as "Scientific.net", "Biomat.net" and others, that help spread results, exchange opinions and publicise meetings and events on this subject. Regarding the promotion of active materials for medical device development it is interesting to consider ways to exchange information and enhance teaching, like those listed below:

- It is highly beneficial to set up a specific forum on active materials and their medical applications, with a specific section devoted to active materials and medical applications, where researchers, universities and companies can get in contact to match technological supply to market requirements, of major importance to the Medical Industry. As a starting point, we have designed a web page on active materials, part of the website of the Machine Engineering Division of Madrid Technical University (www.dim.etsii.upm.es/ldpdim), which it is intended to update with each new future development based on the use of active materials.
- Congresses and scientific meetings are very useful instruments for bringing together the main researchers in an area of knowledge, particularly when this is done according to a fixed schedule to discuss specific topics. Recently, certain thematic conferences focused on the industrial applications of active materials have emerged, such as the "SMART conference: Smart Structures and Materials", the "ASME conference – Smart Materials, Adaptative Structures and Intelligent Systems" and others that contribute to sharing knowledge on these topics. Aware of the need to focus on the medical uses of these active materials, the editor has already organised and chaired the "Special Session on Active Materials for Medical Devices – AMMD 2009", sponsored by "Biomat.net - The Biomaterials

Network", as part of the "International Conference on Biomedical Electronics and Devices – Biodevices 2009" from 14 to 17 January in Oporto. In future years it is hoped to continue with these events after the even more positive results of the second experience, concretely with the organisation of the "Special Session on Rapid Prototyping for Improving Biodevices", part of the "International Conference on Biomedical Electronics and Devices – Biodevices 2010" from 20 to 23 January in Valencia.

- The development of properties data bases for different materials (e.g., "Campus Plastics" or "Polymers: A Properties Database") has proved highly useful when selecting commercial formulations for conventional products made of polymeric materials. Many active material formulations are the result of developments carried out in small companies and research centres and are not commercially available. On the other hand, these companies and research centres are not usually included in the commercial materials data bases mentioned. It would be a great help if information concerning any new active material developments, the results of different characterisation tests and the manufacturers of these materials, were to be progressively added to the most used data bases.
- Creating performance models to evaluate the responses of different classes of multi-purpose material when exposed to different external stimuli is very helpful for simplifying future developments that may also use this type of material. The design of simulators like "Matlab – Simulink", as has been shown throughout this handbook, enables a fast exchange of information with other researchers. Moreover, using "Simulink" to create complex block structures based on small sub-systems makes it easier to integrate work to evaluate device and systems performance from a global point of view. This is also useful for designing devices that can benefit from the use of various active materials by making the task of choosing materials easier and helping to analyse the different factors that influence the end performance.
- To encourage the use of these materials in Industry it is important to make known the advantages expected from their use and teach people to make designs that are based on

their special properties. Therein lays one of the basic benefits of carrying out research work in the University, since the discoveries made encourage changing and gradually updating the syllabuses of the various subjects. This helps to promote and maintain students' interest and to increase the transfer of knowledge arising from research to Society as a whole.

As an additional source of information to aid the future development of devices based on the use of active or "intelligent" multi-purpose materials, included in the section on the annexes to the handbook is a list of the main manufacturers of this type of material and certain additives that can enhance these materials.

References

Díaz Lantada, A. "Metodología para el desarrollo de dispositivos médicos activos basados en el empleo de polímeros activos como sensores y actuadores". PhD Thesis, Universidad Politécnica de Madrid, 2009.

Díaz Lantada, A.; Lorenzo Yustos, H.; Lafont, P.; *et al.* "Teaching applications for rapid prototyping technologies". International Journal of Engineering Education, 23(2), 411–418, 2007.

Freitag, D.; Wohlers, T. "Rapid prototyping: State of the Art". Manufacturing technology information analysis centre. Chicago Illinois, 2003.

Jiménez, J.; Molina, P.; Grandal, J.; *et al.* "El modelo europeo de gestión de la calidad total como sistema de gestión hospitalaria; experiencia y resultados tras dos años de implantación en un hospital público". Revista de Calidad Asistencial, 15, 135–141, 2000.

Kucklick, T.R. "The medical device R&D handbook". CRC Press, Taylor and Francis Group. Florida, 2006.

Lafont Morgado, P.; Lorenzo Yustos, H.; *et al.* "Rapid tooling: Moldes rápidos a partir de estereolitografía". Revista de plásticos modernos, 524, 150–157, 2000.

Pahl, G., Beitz, W. "Engineering design: A systematic approach". 2nd Revised Edition (Ed. Wallace) Edición Revisada. Springer Verlag. London, 1996.

Roozenburg, N.; Eeckels J. "Product design: Fundamentals and methods". John Wiley & Sons. New York, 1995.

Ruiz, U.; Simón, J. "La mejora continua de la Calidad en el Sistema Sanitario: Resultados de la 1ª fase de implantación del Plan de Calidad en España

(1986–1992)". Revista de Sanidad e Higiene Pública, 68, 535–548, 1994.

Ruiz, U.; Simón, J. "Quality management in health care: A 20-year journey". International Journal of Health Care Quality Assurance, 17(6), 323–333, 2004.

Saaksvuori, A.; Immonen, A. "Product lifecycle management". 3rd Edition, Springer Verlag. Berlin, Heidelberg, London, New York, 2008.

Saiz Morón, A.; Lantada Ruiz de Castañeda, P.; Díaz Fernández, A.; *et al.* "Internal Medicine: Fundamental link for the coordination between Primary Care and Specialized Attention". 29th World Congress of Internal Medicine. Buenos Aires, 2008.

Simón, J.; Ruiz, U. "Actividades de Garantía de Calidad en 62 hospitales del Sistema Nacional de Salud". Revista Española de Salud Pública, 69, 341–348, 1995.

Simón, J.; Ruiz Ferrandiz, U.; Orbea Celaya, T.; Díez Laguna, P. "La Norma ISO 9000 en el sector sanitario: Seguridad y mejora del sistema". UNE, 155, Octubre, 9–12, 2001.

Stark, J. "Product lifecycle management: 21st Century paradigm for product realisation". Springer Verlag. Berlin, Heidelberg, New York, 2004.

Ulrich, K.; Eppinger, S. "Product design and development". 4th Edition, Mc-Graw Hill / Irwin. New York, 2007.

Standards Summary

Main organizations

- International Organization for Standarization "ISO" (www.iso.org)
- The World Medical Association (www.wma.net)

"New approach" Directives related to the Medical Industry

- Directive 93/42/EEC related to "Medical devices"
- Directive 90/385/EEC related to "Active implantable medical devices"
- Directive 98/79/EC related to "Medical devices for *in vitro* diagnosis".

Standards related to the development of medical devices

- ISO 10993 standard on "Biological evaluation of medical devices"
- ISO 13485 standard on "Sanitary products. Quality management and regulatory affairs"
- ISO 13488 standard on "Quality systems. Medical devices, sanitary products and especial requirements for applying ISO 9002 standard"

- ISO 14971 standard on "Application of risk management to medical devices and sanitary products"
- ISO 15223 standard on "Symbols used for labelling and information provided together with medical devices"

Standards and associations related to medical imaging

- DICOM standard – Digital Imaging and Communications in Medicine: Strategic Document (http://medical.nema.org)
- Medical Imaging and Technology Alliance (www.medicalimaging.org)
- NEMA – The Association of Electrical and Medical Imaging Equipment Manufacturers (www.nema.org)

Additional documents of interest

- Council of Europe "Convention for the protection of Human Rights and dignity of the human being with regard to the application of biology and medicine: Convention on Human Rights and Biomedicine" (1994)
- UNESCO "Universal Declaration on the Human Genome and Human Rights" (1997) and "Guidelines for Implementation" (1999)
- World Medical Association "Declaration of Helsinki. Ethical principles for medical research involving human subjects" (current revised edition 2008)

Appendix A

Brief Comparison Between Several Families of Active Materials for Actuation Purposes

This appendix includes a brief graphic comparison, in Fig. A.1, between several families of active materials used as actuators, taking into account aspects such as stress generated during actuation[1] and speed of response, according to most references on these matters.

Some areas of application may vary in the following years, as continuous research is improving their properties as actuators; however, we believe such graphic provides a good idea related to current capabilities. Additional information related to the use of similar comparison graphics, for conventional materials, can be found in Michael Asby's "Materials Selection in Mechanical Design", important reference for all engineers and scientists devoted to Materials Science.

[1] Please note that the concept of "stress generated during actuation" is not of application when talking about "optical traps"; as actuation in such a case is not linked to a material, but to the use of electromagnetic waves (light). Optical traps are currently capable of actuation forces in the scale of millinewton.

Handbook of Active Materials for Medical Devices: Advances and Applications
Edited by Andrés Díaz Lantada

www.panstanford.com

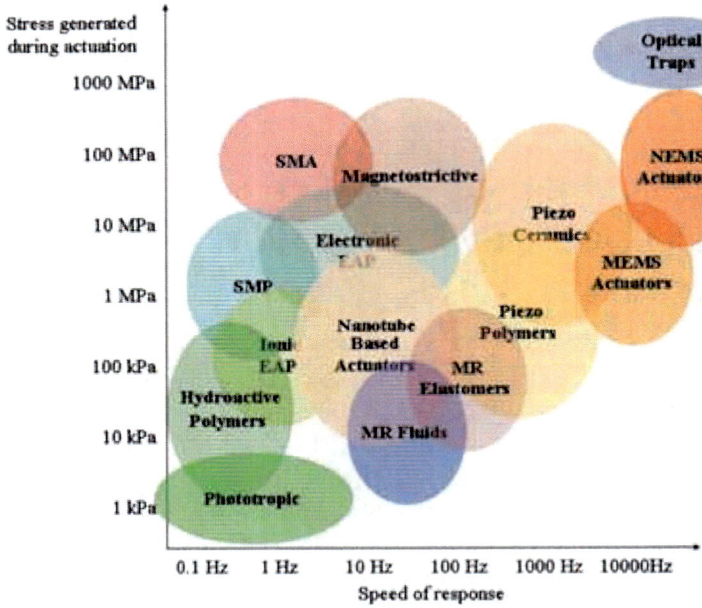

Figure A.1 Comparison between active materials as actuators.[2]

[2] Please note that during the actuation process of MEMS and NEMS actuators, important stresses are deployed but related forces are usually in the range of micro- to millinewton, due to the reduced size of such micro and nanosystems. Many related developments are now linked to using matrixes with great quantities of MEMS and NEMS actuators, for improving the forces attainable.

Appendix B

Remarkable Research Proposals Linked to Possible Medical Solutions Based on Active Materials

Some main challenges of 21st Century Medicine can only be tackled by bringing together solutions from different fields of knowledge and promoting collaboration between worldwide research teams. We would like to expose here some possible developments (and areas of study) for improving the diagnosis and therapeutics linked to multidisciplinary problems, as research roadmap for active materials in medical devices, at least for the next couple of years.

Most of them are based on the combination of different types of novel active materials as transducers for detecting different stimuli or producing alternative responses for a more precise and efficient operation, as has been analysed in several chapters of the handbook.

- Integral management of surgical procedures by combining haptic devices for remote handling, intelligent tools and equipment with feedback capabilities, as well as several solutions for intelligent catheters and minimally invasive active implants.
- Improved diagnosis based on intelligent lab-on-a-chip devices, with optimised operation, thanks to the use of several transducers, capable of carrying out rapid and very efficient chemical analysis and studies.
- Precise control of physiological magnitudes, thanks to implantable sensor networks linked to intelligent drug-

Handbook of Active Materials for Medical Devices: Advances and Applications
Edited by Andrés Díaz Lantada

www.panstanford.com

delivery devices, capable of providing the necessary doses according to patients' requirements.

- Organ replacement based on active implantable biomimetic prosthesis, directly connected to the nervous system of the patient, in order to obtain improved control of the artificial organ's response.
- Novel use of electromechanical couplings from corporal materials and tissues (such as piezoelectricity of bones, ligaments and tendons, etc.) so as to monitor patients' activities and evaluate effectiveness of treatments for multiple pathologies.
- Integral management of cancer based on a combined use of several active materials, so as to provide an easier access to dangerous cells, to help with precise drug delivery and to assist surrounding health tissues after destruction of cancerous cells.

Advances on aspects such as synthesis, processing, characterisation, modelling, simulation and prototyping of active materials and related devices will prove to be of great help for promoting the proposed developments. Such research combined with current information technology capabilities can provide additional solutions to telemedicine approaches and remote patient handling.

Some suppliers, publications and conferences are included in the following appendixes, with the intention of helping researchers in development projects linked to development of active devices.

Appendix C

Remarkable Suppliers of Active Materials

Listed below (in alphabetical order) are some main suppliers of different active materials families with possible application in the development of sensors and actuators for active medical devices.

Please note that many of them are technology-based enterprises in continuous evolution, therefore prone to changing their names (and related websites) as a consequence of strategic fusions.

Active ceramics:

- APC International Limited (www.americanpiezo.com)
- Ceram Tec AG (www.ceramtec.de)
- Ceramic Magnetics Inc. (www.cmi-ferrite.com)
- Ferroperm Piezoceramics A/S (www.ferroperm-piezo.com)
- Kinetic Ceramics Inc. (www.kineticceramics.com)
- Materials Systems Inc. (www.matsysinc.com)
- PI Ceramic GmbH (www.piceramic.de)
- Piezokeramika - European Piezoceramics Limited (www.piezokeramika.com)
- Sparkler Ceramics Pvt. Ltd. (www.sparklerceramics.com)
- TRS Technologies Inc. (www.trsceramics.com)

Bimetals:

- Bimetalle.de (www.bimetalle.de)
- Kanthal (www.kanthal.com)
- Vacuumschmelze (www.vacuumschmelze.de)
- Zapp Gruppe (www.zapp.com)

Handbook of Active Materials for Medical Devices: Advances and Applications
Edited by Andrés Díaz Lantada

www.panstanford.com

- Zodiac Metal Strips Inc. (www.zodiacmetal.in)

Carbon nanotubes:

- Bayer MaterialScience (www.baytubes.com)
- Fibermax Composites (www.fibermax.eu)
- Helix Material Solutions Inc. (www.helixmaterial.com)
- Mknano Impex (www.mknano.com)
- Nano-C Inc. (www.nano-c.com)
- Nanoshel - A Nanotechnology Company (www.nanoshel.com)
- Nanostructures & Amorphous Materials Inc. (www.nanoamor.com)
- Nanothinkx R&D (www.nanothinx.com)
- SES Research (www.sesres.com)
- Timesnano Chengdu Organic Chemicals Limited (www.timesnano.com)

Electroactive polymers (both sensors and actuators):

- Artificial Muscle Inc. (www.artificialmuscle.com)
- Ashashi Glass Corporation (www.agp.co.jp)
- Danfoss Polypower A/S (www.polypower.com)
- EAMEX Corporation (www.eamex.co.jp)
- EMPA Materials Science and Technology (www.empa.ch/eap)
- Envinonmental Robots Inc. (www.environmental-robots.com)
- KTech Corporation (www.ktech.com)
- MCNC Research and Development Institute (www.mcnc.org/rdi)
- Micromuscle AB (www.micromuscle.com)
- Molecular Mechanisms (www.molecularmechanisms.com)
- Nanosonic Inc. (www.nanosonic.com)
- Optotune LLC (www.optotune.com)
- Piezotech S.A. (www.piezotech.fr)
- Quantum Technology Limited (www.quantech.com.au)
- SRI International (www.sri.com/artificialmuscle)

Electrochromic polymers and other chromoactive polymers:

- Lawrence Berkley National Laboratory (http://windows.lbl.gov)
- MUTR Teaching Resources (www.mutr.co.uk)

- Saint - Gobain Sekurit (www.saintgobain.com)
- Switch Lite Privacy Glass (www.switchlite.com)
- Sensor Products Inc. (www.sensorprod.com)
- Velux Sageglass (www.veluxusa.com)

Hydroactive polymers:

- BASF Performance Chemicals (www.performancechemicals.basf.com)
- DuPont: The Miracles of Science (www2.dupont.com)
- Mitsubishi International Corporation (www.micchem.com)
- MUTR Teaching Resources (www.mutr.co.uk)
- Wego Chemical & Mineral Corp. (www.wegochem.com)

Magnetoelastic materials:

- ABB Austrália (www.abbaustralia.com.au)
- IMEGO Swedish ICT (www.imego.com)
- Magna Lastic Devices Inc. (www.mdi-sensor.com)

Magnetorheological fluids:

- Liquids Research Limited (www.liquidsresearch.com)
- Lord Corporation (www.lord.com)
- Magna International Inc. (www.magna.com)
- Wuhan Pangu Damper Technology (www.pangumrf.com)

Magnetostrictive materials:

- Active Signal Technologies (www.activesignaltech.com)
- Etrema Products Inc. (www.etrema.com)
- Marlborough Communications Limited (www.marlboroughcomms.com)
- Metall Rare Earth Limited (www.metall.com.cn)

Pyroelectric transducers:

- Coherent Inc. (www.coherent.com)
- Flir Systems (www.flir.com)
- KTech Corporation (www.ktech.com)
- Murata Manufacturing Corporation (www.murata.com)
- Silverlight Ltd. (www.silverlight.ch)

Quantum tunnelling composites:

- MUTR Teaching Resources (www.mutr.co.uk)

- Peratech Ltd. (www.peratech.com)
- Qio Systems Ltd. (www.qiosystems.com)
- Shadow Robot Company (www.shadowrobot.com)

Shape-memory alloys:

- Bricad Associates Sàrl (www.bricad.com)
- Dynalloy Inc. (www.dynalloy.com)
- Memometal Technologies (www.memometal.com)
- Memry Corporation (www.memry.com)
- Nitinol Devices & Components (www.nitinol.com)
- Nitinol Medical Technologies Inc. (www.nmtmedical.com)
- Nimesis Intelligent Materials (www.nimesis.com)
- SAES Smart Materials (www.shape-memory-alloys.com)
- Special Metals Corporation (www.specialmetals.com)
- TiNi Alloy Company (www.tinialloy.com)

Shape-memory polymers:

- Composite Technology Development Inc. (www.ctd-materials.com)
- Cornerstone Research Group (www.crgrp.net)
- CRG Industries (www.crg-industries.com)
- Diaplex Company (www.diaplex.com)
- MCP Iberia (www.mcp-group.com)
- Mitsubishi Heavy Industries Limited (www.mhi.co.jp)
- MnemoScience GmbH (www.mnemoscience.de)
- MUTR Teaching Resources (www.mutr.co.uk)
- Polymer Expert (www.polymerexpert.fr)

Thermocouples and thermistors:

- ARI Industries Inc. (www.ariindustries.com)
- GEC Instruments (www.gecinstruments.com)
- Goodfellow (www.goodfellow.com)
- Industrial Process and Sensor (www.ipscustom.com)
- Pyro Electric Inc. (www.pyro-electric.com)
- RS Amidata (www.rsonline.es)
- Sensortec Inc. (www.sensortecinc.com)

Appendix D

List of Related Scientific Journals

Listed below are several high-quality scientific journals, linked to the different topics covered within the handbook, where researchers can find additional information on biodevices and medical devices, as well as on the use of active materials for sensing and actuating purposes, especially when associated to the development of "intelligent" devices.

- Acta Biomaterialia – Elsevier
- Annals of Biomedical Engineering – Springer
- Annual Review of Biomedical Engineering
- Annual Review of Materials Research
- Biofabrication – IOP Publishing
- Bioinspiration & Biomimetics – IOP Publishing
- Biomaterials – Elsevier
- Biomedical Engineering Systems and Technologies – Springer
- Computer Methods in Biomechanics and Biomedical Engineering – Taylor & Francis
- IEEE Transactions on Biomedical Engineering
- International Journal of Biomedical Engineering and Technology – Inderscience
- International Journal of Mechanics and Materials in Design – Springer
- Journal of Applied Physics – American Institute of Physics
- Journal of Biomedical Engineering – Elsevier
- Journal of Biomimetics, Biomaterials and Tissue Engineering – Scientific.net

Handbook of Active Materials for Medical Devices: Advances and Applications
Edited by Andrés Díaz Lantada

www.panstanford.com

- Journal of Intelligent Material Systems and Structures – SAGE Publications
- Journal of Materials Science: Materials in Medicine – Springer
- Journal of Microelectromechanical Systems – IEEE ASME
- Journal of Nano Research – Scientific.net
- Journal of Physics D: Applied Physics
- Journal of Tissue Engineering and Regenerative Medicine – Wiley & Sons
- Materials & Design – Elsevier
- Nature Materials – Nature Publishing Group
- Nature Nanotechnology – Nature Publishing Group
- Rapid Prototyping Journal – Emerald
- Science Translational Medicine – Science AAAS
- Science Signalling – Science AAAS
- Sensors – MDPI Publishing
- Sensors and Actuators A: Physical – Elsevier
- Sensors and Actuators B: Chemical – Elsevier
- Smart Materials and Structures – IOP Publishing
- The Open Biomedical Engineering Journal – Bentham Open
- Tissue Engineering: Parts A, B & C – Mary Ann Liebert Inc.

Appendix E

List of Related Conferences and Meetings

Listed below are several high-impact congresses and conferences, linked to the different topics covered within the handbook, where researchers can find additional information on biodevices and medical devices, as well as on the use of active materials for sensing and actuating purposes, especially when associated to the development of "intelligent" devices.

Such series of conferences and their promoters pay special attention to bringing together researchers from different technological and biomedical backgrounds for providing novel multidisciplinary solutions to complex problems.

- BioMEMS and Biomedical Nanotechnology World Congress
- BIOSTEC International Joint Conference on Biomedical Engineering Systems and Technologies - INSTICC:
    - Biodevices
    - Bioinformatics
    - Biosignals
    - Healthinf
- CIMTEC International Conferences on Modern Materials and Technologies
- Conference on Smart Materials, Adaptive Structres and Intelligent Systems - ASME
- Congress of the European Society of Biomechanics - ESB

Handbook of Active Materials for Medical Devices: Advances and Applications
Edited by Andrés Díaz Lantada

www.panstanford.com

- ECCOMAS Thematic Conference on Smart Structures and Materials
- Electroactive Polymer Actuators and Devices (EAPAD Conference) – SPIE
- European Conference on Biomaterials – ESB
- European Conference on Smart Structures and Materials
- European Congress on Advanced Materials and Processes (EUROMAT)
- Eurosensors – IEEE Sponsored
- ICST Conference on Pervasive Health
- International Conference on Intelligent Materials
- International Materials Research Congress
- MEMS Executive Congress – memsindustrygroup.org
- Smart Structures/NDE Conference – SPIE
- World Biomaterials Congress
- World Congress of Internal Medicine – International Society of Internal Medicine
- World Congress on Bioengineering – IEEE EMB
- World Congress on Biomechanics – IFMBE
- World Congress on Medical Physics and Biomedical Engineering – IFMBE/WHO
- World Congress on Tissue Engineering and Regenerative Medicine

Index